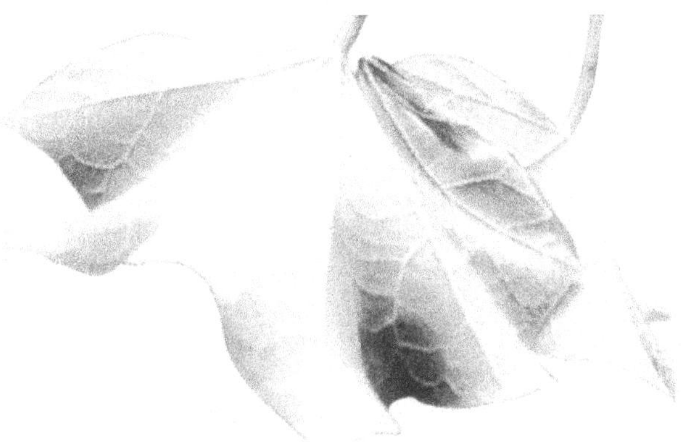

Traditional, Complementary And Alternative Medicine

Policy and Public Health Perspectives

Traditional, Complementary and Alternative Medicine

Policy and Public Health Perspectives

editors

Gerard Bodeker
Gemma Burford

Oxford University, UK

Imperial College Press

Published by

Imperial College Press
57 Shelton Street
Covent Garden
London WC2H 9HE

Distributed by

World Scientific Publishing Co. Pte. Ltd.
5 Toh Tuck Link, Singapore 596224
USA office: 27 Warren Street, Suite 401-402, Hackensack, NJ 07601
UK office: 57 Shelton Street, Covent Garden, London WC2H 9HE

Library of Congress Cataloging-in-Publication Data
Traditional, complementary, and alternative medicine : policy and public health
    perspectives / editors, Gerard Bodeker, Gemma Burford.
      p. cm.
    Includes bibliographical references and index.
    ISBN-13 978-1-86094-616-5
    ISBN-10 1-86094-616-X
  1. Alternative medicine. 2. Traditional medicine. 3. Public health--Political aspects.
    4. Complementary Therapies. 5. Health Policy. 6. Public Health.
    I. Bodeker, Gerard. II. Burford, Gemma. III. Title.
    R733.T72 2007
    362.1--dc22

                            2007280419

British Library Cataloguing-in-Publication Data
A catalogue record for this book is available from the British Library.

First published 2007 (Hardcover)
Reprinted 2016 (in paperback edition)
ISBN 978-1-911299-69-1

Typeset by Stallion Press
Email: enquiries@stallionpress.com

CONTENTS

PUBLIC HEALTH ISSUES: PRIORITY DISEASES AND HEALTH CONDITIONS

CONTRIBUTORS

Joanne Barnes
Associate Professor in Herbal Medicines
School of Pharmacy
Faculty of Medical and Health Sciences
University of Auckland
Grafton Campus
Private Bag 92019
Auckland, New Zealand

Gerard Bodeker
University of Oxford Medical School, UK
and Adjunct Professor of Epidemiology,
    Mailman School of Public Health
Columbia University, New York, USA
Chair, Global Initiative For Traditional Systems (GIFTS) of Health
Oxford OX2 6HG, UK

Gemma Burford
Senior Associate
Global Initiative For Traditional Systems (GIFTS) of Health
Oxford, UK
and International Programme Manager
Aang Serian (House Of Peace)
P.O. Box 13732, Arusha, Tanzania

George Carter
Director
Foundation for Integrative AIDS Research (FIAR)
62 Sterling Place, Suite 2
Brooklyn, NY 11217, USA

Ranjit Roy Chaudhury
Professor and Chairman, The INCLEN Trust and INCLEN Inc
161-L Hans Mansion
1st Floor, Left Wing
Gautam Nagar
New Delhi 110 048, India

Jonathan Cohen
Specialist Registrar
Department of Paediatric Infectious Diseases
Great Ormond Street Hospital
Great Ormond Street
London WC1N 3JH, UK

Mark Dvorak-Little
Stanford Graduate School of Business
350 Memorial Way
Stanford, CA 94305-5015, USA

Govindaswamy Hariramamurthi
Convenor, Medicinal Plants Conservation Network
Foundation for Revitalization of Local Health Traditions (FRLHT)
74/2 Jarakbande Kaval, Attur. P.O, Yelahanka
Bangalore 560 064, India

Fredi Kronenberg
Director, The Rosenthal Center for Complementary and
    Alternative Medicine
Columbia University, College of Physicians and Surgeons
630 W. 168th Street, Box 75
New York, NY 10032, USA

Jianping Liu
Professor and Director
Evidence-Based Chinese Medicine Center for Clinical Research
    and Evaluation
School of Preclinical Medicine
Beijing University of Chinese Medicine
Bei San Huan Dong Lu 11
Chaoyang District
Beijing 100029, China

Patrick Mbindyo
Newborn and Child Health Group
Kemri-Wellcome Trust-University of Oxford Collaborative Programme
P.O. Box 43640-00100
Nairobi, Kenya

Cora Neumann
Department of International Development
Queen Elizabeth House
University of Oxford
Oxford OX1 3TB, UK

Barry Noller
National Research Center for Environmental Toxicology
The University of Queensland
39 Kessels Road
Coopers Plains, QLD 4108
Australia

Chi-Keong Ong
Head of Service Development and Palliative Care Studies
The Shakespeare Hospice
Church Lane, Shottery
Stratford-upon-Avon, CV37 9UL
and Associate Research Fellow
Centre for Primary Health Care Studies
Warwick Medical School
University of Warwick
Coventry CV4 7AL, UK

Allan Rosenfield
Dean, Mailman School of Public Health
Columbia University
722 West 168th Street, Suite 1408
New York, NY 10032, USA

Terence J. Ryan
Emeritus Professor of Dermatology
University of Oxford and Oxford Brookes University
Hill House, Abberbury Avenue
Iffley, Oxon OX44EU, UK

Darshan Shankar
Director
Foundation for Revitalization of Local Health Traditions (FRLHT)
74/2 Jarakbande Kaval, Attur. P.O, Yelahanka
Bangalore 560 064, India

Gilbert Shia
Clinical Fellow
Chinese Medicine Advisory Service
Medical Toxicology Unit
Guy's and St. Thomas' Hospital Trust
Avonley Road
London SE14 5ER, UK

Urmila Thatte
Professor and Head
Department of Clinical Pharmacology
TN Medical College and BYL Nair Hospial
Mumbai Central
Mumbai 400 008, India

Unnikrishnan Payyappallimana
Senior Program Officer
Traditional Systems of Medicine Unit
Foundation for Revitalisation of Local Health Traditions (FRLHT)
74/2 Jarakbande Kaval, Attur. P.O, Yelahanka
Bangalore 560 064, India

Padma Venkatasubramanian
Joint Director
Foundation for Revitalisation of Local Health Traditions (FRLHT)
74/2, Jarakabande Kaval
Attur Post via Yelahanka
Bangalore 560 064, India

Merlin L. Willcox
Honorary Secretary
Research Initiative for Traditional Antimalarial Methods (RITAM)
36 Hare Close
Buckingham MK18 7EW, UK

FOREWORD

In many parts of the world, where medicines are not readily available or affordable, the public continue to rely on medicines used traditionally in their cultures. At the same time, affluent consumers in the industrialized world are spending their own money on healthcare approaches that fall outside what has been considered mainstream medicine. A growing body of national and international studies highlight the reality that there is exponential growth of global interest in and use of traditional (i.e. indigenous), complementary and alternative medicine (TCAM). The scale of this is so sizeable that it constitutes a public health phenomenon in itself.

There is considerable use of traditional medicine in many developing countries: 40% in China and Colombia; 71% in Chile; and up to 80% in some African countries (World Health Organization Global Atlas on Traditional, Complementary & Alternative Medicine, Bodeker *et al.*, 2005). In a number of industrialized countries, almost half of the population now regularly uses some form of CAM, while the figures for Canada and Germany are 70% and 71–75% respectively, and Australians spend more on complementary medicines than on pharmaceutical drugs. In the US, Americans now make more visits to complementary practitioners than to primary care physicians and spend more on complementary therapies than on hospitalizations.

Individuals seek to avoid long-term use of pharmaceuticals, with their potential for side effects. Thus, chronic conditions including pain conditions are a major reason that people seek the help of CAM practitioners. Women outnumber men in their use of CAM, often by 2:1. CAM use is also associated with higher education, higher income and strong environmental values.

Naturally, governments have become increasingly focussed on the public's need to be assured of safety, reliability and a beneficial therapeutic outcome from the healthcare choices that they make. Accordingly, these societal trends have been matched in the past decade by a growing momentum in regulation, research, policy development and professional education.

Drawing on data from policy studies, and in areas of priority in international health, such as malaria and HIV, as well as in the areas of common ailments such as skin conditions and fractures, this book provides a unique and important overview of the major trends of relevance to public health and health policy. After almost two decades of international research into the clinical and experimental dimensions of complementary and traditional therapies, this newer focus on the public health and policy dimensions will bring research and policy attention to a new and wider set of questions. These include: evidence based decision-making, the cost-effectiveness of TCAM treatments compared with other more mainstream approaches to managing health and disease; how the health and safety of populations is impacted by TCAM use; and how TCAM providers can best partner with mainstream healthcare colleagues to deliver AIDS and malaria prevention messages and to communicate information on healthy lifestyles.

The focus on population trends in self-medication, expenditures on alternative healthcare modalities, healthcare outcomes for TCAM and chronic disease, and the prospects for low-cost and locally available methods of disease prevention and management is timely. Indeed, it is overdue in view of the widespread and long-standing use of TCAM globally.

By providing a public health and policy perspective, the various chapters in this book illustrate a basis for effective integration of services for the benefit of the public, and potentially for cost-savings to governments through effective means of prevention and affordable methods of health maintenance and disease control. The book brings together a global overview of the challenges, promise and professional requirements of a vast area of health care practice that is now international in scope and worthy of increased attention and analysis. The single most important challenge for the future is to provide solid evidence-based decision making, as has been done recently in the area of malaria therapy.

Allan Rosenfield, MD, FACOG
DeLamar Professor of Public Health and Ob/Gyn
Dean, Mailman School of Public Health
Columbia University
New York, USA

POLICY

INTRODUCTION

Gerard Bodeker and Gemma Burford

It is now well established that interest in traditional, complementary and alternative medicine (TCAM) is rising rapidly throughout the world. Policy-makers, consumers and professional organisations have been calling variously for greater evidence, integration of TCAM and modern medical services; public sector support for TCAM services; and comprehensive national policy for what has been a consumer-led trend in most countries. Some countries, notably China, India and a number of other Asian nations, have been working actively to build the TCAM sector for the combined motives of perpetuating tradition and promoting cost–effectiveness in health services. In addition, there has been a dawning awareness of the significant export potential of traditional medicines in a burgeoning global marketplace for herbal medicines. This economic incentive has strengthened the drive for increased levels of production and quality control.

At the same time as consumer demand is rising and policy-makers are beginning to respond with moves to formalise TCAM within national policy, it is widely recognised that the indigenous sources of medical knowledge are disappearing and that there is a substantial inter-generational loss of traditional medical knowledge, especially within the oral traditions of the world (Posey, 2000). In these traditions, health knowledge extends to an appreciation of both the material and non-material properties of plants, animals and minerals. Their classificatory systems range in scope from the cosmological to the particular in addressing the physiological makeup of individuals and the specific categories of *materia medica* needed to enhance health and well-being. Mental, social, emotional, spiritual, physical and ecological factors are all taken into account. In establishing policy, these fundamental theoretical underpinnings of traditional health systems may either be respected and perpetuated, or converted into a biomedical expression and agenda. These approaches result in very different prospects for traditional medical knowledge and its continuity as a cultural health care resource.

With such a wide spectrum of approaches to TCAM at national and local levels, and the growing trend towards global and regional analysis of utilisation patterns and formalisation, there is now a clear need for a set of public health and policy perspectives to provide models and reference points for planners, policy-makers, programme developers and practitioners.

A broad policy overview and study of trends in utilisation and regulatory and policy development can be found in the World Health Organisation's Global Atlas of Traditional, Complementary and Alternative Medicine (Bodeker *et al.*, 2005). Based around a set of standardised core indicators, the WHO Global Atlas on TCAM provides information on the context, levels of use, structure and processes of TCAM at national, regional and global levels.

The Atlas, coordinated and edited by teams at Oxford University and the London School of Hygiene and Tropical Medicine, draws on data gathered by regional teams from Africa, the Americas, the Eastern Mediterranean, Europe, the Western Pacific, and South and South-East Asia. It comprises a map volume and a text volume. Through global and regional maps and tables, the former provides a visual representation of topics such as the popularity of herbal/traditional medicine, Ayurveda, Siddha, Unani, traditional Chinese medicine, homeopathy, acupuncture, chiropractic, osteopathy, bone-setting, spiritual therapies, and others; national legislation and traditional medicine policy; public financing; legal recognition of traditional medicine practitioners by their area of therapy; education and professional regulation; conventional health care practitioners who are entitled to provide various traditional, complementary and alternative therapies; and many other aspects. The text volume expands and supplements the map volume through detailed accounts of the development of traditional, complementary and alternative medicine in 23 countries across the world, as well as overviews of their status in each of the six WHO Regions.

Through these two volumes, a global picture of the development of traditional, complementary and alternative medicine becomes evident, revealing people's belief in and dependence on different traditional health systems around the world.

In the context of producing this first attempt at generating a systematic global overview of TCAM, what became apparent was that there is less data available on TCAM than the coordinating or regional teams would have wished, thus making mapping and policy analysis a more approximate exercise than was considered ideal. What this data collection exercise did reveal, however, is the wide spectrum of stages of policy development across regions, and among countries within regions. Interestingly, the global trend has shifted from being led by consumers and advocacy groups of practitioners, to a situation in most countries where governments are now working towards establishing a full regulatory context for the practice and use of TCAM. At one end of the spectrum, there are countries that formally promote and finance TCAM development, while at the other end, there are countries where the process of national recognition and regulation has not yet begun. For the countries in between, the picture is one of emerging policy, legislation and investment, with varying degrees of autonomy for the different TCAM professions. What is little known, other than in a very few industrialised countries, is the full extent of TCAM use by the public. At a global level, the often-cited 1983 estimate by Bannerman *et al.* that 'over 80% of the world's population relies on traditional medicine for its primary health care needs' has neither been updated, nor analysed in detail. In particular, little research has been conducted on the differing patterns of TCAM utilisation according to disease, income, gender, geography and culture.

Our work on the WHO Global Atlas on TCAM led to the realisation that, in addition to gaps in comparative policy studies of this sector, there was also a dearth of public health models for countries to draw on in planning health services and in integrating TCAM — either fully or selectively — into national health care.

Accordingly, drawing in part on data from the WHO Global Atlas, with permission of WHO Kobe, the sponsor of this project, we have assembled a set of policy-related chapters that analyse trends across a set of key policy issues such as regulation, education, safety, and finance within the TCAM sector.

We extend our appreciation and recognition to all who participated in the massive global data collection exercise and who are listed by name in the WHO Global Atlas. It is this data that has been analysed and commented on in the first four chapters of this volume.

At the same time, we were also aware that there exist important public health models, policy examples, NGO programmes and other TCAM innovations which highlight more fundamental principles of health planning, service development and public health outcomes. Accordingly, this volume brings together a sample of these. These include a model for self-sufficiency in family medicines through the production of home herbal gardens and data on significant public health benefits that have resulted; and an approach to harnessing the indigenous health knowledge and provider networks in refugee communities as a means of providing basic health needs and mental health through the use of locally available and culturally familiar strategies in an environment where most links with heritage and home have been shattered. Priority diseases such as malaria and HIV/AIDS are also considered from the perspective of TCAM as are common ailments such as skin conditions. Finally, resource rights issues are addressed through discussions of sustainability in medical plant use and in the intellectual property issues associated with the development of traditional medical knowledge for commercial purposes.

It is an intentionally eclectic and broad-based set of perspectives, designed to illustrate the wide range of work being done in this field. It is simply a beginning. Future work will inevitably build on, differentiate and diverge from these perspectives to create new directions, analytic frameworks and frames of reference for service development and integrated health care delivery in TCAM.

We would like to thank all of the contributors to the book, to WHO Kobe for allowing the use of data from the WHO Global Atlas in the first four chapters, and all who generated this data in the production of the WHO Global Atlas. We also recognise the work of many NGOs and community groups who are pioneering important public health initiatives at the local level in combating major diseases and common ailments through the use of TCAM.

References

Bannerman RH, Burton J, Wen-Chieh C. *Traditional Medicine and Health Care Coverage: A Reader for Health Administrators and Practitioners*. Geneva: World Health Organization, 1983.

Bodeker G. Lessons on integration from the developing world's experience. *Br Med J* 2001;322:164–167.

Bodeker G. Planning for cost-effective traditional health services. In: *Traditional Medicine: Better Science, Policy and Services for Health Development. Proceedings of a WHO International Symposium, Awaji Island, Hyogo Prefecture, Japan, 11–13 September 2000*. Kobe: WHO Centre for Health Development, 2001, pp. 31–70.

World Health Organization. *WHO Traditional Medicine Strategy 2002–2005*. Geneva: World Health Organization, 2002 (WHO/EDM/TRM/2002.1).

World Health Organization Centre for Health Development. *Traditional Medicine: Better Science, Policy and Services for Health Development. Proceedings of a WHO International Symposium, Awaji Island, Hyogo Prefecture, Japan, 11–13 September 2000*. Kobe: WHO Centre for Health Development, 2001.

World Health Organization Centre for Health Development. *Global Information on Traditional Medicine/Complementary and Alternative Medicine: Practices and Utilization. Proceedings of WKC International Consultative Meeting, Kobe, Japan, 19–21 September 2001*. Kobe: WHO Centre for Health Development, 2002.

Widespread global use of herbal/traditional medicine. [*Source*: WHO Global Atlas of Traditional, Complementary & Alternative Medicine (TCAM) (Bodeker *et al.*, 2005).]

CHAPTER 1

POLICY AND PUBLIC HEALTH PERSPECTIVES ON TRADITIONAL, COMPLEMENTARY AND ALTERNATIVE MEDICINE: AN OVERVIEW

Gerard Bodeker, Fredi Kronenberg and Gemma Burford

1.1. Introduction

The growth of public interest in, and use of, traditional, complementary and alternative medicine (TCAM) has been well documented. In a number of industrialised countries, almost half of the population now regularly uses some form of TCAM, while the figures for Canada and Germany are 70% and 71–75% respectively (Table 1.1). Considerable use of TCAM also exists in many developing countries: 40% in China and Colombia, 71% in Chile, and up to 80% in some African countries (Kasilo *et al.*, 2005). In this book, the term 'traditional medicine' is used when there is a need to refer exclusively to the indigenous health traditions of the world, in their original settings, while 'complementary and alternative medicine' (CAM) refers to health care approaches outside the biomedical mainstream in industrialised countries. More often, 'TCAM' is used to encompass both of the above.

The WHO Global Atlas on Traditional, Complementary and Alternative Medicine, a large international collaborative effort to document current

Table 1.1. Utilisation of TCAM in Industrialised Countries.

Country	Utilisation (% of Population)	Reference
Australia	48	MacLennan *et al.*, 1996
Canada	70	Health Canada, 2001
Denmark	33	Dansk Institut for Klinisk Epidemiologi, 1995
France	49	Fisher & Ward, 1994
Germany	71	Melchart *et al.*, 1995
	75	Marstedt & Moebus, 2002
United Kingdom	47	Thomas *et al.*, 2001
United States	62%/36%*	Barnes *et al.*, 2004

*Note: 62% when definition included prayer specifically for health reasons; 36% when prayer was excluded.

trends in utilisation, sectoral growth and policy in TCAM, highlights the trend of high TCAM use around the world and the accompanying policy and research response (Bodeker *et al.*, 2005). Popular use of TCAM and increasing consumer demand has been accompanied by a growth in research and associated literature, with an increase in an evidence-based approach over the past decade (Barnes *et al.*, 1999). Research and policy developments to date have, however, largely addressed clinical, regulatory and supply-oriented issues, to the general neglect of wider public health dimensions. Typically, research has focused on efficacy, mechanisms of action and safety of complementary and traditional therapies.

In certain developing countries, where there is long-term practice of TCAM both within and outside the dominant health care system, interest has been building over the past decade or more for a policy framework for TCAM within national health care systems, and some guidelines have been developed (Nelson, 1998; Bodeker, 2001a). However, in industrialised countries, regulation of CAM practitioners, establishment of standards of practice, guidelines for licensing and self-regulation, while occurring within a small number of the licensed professions (massage; acupuncture; chiropractic), have only recently been considered on a broader national scale (House of Lords Select Committee on Science and Technology, 2000; White House Commission on Complementary and Alternative Medicine Policy, 2002). Education and training efforts in these countries have largely focused on medical students and conventional health care practitioners (Bhattacharya, 2001; Marcus, 2001; Berman, 2001).

1.1.1. *Cultural and Spiritual Origins*

In most developing countries, traditional health systems are grounded in long-standing cultural and spiritual values. Traditional health knowledge extends to an appreciation of both the material and non-material properties of plants, animals and minerals. Its classificatory systems range in scope from the cosmological to the particular, in addressing the physiological makeup of individuals and the specific categories of *materia medica* (the materials used for therapeutic purposes) needed to enhance health and well-being. Mental, social, spiritual, physical and ecological factors are all taken into account.

A fundamental concept found in many systems is that of balance — the balance between mind and body, between different dimensions of individual bodily functioning and need, between individual and community, individual/community and environment, and individual and the universe. The breaking of this interconnectedness of life is a fundamental source of *dis-ease*, which can progress to stages of illness and epidemic. Treatments, therefore, are designed not only to address the locus of the disease, but also to restore a state of systemic balance to the individual and his or her inner and outer environment (Bodeker, 2000). They often involve other members of the family or community, and may be associated with specific places, such as ancestral shrines (Neumann & Bodeker, this volume) or sacred groves (Lebbie & Guries, 1995).

There is an emerging trend for certain elements of traditional health care to be removed from their original context and subsequently incorporated into formal health systems, or developed as part of a parallel 'complementary and alternative medicine' (CAM) sector. This is not a new process—the CAM disciplines of chiropractic and osteopathy both evolved from earlier traditions of bone setting (Hemmila *et al.*, 2002) — but it appears to be on the increase. In several industrialised countries, for example, acupuncture is offered in clinical settings as a pain relief technique, with no reference to the theories of energy (*qi*) flow that underlie its use in Traditional Chinese Medicine. In Belgium, 74% of acupuncture treatments are given by conventional allopathic physicians (Monckton *et al.*, 1999), while in Iceland, nurses and physiotherapists can be licensed to provide acupuncture after an 18-month training course (Veal, 2001).

In establishing policies, it is important that the fundamental theoretical underpinnings of traditional health systems be respected and perpetuated, in order to ensure their continuity in an intact form. It is also important to acknowledge that the social contexts of traditional health care often differ from those of the allopathic (modern, biomedical or 'Western') health sector, particularly with regard to family involvement and the economics of treatment.

1.1.2. *World Health Organization Policy*

The WHO Traditional Medicines Strategy 2002–2005 focused on four areas identified as requiring action, in order to maximise the potential of TCAM to play a role in public health: namely policy; safety, efficacy and quality; access; and rational use. Within these areas, WHO 2002–2005 identified respective challenges for action:

National policy and regulation

- Lack of official recognition of TCAM and TCAM providers
- Lack of regulatory and legal mechanisms
- TCAM not integrated into national health care systems
- Equitable distribution of benefits in indigenous knowledge and products
- Inadequate allocation of resources for TCAM development and capacity building

Safety, efficacy and quality

- Inadequate evidence base for TCAM therapies and products
- Lack of international and national standards for ensuring safety, efficacy and quality control
- Lack of adequate regulation of herbal medicines
- Lack of registration of TCAM providers
- Inadequate support of research
- Lack of research methodology

Access

- Lack of data measuring access levels and affordability
- Lack of official recognition of role of TCAM providers
- Need to identify safe and effective practices
- Lack of cooperation between TCAM providers and allopathic practitioners
- Unsustainable use of medicinal plant resources

Rational Use

- Lack of training for TCAM providers
- Lack of training for allopathic practitioners on TCAM
- Lack of communication between TCAM and allopathic practitioners, and between allopathic practitioners and consumers
- Lack of information for the public on rational use of TCAM

Considerable progress has been made in the development of national policies. At the launch of the Strategy in 2002, only 25 of WHO's 191 Member States had a national policy on TCAM (WHO, 2002), but the recent Global Atlas on Traditional, Complementary and Alternative Medicine commissioned by the WHO Centre for Health Development shows that there are now 66 out of a total of 213 Member States with TCAM policies (Bodeker *et al.*, 2005). A further 43 Member States have at least some specific legislation relating to TCAM, even in the absence of an official national policy, while 20 Member States are currently in the process of developing policies and/or legislation.

In the absence of baseline data, the extent to which the Strategy's other objectives have been achieved is unclear. The development of the WHO Global Atlas on TCAM has highlighted the urgent need for systematic policy-related research, utilisation studies and public outcomes research at the regional, national and international levels. The standardisation of data collection initiatives would allow for international and inter-regional comparisons, as well as the monitoring of progress, and the development of a systematic framework for such research would provide a firm foundation for future WHO Strategies.

1.2. Contexts for Integration and Evaluation: Shaping Questions and Establishing Priorities for Action

1.2.1. *Health Service Utilisation and Evaluation*

As noted above, the public of many countries is using health care services that are outside the purview and understanding of the dominant medical system. Complementary and traditional medical services are often used alongside conventional medical treatment, but many patients avoid disclosing their use of TCAM to their conventional health care providers: some recent studies have found the rate of non-disclosure to be as high as 77%. The main reasons for non-disclosure were concern about negative responses by medical practitioners; a belief that the practitioners did not need to know about their TCAM use; and the fact that the practitioners did not ask (Robinson & McGrail, 2004).

Thus, a vast, informal, and until recently, 'silent' health care sector exists in all countries, and no comprehensive picture of this exists as yet in any country. Most estimates of the extent of TCAM use have not been population-based, particularly in African countries, where estimates of use range from very low to very high (Bodeker, 2001b). Even in the few countries — mostly industrialised — where population-level TCAM utilisation studies have been conducted, methodological differences make comparisons extremely difficult. Some surveys specify visits to TCAM providers only, others focus on self-medication with TCAM products, and others include both. Lists of eligible therapies are provided in some surveys, whereas in others, the respondents themselves are left to define what constitutes TCAM. The interview technique (questionnaire, telephone or face-to-face) may affect the findings. Even the period of recall varies from one survey to another: some studies are concerned with TCAM utilisation in the past year, or a shorter period such as the past three months, while others relate to lifetime use (WHO Centre for Health Development, 2001).

In particular, what is lacking is a detailed understanding of the differing patterns of use according to disease, income, gender, age, geography and culture. Other research questions include: What are the emerging trends of TCAM use? What is the quality of services being offered to the public? What models exist for partnering the best of TCAM along with the best of conventional medicine to provide effective and affordable health care?

1.2.2. *Social and Cultural Dimensions*

Social, cultural and political values, as well as socio-economic factors, influence TCAM use in industrialised societies (Astin, 1998; Ong *et al.*, 2002; Eskinazi & Mindes, 2001; Eskinazi, 2001). Predictors of TCAM use in the United States, in a 1998 survey, included commitment to environmentalism, commitment to feminism, and interest in spirituality and personal growth psychology. Members of such groups tend to perceive TCAM as more congruent with their values, worldview and beliefs than the dominant health care system (Astin, 1998).

Ethnic minorities in industrialised countries often continue to use the traditional medicine from their culture alongside, or even in place of, conventional medicine (Ma, 1999; Kronenberg *et al.*, 2002; Factor-Litvak *et al.*, 2001; Reiff *et al.*, 2003). This can apply even in settings where conventional health care is provided free of charge, but traditional health care services must be paid out of pocket, as in the case of Chinese communities in the United Kingdom (Ong *et al.*, 2001; Green *et al.*, 2002). As in developing countries, the affordability, availability and cultural familiarity of traditional medicine, together with family influence (Vissandjee *et al.*, 1997), contribute to the continued use of traditional medical providers and medicines in 'ethnic enclaves'. Ethnic minority patients may be reluctant to seek treatment via the conventional system, or may fail to return for follow-up, due to linguistic barriers and the corresponding absence of shared concepts about health and illness. This is particularly true in the case of patients with mental health problems (Green *et al.*, 2002).

In both ethnic enclaves in industrialised countries and in developing countries, the 'disease' perspective of conventional biomedicine, with its emphasis on quantifiable physical data and on the individual patient, often excludes other dimensions of meaning — psychological, moral and social — that are relevant to patients and their families. Thus, a patient may be told after a physical examination and tests that 'nothing is wrong' physically, but continue to feel unwell or unhappy (Helman, 1994: 137–138). 'Soul loss' may not be recognised as a possible cause of illness, yet may lead to serious problems (O'Connor, 1995). In these situations, a culturally familiar TCAM practitioner, or 'vernacular specialist', can often provide a way of addressing the experience of illness, rather than the physical presence of disease, within the context of the patient's family or wider community.

Policy and research questions in this arena include: In industrialised societies, can ethnic preferences for traditional medicine be built into conventional health service design, to create greater consumer-friendliness in services? What combination of TCAM and conventional services will enhance the health of ethnic minorities? In developing countries, where the number of traditional health practitioners can be hundreds of times greater than that of modern medical practitioners (WHO, 2002), can this vast informal sector be brought into a partnership for addressing national health care goals in an improved model of health care, ensuring that important primary care services are delivered to all those who need them? How can attention to cultural aspects of health and health care be a bridge rather than a barrier to increased health service utilisation and improved levels of health in developing societies?

1.2.3. *Economic Factors*

In most countries, patients are paying out-of-pocket, sometimes on a large scale, for TCAM services still largely not covered by insurance. Of 213 WHO Member States surveyed for the recent Global Atlas (Bodeker *et al.*, 2005), only 58 (27%) are known to have any form of public financing for TCAM, whether full or partial. Reimbursement of TCAM costs by public health insurance is often restricted to specific therapies, or to certain categories of practitioners, and only in a few countries — such as China, Korea and Viet Nam — are traditional treatments and products fully covered by public health insurance. Dedicated public-sector hospitals for TCAM (not necessarily all therapies) are found only in China, Viet Nam, Pakistan, Cuba and the United Kingdom, although individual therapies are offered in public-sector general hospitals in a number of other countries (Bodeker *et al.*, 2005), and in Britain there is a growing trend for the National Health Service to pay for the services of complementary providers (House of Lords Select Committee on Science and Technology, 2000).

Adequate government funding is a prerequisite for effective traditional health care services. Under-investment risks perpetuating poor standards of practice and products, and also contributes to maintaining old stereotypes of inferior services and knowledge in traditional medicine.

In rural areas of many developing countries, self-medication with herbal remedies or dietary therapies is the first-line approach to treating common diseases, with traditional healers consulted only after home remedies have failed. Increasing regulation and professionalisation of traditional medicine in these countries may result in rising costs, with the risk that the poor may eventually be deprived of services that have historically been their first and last resort for health care. Even if the cost of treatment does not rise in real terms, formalisation processes that disallow flexible methods of payment—such as instalments, and payments in kind—may compromise affordability.

As growing TCAM markets lead to new economic possibilities, research and business interests may shift from providing affordable health care to developing products that can be marketed. The commercial production of botanical medicines can further complicate issues of availability and affordability. As an example, *Artemisia annua* grown in Tanzania is exported to Europe for processing into anti-malarial drugs, with dihydroartemisinin as the active ingredient; the finished products are re-imported to Tanzania and sold for US$6–7 per dose, far beyond the reach of most people who need them. A feasibility study conducted by Tanzania's National Institute of Medical Research recommended the commercial production of dihydroartemisinin products within the country, at a cost of around $2 per dose. The WHO Regional Director for Africa has already announced technical support for the programme, including the provision of pure dihydroartemisinin as a reference standard (WHO/AFRO, 2003). An alternative approach could be to fund research into appropriate methodologies for sustainable cultivation and processing of *A. annua* at the local level, with a focus on maximising safety and efficacy while minimising costs. The utilisation of a whole-plant product such as herbal tea, rather than a pharmaceutical with a single 'active' ingredient, may also reduce the potential for the development of parasite resistance (Willcox *et al.*, 2004).

Questions relevant to the economics of TCAM include: Is the public getting value for its money? What modalities are safest and most cost-effective for managing the conditions that are the largest burden on national health budgets? Do TCAM modalities contribute to cost savings through preventing illness, and if so, how can they be expanded? Why are people paying out-of-pocket, as in the UK, for complementary health care services when they have free conventional health services available, or in the US when they may have insurance coverage for conventional approaches? What impact does insurance coverage of TCAM have on use? What are sound models of health financing for CAM and traditional medical services? In the developing world, how might international funders such as the World Bank, WHO, the Gates and Rockefeller Foundations, the Global Fund and others evaluate and potentially include traditional medicine within the treatment spectrum for priority diseases in public health programmes that they are supporting?

1.2.4. *Priority Disease Management*

TCAM is being used by the public in the management of chronic conditions that are costly to society, including pain and arthritis, and for more life-threatening diseases such as heart disease, cancer and HIV-related illness (Wootton & Sparber, 2001a; Wootton & Sparber, 2001b; Lengacher *et al.*, 2002; Bodeker *et al.*, 2001). In poorer countries, the search for effective and affordable treatments for such epidemics as malaria and opportunistic infections associated with AIDS is driving renewed interest in traditional medicine (Bodeker *et al.*, 2005; UNAIDS, 2002), although herbal medicines are not always the first treatment choice (WHO, 2002). Yet, adequate data do not exist on current patterns of use and effectiveness of the various treatments being used alone and in combination. Additional information is needed on health concerns of the elderly, women, and children. Increasingly, patients are expecting health professionals to guide them in making differential treatment decisions, based on either formal evidence or clinical experience as to whether TCAM or conventional approaches work better, alone, or together.

There are many other dimensions of public health significance that have yet to receive serious and dedicated research attention, funding, or policy consideration. What is called for now is the generation of public health agendas to guide the development of this field. While such agendas will, of course, vary from country to country, a framework is offered here as a contribution towards the development of a more comprehensive approach by policy makers, research groups and funders.

1.3. A Policy Framework

Important issues for setting national and international public health research priorities have been outlined by the Council on Health Research for

Development (COHRED), an international NGO established to 'promote, facilitate, support and evaluate the Essential National Health Research strategy'. This includes underlying values and operating principles that are sufficiently general to fit the TCAM field as much as any other area of health care (Bodeker *et al.*, 2001). These are: equity; ethics; sustainability; knowledge generation; knowledge management/utilisation; capacity building; and the development of an appropriate research environment. While there are other frameworks for policy development, COHRED's serves as a catalyst for thought and discussion.

1.3.1. *Equity*

Equity issues concern both availability of conventional medicine for those who have access only to traditional medicine, and inability to afford the more researched and increasingly expensive CAM treatments. An equity perspective in developing country health care systems would ensure access to affordable, high quality services for those who currently most rely on traditional medicine or have little or no medical care.

In industrialised societies, complementary medicine use has been found to be associated with higher income and education (Astin, 1998; Eisenberg *et al.*, 1998; Ong *et al.*, 2002). Members of the dominant culture who have lower incomes and educational levels tend not to use complementary medicine: this may be due to less disposable income, and less exposure to information about complementary therapies. Availability of broader choices in health care services in these countries is increasingly becoming an elite service for the educated and well-to-do.

Conversely, traditional medicine use by ethnic minorities in those same societies is substantive at times may be the first line treatment for the poor and for those not speaking the language of the dominant society (Kronenberg *et al.*, in press). Inadequate and expensive conventional medical services are factors in such reliance on traditional medicine. 'Complementary' medicine in these situations is not complementary; rather, since basic conventional medical care may not be accessible, a danger exists of facilitating a 'separate but unequal health care system' (White House Commission on CAM Policy, 2002).

1.3.2. *Ethics*

1.3.2.1. Clinical research

While there are international guidelines for standards of clinical research (Levine & Gorvitz, 2000; Willcox *et al.*, Chapter 16 of this volume), research in TCAM may differ from clinical evaluation of conventional drugs. WHO guidelines for evaluation of herbal medicines consider that for traditional medicines with an established history of use, it is ethical to proceed from basic animal toxicity studies directly to Phase 3 clinical trials (Chaudhury *et al.*, this volume).

Ethical dilemmas can present themselves. In studies to evaluate tropical plants used to prevent and treat malaria, research ethics may require that standard conventional treatment be given to all subjects, so the traditional remedy can only be evaluated in conjunction with conventional treatment (Willcox & Bodeker, Chapter 10 of this volume). Unless alternative models can be developed, the full therapeutic potential of traditional medical treatments may never be known through clinical research.

1.3.2.2. Intellectual Property Rights (IPR)

Exploitation of traditional medical knowledge for drug development without the consent of customary knowledge holders is not acceptable under international law (UN Convention on Biological Diversity, 1993). State parties are required to 'respect, preserve and maintain knowledge, innovations and practices of indigenous and local communities embodying traditional lifestyles … and promote their wider application with the approval and involvement of the holders of such knowledge, innovations and practices and encourage the equitable sharing of the benefits arising from the utilisation of such knowledge, innovations and practices'. Contracting parties should 'encourage and develop models of co-operation for the development and use of technologies, including traditional and indigenous technologies'.

Until recently, the Convention on Biological Diversity (CBD) competed for influence with the more powerful Trade Related Aspects of Intellectual Property Systems (TRIPS) of the World Trade Organisation (WTO). TRIPS makes no reference to the protection of traditional knowledge. Nor does TRIPS acknowledge or distinguish between indigenous, community-based knowledge and that of industry. In November 2001, the declaration of the

Fourth Ministerial Conference in Doha, Qatar, mandated a review of TRIPS provisions and called for a harmonisation between the CBD and TRIPS. The WTO has begun the process to harmonise TRIPS and the CBD, with particular attention to ensuring adequate protection for indigenous intellectual and cultural property rights (World Trade Organization, 2002).

Researchers evaluating traditional medicines need to recognise that under international law, the customary owner — and often the country of origin — holds rights over the knowledge being evaluated. This has implications for patenting. If a patent is sought by a non-indigenous group, prior informed consent and just benefit sharing with customary owners must be established. A challenge here is how to determine who represents a community, and what represents full consent. These issues are explored in more depth by Bodeker (Chapter 17 of this volume).

1.3.3. *Sustainability*

A number of factors need to be addressed if new policies and practices are to become entrenched and endure. Among the most important are regulation of practice and practitioners, and the provision of adequate financing mechanisms.

1.3.3.1. Regulation

In order to achieve incorporation of TCAM into national health care programmes and systems, it is necessary to distinguish qualified practitioners from those without such qualifications, and to differentiate safe TCAM products from potentially hazardous ones (Shia *et al.*, Chapter 4 of this volume). Issues relating to pharmacovigilance (the monitoring of adverse drug reactions, and appropriate responses to ensure the safety of the public) are explored in detail by Barnes (Chapter 5 of this volume) with reference to herbal medicines in the United Kingdom within the broader context of emerging EU-wide legislation.

Some countries have already taken steps to achieve regulation of practitioners. In the United Kingdom, the House of Lords Select Committee on Science and Technology (2000) recommended that self-regulation should be a cornerstone for the formalisation of the complementary professions. Osteopaths and chiropractors have been registered as official health professions in the UK through an Act of Parliament, and the basis for maintenance of professional standards is that of self-regulation. The same principle is being applied to medical herbalists and acupuncturists, both of which professions are on track for registration (Walker & Budd, 2002; McIntyre, 2004). Self-regulation of certain TCAM professions is also emerging in Belgium (Eeckloo, 2001), Norway (Langworthy & Birkelid, 2001) and the Russian Federation (Goryunov, 2003, personal communication).

New Zealand has registered more than 600 Maori traditional healers who provide services within the wider health care system. While the government reimburses their services under health insurance, criteria for registration and oversight of professional practice are the responsibility of Maori traditional health practitioner associations (Scrimgeour, 1996).

In the United States, chiropractors are licensed in all 50 states, and acupuncturists are licensed in 41 states. The National Council for Certification of Acupuncture and Oriental Medicine holds a national exam for Traditional Chinese Herbal Medicine. The Botanical Medicine Academy and the American Herbalists Guild are developing a voluntary national examination in the US for practitioners of Western herbal medicine (Abascal & Yarnell, 2001). The United States conferred greater national attention to the policy arena with the establishment in 2000 of the White House Commission on Complementary and Alternative Medicine Policy, whose mandate was to provide 'legislative and administrative recommendations for assuring that public policy maximised the benefits to Americans of Complementary and Alternative Medicine'.

Asia has seen the most progress in incorporating traditional health systems into national health policy. In China, this began in 1951 with the establishment of a Traditional Chinese Medicine Division within the Ministry of Public Health, upgraded to a Department in 1954. In 1988, the State Council established the State Administration of Traditional Chinese Medicine as an independent administrative body in its own right, with eight major departments. The current Chinese regulatory framework not only promotes integration with modern medicine, but also regards TCAM as a major source of international trade and foreign exchange earnings. The Government's commitment to 'develop modern medicine and Traditional Chinese Medicine' has been written into the National Constitution, and the two are regarded as being of equal importance (Baoyan, 2005).

Integration of TCAM into national health care services also began in the 1950s in Viet Nam, where regulated TCAM provision is now available in the Government sector — including institutes of traditional medicine, hospitals of traditional medicine, and departments of traditional medicine in general hospitals, town and village centres — as well as the non-governmental sector. There are several dedicated agencies for TCAM, regulation of practice and products, research, formal training coursework and associations of practitioners. The official national policy on TCAM was formulated in 2003 (Hien & Truong, 2005).

In India, formal recognition for Indian systems of medicine came with the Indian Medicine Central Council Act of 1970, which established regulatory councils for education and practice. The first steps towards mainstreaming traditional health care systems in national health services were taken in 1983, with the recognition of their potential contribution towards achieving the goal of 'Health for All'. This ultimately led to the establishment of an independent Department headed by a Secretary in the Government of India and, in 2002, to the development of a specific national policy on Ayurveda, Yoga and Naturopathy, Unani, Siddha and Homeopathy (AYUSH). In addition to facilitating the integration of these health care systems into national health programmes, the policy also emphasises affordability, safety, efficacy, and the sustainable use of raw materials — particularly those of plant origin (Lavekar & Sharma, 2005).

1.3.3.2. Financing/Insurance Coverage

Out-of-pocket is the most important means of financing TCAM treatments worldwide, and the *only* available financing mechanism in a large number of developing countries, where neither public funding nor private insurance covers these treatments (Burford *et al.*, Chapter 2 of this volume). Even in industrialised countries, insurance coverage for CAM services is relatively new and incomplete, so out-of-pocket spending is considerable. Americans have been found to spend more on CAM than on all US hospitalisations (Eisenberg *et al.*, 1993; Astin, 1998), while Australians spend more on CAM than on all prescription drugs (MacLennan *et al.*, 1996). In Canada, the total out-of-pocket expenditure on CAM was estimated at US$2.4 billion in 1997 (Health Canada, 2001), while in the United Kingdom it was estimated at £1.47 billion per annum in 2003, with the inclusion of over-the-counter products (Ong & Banks, 2003).

The effect of user fees on health care utilisation and health outcomes was a subject of debate in the 1990s, centred on the ability and willingness of households to pay out-of-pocket for health care. Research indicates that willingness to pay is not always synonymous with ability to pay: the poor may sacrifice other basic needs such as food and education in order to pay for health care, often with serious consequences (Bodeker, 2002).

Public health insurance is an important funding mechanism for TCAM services in a number of countries of the European Region, with 22 European countries offering full or partial reimbursement for selected TCAM therapies (Burford *et al.*, Chapter 2 of this volume) as well as a few other industrialised countries. Some major American medical insurers confer some benefits for limited complementary medical services, primarily through employer-sponsored health plans (Pelletier & Astin, 2002). In the year 2000, 70% of employee-sponsored programmes covered chiropractic; 17% covered acupuncture, 12% covered massage, and the numbers dwindled from there for other CAM services (White House Commission on CAM Policy, 2002). In the United Kingdom in 1995, 40% of GP practices provided access to CAM, with 10% of the cost being met by the National Health Service (Thomas *et al.*, 2001). In Australia, since the introduction of a Medicare rebate for acupuncture in 1984, use of acupuncture by medical practitioners has increased greatly. Claims rose from 655,000 in the financial year 1984–85 to 960,000 in 1996–97, and Medicare reimbursements to doctors for acupuncture rose from $7.7 million to $17.7 million (Easthope *et al.*, 1998).

In the few developing countries where insurance exists, those who can afford the insurance payments will tend to be beneficiaries of a more regulated and safe traditional medicine practice, while the poor continue to purchase unregulated drugs from unlicensed vendors. This creates the skewing of services towards the more affluent that is found with complementary medicine use in industrialised societies, in contrast to the customary role of traditional medicine serving as the first and last resort for health care for the poorer members of society. There is also a risk that improved regulation and training may have the unwanted 'side effect' of destroying the flexibility and community-centred focus inherent in many traditional health systems, which permits the poorest clients to pay by instalments or make a gift in kind to the practitioner. Careful planning by policy-makers is required to ensure that, in becoming 'modernised' and 'professionalised', traditional health care services do not lose the advantages that currently make them an attractive option for millions around the world (Burford *et al.*, Chapter 2 of this volume).

In the case of ethnic minorities in industrialised societies, health insurance coverage can lead to a substantial increase in the use of traditional medical services (Pourat *et al.*, 1999). Again, there is creation of an elite programme through the requirement of insurance coverage, with the poor being less likely to have access to their traditional health care services.

Evaluating health insurance records can be an effective way of estimating whether there are cost savings from using traditional or complementary health care. A retrospective study of Quebec health insurance enrollees compared a group of 1418 Transcendental Meditation (TM) practitioners with 1418 non-meditators. The yearly rate of increase in payments in both groups was not significantly different before learning meditation. After learning, the annual change in mean payments was a decline of 1–2% for the TM group, and an increase of up to 12% for non-meditators. The estimated cost saving was as much as $300 million per year (Herron & Hillis, 2000).

Cost-benefit research could assess outcomes when traditional or complementary approaches are compared, or combined, with conventional care. This would assist health authorities in making informed choices about the selection of treatments and services to be incorporated into integrated health care programmes.

1.3.4. *Knowledge Generation*

The initiative taken by the United States Congress a decade ago to establish at the National Institutes of Health an Office of Alternative Medicine (now the National Center for Complementary and Alternative Medicine, NCCAM) has led to a focused programme of clinical and basic science research, now seen internationally as a model for how to proceed in conventional scientific research in TCAM (Bodeker & Kronenberg, 2002). NCCAM's mandate is to support rigorous research into efficacy and safety, and thereby establish the evidence base needed for integration of TCAM into standard medical care (Brixey *et al.*, 2005). A public health agenda is now required, in addition to the focus on experimental and clinical research. While some progress has already been made towards this goal in the United States, with the establishment of a Committee on the Use of Complementary and Alternative Medicine by the American Public under the Institute of Medicine (IOM, a non-profit non-governmental organisation) to explore scientific, policy and practice questions arising from the significant and increasing use of CAM within the country (Institute of Medicine, 2005), efforts must be increased, both within the US and globally. Public health professionals themselves need to be involved in defining the public health dimensions of traditional and complementary medicine.

Adequate funding is of central importance. In the US, funding was initially provided by private donors whose contributions resulted in programmes at academic medical centres (Kronenberg, 2001a). The advent of NCCAM at the NIH substantially legitimised CAM research, and has been followed by funding initiatives from national and international foundations. The biomedical community's response has escalated research momentum. This wave has yet to reach public health research. In the absence of a significant voice from the public health research community, funders have remained focused on issues of safety, efficacy and the mechanisms of action of complementary and traditional medicine. Priority should now be assigned to strengthening the public health research agenda if knowledge generation is to keep abreast of consumer demand for cost-effective services, and government and insurer demands for policy information.

In addition, mainstream research funds should encourage a component of research into traditional ways of treating specific conditions, and the contribution of TCAM therapies to disease prevention and general health maintenance. While research into prevention is long-term, methodologically difficult and often expensive, the potential benefits could be substantial (Herron & Hillis, 2000). Other important areas of research include the extent to which therapeutic outcomes are based on belief, attitude and expectations; the contribution of TCAM therapies to the spiritual dimensions used in assessing an individual's quality of life; and the effects of combining therapies, as when traditional Chinese medicine and allopathic medicine are used simultaneously in treating a condition.

1.3.5. *Knowledge Management and Utilisation*

In order to ensure sound standards of practice based on recognised levels of training and the use of TCAM therapies that are safe and effective, information generation and dissemination is needed across a wide range of professional and commercial areas. Comprehensive information resources will be fundamental to the evolution of research and policy activities, but developing them will be challenging to accomplish. Material currently accessible online is limited in scope. Much of it consists of commercial sites containing information related to products being marketed. Only a small number of bibliographic databases (e.g. MEDLINE from the US, and the British Library's AMED) allow free access to information, albeit from a limited sample of journals. Full papers are available free of charge only in rare cases; more usually, the abstract or even just the citation is given. Most relevant scientific databases are accessible on a fee-paying basis. Each database is compiled in a unique format and style. Data structure, indexing methods and terminology used for data retrieval are also vary widely. Much of the material is not available in English (Kronenberg, 2001b).

A freely available, comprehensive, web-based resource on complementary and traditional medicine could provide accurate and authoritative information on safety and efficacy, legal and regulatory policies, research resources, education and training programmes, trade statistics, intellectual property guidelines, among other content. It would also allow for rapid, global updating of information in a field of growing significance worldwide. Initiatives have been proposed to make significant investments of time, but would need substantive funding to establish this — e.g. by the Commonwealth countries (Reuters, 2001) and others (Noller *et al.*, 2001; Kronenberg, 2001a).

1.3.6. *Capacity Building*

What constitutes capacity in public health with respect to complementary and traditional medicine, and how should capacity be strengthened? Strengthening is needed in safety, efficacy, standardisation, current utilisation, cost-effectiveness, customer satisfaction, priority diseases (communicable and degenerative), disease prevention, and the maintenance of overall well-being.

Investment in professionals will result in leaders who will contribute to implementing public health responses to the growth in complementary and traditional medicine. Schools of public health can contribute by offering training for students in areas of TCAM, encouraging masters and doctoral research projects, and providing continuing education programmes. Wherever biomedical health care providers, such as physicians, nurses, pharmacists and midwives, are permitted to offer TCAM therapies, they must receive adequate training in the fundamentals of the relevant TCAM modalities as well as in conventional medicine. A matter of some concern is the number of countries in which physicians and/or allied health professionals are legally entitled to provide TCAM treatments with only limited training, or without receiving any specific training in these health care approaches (Bodeker *et al.*, Chapter 3 of this volume).

Expanded capacity would include greater understanding of the potential for benefit, risks, and the costs of these health care approaches. It would include systems for harnessing potential contributions to meeting major public health challenges — both in terms of practitioners as a resource for disseminating health information, and through tested modalities offering potential cost-effective choices.

An often-quoted statistic is that only 10% of the funding for health care research and development is spent on 90% of the world's health problems (Global Forum for Health Research, 2004). Traditional health care systems can make a significant contribution to the fight against priority diseases affecting the developing world, including HIV/AIDS, malaria and tuberculosis, and against the unacceptably high levels of maternal and perinatal mortality that currently exist in many countries (Bodeker *et al.*, Chapter 3 of this volume). There are notable examples in Africa of traditional health practitioners being involved in HIV prevention programmes. Each trained practitioner is able to deliver a prevention message to around 1000 people in less than a year (Green, 1997). Emerging research is focusing on the role that traditional herbal medicines might play in alleviating the symptoms of HIV/AIDS, for those unable to afford or obtain even subsidised anti-retroviral drugs (Liu, Chapter 12 of this volume; Bodeker *et al.*, Chapter 11 of this volume; Bodeker *et al.*, 2000). Similarly, in the field of malaria, an international research collaboration coordinated by the Global Initiative for Traditional Systems of Health is addressing both prevention — through traditional methods for repelling and controlling mosquitoes — and treatment (Willcox & Bodeker, Chapter 10 of this volume; Bodeker & Willcox, 2000, Willcox *et al.*, 2001; Willcox *et al.*, 2004).

Despite the growing number of small and medium-sized initiatives to involve traditional health care providers in the management of priority health problems, their potential has been almost entirely overlooked in the large-scale international programmes for combating these problems, such as those funded by the World Bank, Gates Foundation, Global Fund and other major donors. If these large global programmes are to achieve their goals, however, there is also a need for them to consider factors such as cultural familiarity and acceptability, affordability, accessibility, and the potential for local production in order to generate long-term sustainability after the withdrawal of funding. Effective capacity building can raise awareness of such issues and help traditional health care systems, which offer all of these advantages, to find a place across disease categories in the respective agendas of large funders.

1.3.7. *Research Environment*

Further development of TCAM services is predicated on a broad base of quality research. The NIH/NCCAM experience in the US has shown that when funds are available and priorities are set, TCAM research will grow exponentially. As noted in Section 1.3.4 above, the need now is to expand beyond just basic, clinical and experimental research to a fully articulated programme of public health research.

Donors, policy-makers, patients, and health care providers worldwide have all called for evidence of what constitutes the 'best' treatments. The randomised controlled clinical trial (RCT) is considered by the biomedical establishment to be the core of biomedical evidence, but considerable preliminary work is essential, particularly in areas of traditional systems of medicine, before one can even design the appropriate RCT. Respecting the basic concepts and principles of traditional health care systems, while developing trials according to rigorous clinical pharmacological principles, is an important challenge. The question of how 'gold standard' RCT methodology can be adapted to meet the needs of these systems, or other scientific methodologies used, is already being addressed, both within the Indian context and in Traditional Chinese Medicine (Chaudhury *et al.*, Chapter 15 of this volume). It should also be recognised that while providing valuable information, RCTs have limitations that can be addressed by social science and public health research methodologies. RCTs are inadequate for measuring infrequent adverse outcomes, such as rare side-effects of drugs, and there are also limitations in adequately evaluating the long-term consequences of therapy, such as toxicity from chronic, low-level exposure to medications. Ethnographic, epidemiological, observational, survey and cohort methodologies can contribute, and fall within the public health domain (Margolin, 1999).

Unmet health needs of ethnic minorities, women, children, the poor, the elderly and those with special medical conditions must be considered in the establishment of a public health research framework and priorities for action. Also needing attention are diseases for which current conventional treatment regimens are unsatisfactory, e.g. many cancers and chronic debilitating conditions, for which the public are turning to TCAM.

Prevention of disease is a cornerstone of many traditional and complementary health systems, with diet and nutrition as well as traditional forms of exercise (e.g. yoga, Tai Chi) and stress reduction being used in combination to promote balanced health (Schneider *et al.*, 2002). While research into illness prevention is long-term, methodologically difficult and often expensive, the potential benefits could be substantial (Herron & Hillis, 2000).

Belief and attitude have an influence on treatment outcomes in all therapeutic settings, western and other traditions. A 'placebo' or 'meaning response' effect is an important component of many therapies. The extent to which therapeutic outcomes are based on expectancy is an important area of study.

WHO's Quality of Life Assessment includes spiritual dimensions in assessing an individual's quality of life. Here, 'spiritual' relates to the sense of meaning regarding the self or extending beyond the self. The spiritual dimension of life and well-being is central to many traditional and complementary health systems. In Britain, 12% of those who use CAM providers use the services of 'spiritual healers' (Ong *et al.*, 2002). This trend, its origins and outcomes are important areas of research.

Comparative evaluation of complementary and conventional medicine approaches to treating specific health conditions is needed. This may include study of cross-cultural healing practices to identify common treatments and/or to combine evidence for a specific herb or treatment regimen. Comparative studies could assess feasibility, cost-effectiveness, and environmental impact as well as specific biomedical outcomes.

Combinations of therapies should also be studied. For example modern medicine and traditional systems (such as Ayurveda in India and Traditional Chinese medicine) are often used simultaneously in the treatment of certain diseases in Asian countries. Caution should be exercised to identify and address cultural biases in the assumptions, methodologies and concepts when conducting comparative research.

A range of methodologies, then, can and should be employed in evaluating traditional and complementary therapies. These should be applied in a manner that is sensitive to the theoretical, clinical, and cultural assumptions of the modality/systems being evaluated in order to ensure that the research design adequately measures what one thinks is being studied (Chaudhury *et al.*, Chapter 15 of this volume).

New directions must be forged by researchers who are able to transcend limitations in research orthodoxy in the interests of providing sound information to the public on what constitutes good health care.

1.4. Conclusion

As governments, the World Health Organization, and other international bodies begin to address the complexities of establishing regulatory and policy guidelines for ensuring the safety and quality of complementary and traditional health services, a broad public health capacity is called for. As discussed here, this should evolve with an awareness of social, cultural and political dimensions, and should address values (equity, ethics), sustainability (regulation, financing, knowledge generation, knowledge management, capacity building) and the research environment.

Such a broad-based strategy is required if complementary and traditional medicine is to shift from the marginal status it holds in most countries, to having a significant role in national health care. Political will as well as scientific will and data are needed to support such an agenda. Ultimately, nothing would be considered complementary or alternative, orthodox or conventional. Rather, all possible contributions to health would be evaluated for their promise, and harnessed for the good of the public's health.

Acknowledgements

This work was funded in part by the Global Initiative for Traditional Systems of Health (Dr. Bodeker); the WHO Centre for Health Development, Kobe, Japan, for work on the WHO Global Atlas on Traditional, Complementary and Alternative Medicine (Dr. Bodeker and Ms. Burford) and the NIH National Center for Complementary and Alternative Medicine, grant P50-AT00090 (Dr. Kronenberg). The chapter builds on an earlier publication, Bodeker G, Kronenberg F. A public health agenda for complementary, alternative and traditional (indigenous) medicine. Am J Public Health 2002;92(10):1582–1591. Thanks to Christine Wade and Janet Mindes for their helpful comments on early drafts of the manuscript.

References

Abascal K, Yarnell E. Certifying skill in medicinal plant use. *HerbalGram* 2001;52:18–19.

Astin JA. Why patients use alternative medicine: results of a national study. *JAMA* 1998;279:1548–1553.

Baoyan L. People's Republic of China. In: Bodeker G, Ong C-K, Grundy C, Burford G, Maehira Y (eds.) *WHO Global Atlas of Traditional, Complementary and Alternative Medicine: Text Volume.* Kobe, Japan: World Health Organization Centre for Health Development, 2005, pp. 187–192.

Barnes J, Abbot NC, Harkness EF, Ernst E. Articles on complementary medicine in the mainstream medical literature: an investigation of MEDLINE, 1966 through 1996. *Arch Intern Med* 1999;159(15):1721–1725.

Barnes P, Powell-Griner E, McFann K, Nahin R. *2004. CDC Advance Data Report #343.* Complementary and alternative medicine use among adults: United States, 2002.

Berman B. Complementary medicine and medical education. *Br Med J* 2001;322:121–122.

Bhattacharya B. Programs in the United States with complementary and alternative medicine education: an ongoing listing. *J Altern Complement Med* 2001; 6:77–90.

Bodeker G. Traditional health systems: valuing biodiversity for human health and well being. In: Posey DA (ed.) *Cultural and Spiritual Values of Biodiversity*. A Complementary Contribution to the Global Biodiversity Assessment. Nairobi: Intermediate Technology Publications and UN Environment Programme, 2000, pp. 261–284.

Bodeker G. Planning for cost-effective traditional health services. In: WHO Centre for Health Development, *Traditional Medicine. Better Science, Policy and Services for Health Development. Proceedings of a WHO International Symposium Awaji Island, Japan 11–13 September 2000*. Kobe, Japan: World Health Organization Centre for Health Development, 2001a, pp. 31–70.

Bodeker G. Lessons on integration from the developing world's experience. *Br Med J* 2001b;322:164–167.

Bodeker G. In: *Traditional Medicine in Asia*. Chaudhury RR, Rafei UM (eds.) New Delhi: WHO Regional Office for South-East Asia, 2002.

Bodeker G, Jenkins R, Burford G. International Conference on Health Research for Development (COHRED), Bangkok, Thailand, 9–13 October 2000: report on the symposium on traditional medicine, 9 October 2000. *J Altern Complement Med* 2001;7:101–108.

Bodeker G, Kabatesi D, Homsy J, King R. A regional task force on traditional medicine and AIDS in East and Southern Africa. *Lancet* 2000;355:1284.

Bodeker G, Kronenberg F. A public health agenda for complementary, alternative and traditional (indigenous) medicine. *Am J Public Health* 2002;92(10): 1582–1591.

Bodeker G, Ong C-K, Grundy C, Burford G, Maehira Y (eds.) *WHO Global Atlas of Traditional, Complementary and Alternative Medicine: Text Volume*. Kobe, Japan: World Health Organization Centre for Health Development, 2005.

Bodeker G, Willcox ML. Conference report: the first international meeting of the Research Initiative on Traditional Antimalarial Methods (RITAM). *J Altern Complement Med* 2000;6(2):195–207.

Brixey RJD, Kun KE, Killen J. United States of America. In: Bodeker G, Ong C-K, Grundy C, Burford G, Maehira Y (eds.) *WHO Global Atlas of Traditional, Complementary and Alternative Medicine: Text Volume*. Kobe, Japan: WHO Centre for Health Development, 2005, pp. 63–74.

Chaudhury R. *Herbal Medicine for Human Health*. New Delhi: WHO Regional Office for South-East Asia, 1992.

Dansk Institut for Klinisk Epidemiologi. *DIKES sundheds- og sygelighedsunder-søgelsen 1994 [DIKE's Health and Morbidity Studies 1994. Preliminary Results]*. Copenhagen: Danish Institute for Clinical Epidemiology, 1995.

Easthope G, Beilby JJ, Gill GF, Tranter BK. Acupuncture in Australian general practice: practitioner characteristics. *Med J Aust* 1998;169:197–200.

Eeckloo K. *Regulation and Registration of Unconventional Practitioners: The Case of Belgium, Paper Commissioned by Department of Health and Children*. Dublin: Department of Health and Children, 2001 (unpublished paper). Cited in: O'Sullivan T. *Report on the Regulation of Practitioners of Complementary and Alternative Medicine in Ireland*. Dublin: Institute of Public Administration, Health Services Development Unit, 2002.

Eisenberg DM, Davis RB, Ettner SL *et al.* Trends in alternative medicine use in the United States, 1990–1997: results of a follow-up national survey. *JAMA* 1998;280:1569–1575.

Eisenberg DM, Kessler RC, Foster C, Norlock FE, Calkins DR, Delbanco TL. Unconventional medicine in the United States. Prevalence, costs, and patterns of use. *N Engl J Med* 1993;328:246–252.

Eskinazi D. Factors that will shape the future of alternative medicine: an overview. In: Eskinazi D (ed.) *What Will Influence the Future of Alternative Medicine? A World Perspective*. Singapore: World Scientific Publishers, 2001, pp. 1–22.

Eskinazi D, Mindes JJ. Alternative medicine: definition, scope and challenges. *Asia Pac Biotech News* 2001;5:19–25.

Factor-Litvak P, Cushman LF, Kronenberg F, Wade C, Kalmuss D. Use of complementary and alternative medicine among women in New York city: a pilot study. *J Altern Complement Med* 2001;7:659–666.

Fisher P, Ward A. Medicine in Europe: complementary medicine in Europe. *Br Med J* 1994;309:107–111.

Global Forum for Health Research. *10/90 Report on Health Research 2003–2004*. Geneva: Global Forum for Health Research, 2004.

Green EC. The participation of African traditional healers in AIDS/STD prevention programmes. *Trop Doct* 1997;27(Suppl 1):56–59.

Green G, Bradby H, Chan A, Lee M, Eldridge K. Is the English National Health Service meeting the needs of mentally distressed Chinese women? *J Health Serv Res Policy* 2002;7(4):216–221.

Health Canada. Perspectives on complementary and alternative health care. A collection of papers prepared for Health Canada. *Health Canada*, 2001.

Helman CG. *Culture, Health and Illness*, 3rd edn. Oxford: Butterworth-Heinemann.

Hemmila HM, Keinanen-Kiukaanniemi SM, Levoska S *et al.* Long-term effectiveness of bone-setting, light exercise therapy, and physiotherapy for prolonged back pain: a randomized controlled trial. *J Manipulative Physiol Ther* 2002;25(2):99–104.

Herron RE, Hillis SL. The impact of the transcendental meditation program on government payments to physicians in Quebec: an update. *Am J Health Promot* 2000;14:284–291.

Hien TV, Truong CQ. Socialist Republic of Viet Nam. In: Bodeker G, Ong C-K, Grundy C, Burford G, Maehira Y (eds.) *WHO Global Atlas on Traditional, Complementary and Alternative Medicine.* Kobe, Japan: World Health Organization Center for Health Development, 2005, pp. 205–211.

House of Lords Select Committee on Science and Technology. *Sixth Report: Complementary and Alternative Medicine,* 21 November 2000. www.publications.parliament.uk/pa/ld199900/ldselect/ldsctech/123/12301.htm (2000).

Institute of Medicine. *Complementary and Alternative Medicine (CAM) in the United States.* Washington, D.C.: The National Academies Press, 2005, p. 330.

Kasilo OMJ *et al.* Regional overview: African region. In: Bodeker G, Ong C-K, Grundy C, Burford G, Maehira Y (eds.) *WHO Global Atlas of Traditional, Complementary and Alternative Medicine: Text Volume.* Kobe, Japan: World Health Organization Centre for Health Development, 2005.

Kronenberg F. Academic and funding perspective in developing alternative medicine research in the US. In: Eskinazi D (ed.) *What Will Influence the Future of Alternative Medicine? A World Perspective.* Singapore: World Scientific Publishers, 2001a, pp. 105–125.

Kronenberg F. A comprehensive information resource on traditional, complementary, and alternative medicine: toward an international collaboration. *J Altern Complement Med* 2001b;7:723–729.

Kronenberg F, Cushman L, Wade C, Kalmuss D, Chao M. Race/ethnicity and women's use of complementary and alternative medicine in the United States: results of a national survey. *Am J Pub Health,* in press.

Kronenberg F, Wade C, Cushman L *et al.* CAM use among American women in four racial ethnic groups. *Harvard CAM Science Conference held in Boston, MA in April 2002* (Abstract, 2002).

Langworthy JM, Birkelid J. General practice and chiropractic in Norway: how well do they communicate and what do GPs want to know? *J Manipulative Physiol Ther* 2001;24(9):576–581.

Lavekar GS, Sharma SK. Republic of India. In: Bodeker G, Ong C-K, Grundy C, Burford G, Maehira Y (eds.) *WHO Global Atlas of Traditional, Complementary and Alternative Medicine.* Kobe, Japan: World Health Organization Centre for Health Development, 2005, pp. 89–96.

Lebbie AR, Guries RP. Ethnobotanical value and conservation of sacred groves of the Kpaa Mende in Sierra Leone. *Econ Bot* 1995;49(3):297–308.

Lengacher CA, Bennett MP, Kip KE, Keller R, La Vance MS, Smith LS, Cox CE. Frequency of use of complementary and alternative medicine in women with breast cancer. *Oncol Nurs Forum* 2002;29(10):1445–1452.

Levine RJ, Gorvitz S (eds.) *Biomedical Research Ethics: Updating International Guidelines.* World Health Organization: Council for International Organization of Medical Sciences, 2000; p. 295.

Ma GX. Between two worlds: the use of traditional and Western health services by Chinese immigrants. *J Community Health* 1999;24:421–437.

MacLennan AH, Wilson DH, Taylor AW. Prevalence and cost of alternative medicine in Australia. *Lancet* 1996;347:569–573.

Marcus DM. How should alternative medicine be taught to medical students and physicians? *Acad Med* 2001;76:248–250.

Margolin A. Liabilities involved in conducting randomized clinical trials of CAM therapies in the absence of preliminary, foundational studies: a case in point. *J Altern Complement Med* 1999;5:103–104.

Marstedt G, Moebus S. *Gesundheitsberichterstattung des Bundes — Heft 9: Inanspruchnahme Alternativer Methoden in der Medizin* ["Health Reports by the Federal Government — Issue 9: Use of Alternative Methods in Medicine"]. Berlin: Robert-Koch-Institut, Statistisches Bundesamt, 2002.

McIntyre M. British government calls for regulation of herbal and acupuncture practitioners in UK. *HerbalGram* 2004;62:66–67.

Melchart D, Linde K, Weidenhammer W, Worku F, Wagner H. The integration of natural healing procedures into research and teaching at German universities. *Altern Ther Health Med* 1995;1(1):30–33.

Monckton J, Belicza B, Betz W, Engelbart H, van Wassenhoven M. *COST Action B4: Unconventional Medicine in Europe. Final Report of the Management Committee, 1993–1998.* Brussels: European Commission Directorate-General for Science, Research and Development, 1999.

Nelson T. Commonwealth Health Ministers and NGO's seek health for all. *Lancet* 1998;352:1766.

Noller BN, Myers S, Abegaz B, Singh MM, Kronenberg F, Bodeker G. Global forum on safety of herbal and traditional medicine: 7 July 2001, Gold Coast, Australia. *J Altern Complement Med* 2001;7:583–601.

O'Connor BB. *Healing Traditions.* Philadelphia: University of Pennsylvania Press, 1995, pp. 21 and 93.

Ong CK, Banks B. *Complementary and Alternative Medicine: The Consumer Perspective.* London: The Prince of Wales's Foundation for Integrated Health, 2003.

Ong CK, Patterson S, Doll H, Stewart-Brown S, Bodeker GC, Griffiths S. *Do Factors Which Influence Preference for Traditional Chinese Medicine (TCM) in the Oxfordshire Chinese Community Affect Access to GP Care?* University of Oxford: Health Services Research Unit, 2001.

Ong C-K, Petersen S, Bodeker GC, Stewart-Brown S. Health status of people using complementary and alternative medical practitioner services in four English counties. *Am J Public Health* 2002;92(10):1653–1656.

Pelletier KR, Astin JA. Integration and reimbursement of complementary and alternative medicine by managed care and insurance providers: 2000 update and cohort analysis. *Altern Ther Health Med* 2002;8:38–39.

Pourat N, Lubben J, Wallace SP, Moon A. Predictors of use of traditional Korean healers among elderly Koreans in Los Angeles. *Gerontologist* 1999;39: 711–719.

Reiff M, Kronenberg F, Balick M, Lohr P, Roble M, Cortez L, O'Connor B, Fugh-Berman A. Ethnomedicine in the urban environment: Latino healers in New York city. *Hum Organ* 2003;62:12–26.

Reuters. *Commonwealth Backs Plan for $10 Million Traditional Medicine Hub.* http://216.239.33.100/search?q=cache:vzVZOvKAjh0C:www.enn. com/news/wire-stories/2001/11/11302001/reu_45734.asp+reuters+commonwealth+health+ministers&hl=en (20 November 2001).

Robinson A, McGrail MR. Disclosure of CAM use to medical practitioners: a review of qualitative and quantitative studies. *Complement Ther Med* 2004;12(2–3):90–98

Schneider RH, Alexander C, Salerno JW, Robinson DK, Fields JZ, Nidich SI. Disease prevention and health promotion in the elderly with a traditional system of natural medicine. *J Aging Health* 2002;14:57–58.

Scrimgeour D. Funding for community control of indigenous health services. *Aust N Z J Public Health* 1996;20:17–18.

Sparber A, Wootton JC. Surveys of complementary and alternative medicine: Part II. Use of alternative and complementary cancer therapies. *J Altern Complement Med* 2001;7:281–287.

State Administration of Traditional Chinese Medicine of the People's Republic of China. *Anthology of Policies, Laws and Regulations of the People's Republic of China on Traditional Chinese Medicine.* Shangdong: Shangdong University, 1997.

Thomas KJ, Nicholl JP, Coleman P. Use and expenditure on complementary medicine in England: a population-based survey. *Complement Ther Med* 2001;9:2–11.

UNAIDS. *Ancient Remedies, New Disease: Involving Traditional Healers in Increasing Access to AIDS Care and Prevention in East Africa.* UNAIDS/02.16E. Geneva: UNAIDS.

United Nations Convention on Biological Diversity. http://www.biodiv.org (1993).

Veal L. A comparison of the use of complementary therapies in Australia and Iceland. *Complement Ther Nurs Midwifery* 2001;7:72–77.

Vissandjee B, Barlow R, Fraser DW. Utilisation of health services among rural women in Gujarat, India. *Public Health* 1997;997:135–148.

Walker LA, Budd S. UK: the current state of regulation of complementary and alternative medicine. *Complement Ther Med* 2002;10:8–13.

White House Commission on Complementary and Alternative Medicine Policy. *Final Report, March 2002.* www.whccamp.hhs.gov/finalreport.html (2002).

Willcox ML, Bodeker G, Bourdy G *et al. Artemisia Annua.* In: Willcox ML, Bodeker G, Rasoanaivo P (eds.) *Traditional Medicinal Plants and Malaria.* Boca Raton: CRC Press, 2004.

Willcox ML, Cosentino MJ, Pink R, Bodeker G, Wayling S. Natural products for the treatment of tropical diseases. *Trends Parasitol* 2001;17:58–60.

Willcox ML, Bodeker G, Rasoanaivo P. *Traditional Medicinal Plants and Malaria.* Boca Raton: CRC Press, 2004.

Wootton JC, Sparber A. Surveys of complementary and alternative medicine: Part IV. Use of alternative and complementary therapies for rheumatological and other diseases. *J Altern Complement Med* 2001a;7:715–721.

Wootton JC, Sparber A. Surveys of complementary and alternative medicine: Part III. Use of alternative and complementary therapies for HIV/AIDS. *J Altern Complement Med* 2001b;7:371–377.

World Health Organization. *Traditional Medicine Strategy 2002–2005.* http://www.who.int/medicines/organization/trm/orgtrmmain.shtml (May 2002).

World Health Organization, Centre for Health Development (WHO Kobe Centre, WKC). *Proceedings from the WKC International Consultative Meeting, 19–21 September 2001: Global Information on Traditional Medicine/Complementary and Alternative Medicine: Practices and Utilisation.* Kobe: WHO Centre for Health Development, 2001.

World Health Organization, Regional Office for Africa (WHO/AFRO) Press Release, 25 April 2003. *WHO to Support Production of Indigenous Anti-Malarial Medicine in Africa.* Brazzaville: WHO/AFRO. http://www.afro.who.int/press/2003/pr2003042502.html (2003).

World Trade Organization. *Trade Related Aspects of Intellectual Property Systems (TRIPS).* www.wto.org/english/tratop_e/trips_e.htm (2002).

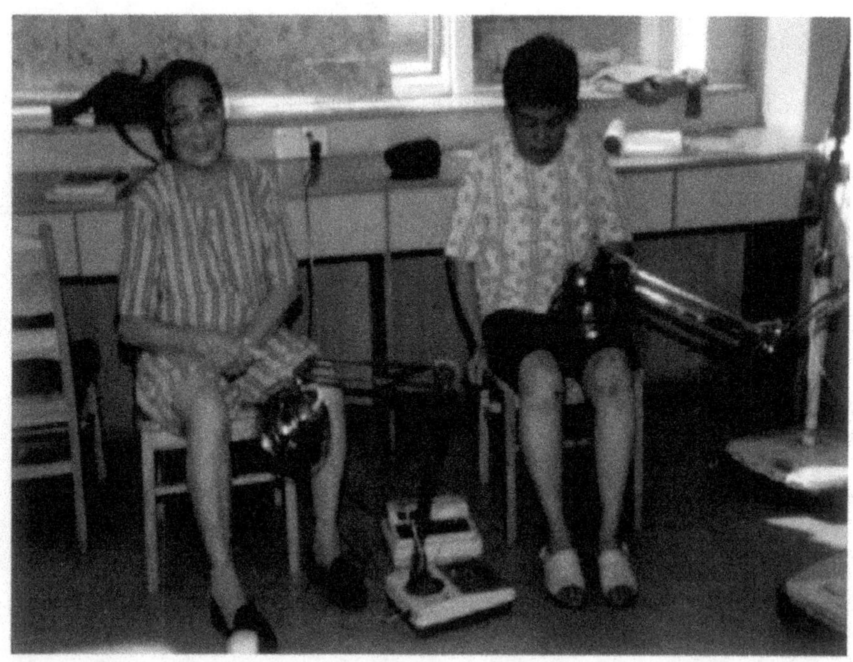

Elderly women receiving electro-acupuncture at a government-funded clinic in Guangzhou, China. (*Photo courtesy of F. Kronenberg.*)

CHAPTER 2

FINANCING TRADITIONAL, COMPLEMENTARY AND ALTERNATIVE HEALTH CARE SERVICES AND RESEARCH

Gemma Burford, Gerard Bodeker and Chi-Keong Ong

2.1. Introduction

In recent years, issues of financing and cost-effectiveness for traditional, complementary and alternative medicine (TCAM) have increasingly been incorporated into policy discussions (Bodeker, 2002). Nonetheless, the newly released WHO Global Atlas on Traditional, Complementary and Alternative Medicine (Bodeker *et al.*, 2005) illustrates that throughout the world, a very high proportion of TCAM expenditure is still covered by out-of-pocket payment or private health insurance. Only 58 of the 212 surveyed countries are known to have public financing mechanisms for TCAM. The majority of these relate to service provision rather than research. No information is available on TCAM financing for a further 103 countries.

As in the case of allopathic health care, there are two distinct public-sector financing mechanisms for TCAM treatments. The first — exemplified by Cuba, the Russian Federation, the United Kingdom and Viet Nam — is the 'national health service' model in which eligible users pay no fee, or a greatly reduced fee, and treatment costs are covered directly from the national health budget. The second mechanism is the full or partial reimbursement of treatment expenses by public health insurance. This method is utilised by 22 countries in the European Region, as well as the United States, the Republic of Korea, Japan, Australia and New Zealand. Some countries, such as Denmark and China, combine both systems.

There is a widespread perception that TCAM is chosen over allopathic health care primarily for economic reasons, and that it is 'the medicine of the poor'. This is often true for countries in which the traditional sector predominates over the 'complementary/alternative' sector, including much of the African Region, Latin America and several Asian countries. In Pakistan, allopathic pharmaceuticals are beyond the reach of over 80% of the population (Gilani & Hannan, 2005). Similarly, an African Development Bank (1995) study of 800 households in Abidjan, Côte d'Ivoire, showed that devaluation of the Ivorian franc was associated with a concurrent shift from modern to traditional medicine by 13.5% of households. Countries with no significant domestic pharmaceutical industry must rely on expensive imports for their allopathic health care services; but traditional medicine, by definition, uses products derived from locally available plant, animal and mineral sources. These products are often harvested from the wild by patients or their families, so that no monetary expenditure is incurred (Ahorlu *et al.*, 1997).

It cannot be assumed, however, that TCAM is always a cheaper option than allopathic medicine. In South Africa, for example, the cost of traditional treatment for a condition such as *umtsebulo* (presumed soul loss) can be as high as US$125 (Kale, 1995). In some countries, governments subsidise the pharmaceutical industry to make allopathic drugs more affordable, but do not subsidise herbal products or materials. Thus, herbal preparations are often more expensive than allopathic drugs. A similar situation exists for complementary and alternative systems of medicine (such as acupuncture, homeopathy, chiropractic and osteopathy). These systems of health care are often excluded from government health subsidies, and practitioners are at liberty to charge whatever they want to. The cost to patients may be several times higher than that of a comparable allopathic treatment, although direct comparisons are difficult because the circumstances of utilisation differ. The result is a consistent trend towards utilisation by patients with a high disposable income. For each of the four CAM therapies listed above, the estimated overall popularity is significantly lower in countries with a gross domestic product (GDP) of less than Int$15,000 than in those with GDP Int$15,000 or more (p < 0.05) (Bodeker *et al.*, 2005).

Higher disposable incomes and higher education levels are both predictors of CAM use in the Netherlands (Menges, 1994) and the United States of America (Astin, 1998). Likewise, a recent survey conducted in the United Kingdom found that patients from professional, clerical, junior managerial and administrative work categories are more likely to be users of CAM. Those from skilled working class groups and unskilled manual workers are more likely to be non-users (Ong *et al.*, 2002).

2.2. Out-of-Pocket Payment

At a global level, out-of-pocket payment is the most important financing mechanism for TCAM. In most African and Middle Eastern countries, as well as a large number of countries in Latin America, the Caribbean and Asia, no public financing mechanisms or private insurance programmes exist, and the costs of traditional health care services are paid entirely out-of-pocket.

Research to quantify out-of-pocket expenditure on TCAM has been conducted in only a few countries. Nonetheless, the available data are striking. In the United Kingdom, out-of-pocket payment represents 79% of the total expenditure on TCAM treatments, with a mean expenditure of £13.62 per person per month (Thomas *et al.*, 2001). With the inclusion of over-the-counter products, expenditure on TCAM in the United Kingdom could be as high as £1.47 billion per annum (Ong & Banks, 2003). In the United States, the total out-of-pocket TCAM expenditure was estimated at US$2.7 billion in 1997, comparable to the projected 1997 out-of-pocket expenditure for all physician services, while in Canada this figure was US$2.4 billion (Health Canada, 2001). In Australia, the 1996 expenditure on TCAM was higher than that for all prescription drugs (MacLennan *et al.*, 1996).

Only two developing countries have statistics on out-of-pocket expenditure. In Indonesia, a 2001 survey estimated that 2.7% of the population uses TCAM for outpatient services, with an average expenditure of US$5.70 per person. The total out-of-pocket spending on TCAM has been estimated at US\$38.6 million (Hayatie Amal & Hardaningsih, 2005). In Cameroon, the annual expenditure on medicinal plant products sold in public markets in Yaounde alone has been estimated at US\$6–8 million (Betti, 2002). This does not include visits to traditional health practitioners.

2.2.1. *Flexibility of Out-of-Pocket Payment for TCAM Services*

As explained by Lantum (2005) with reference to Cameroon, traditional medicine in rural societies is not necessarily viewed as a 'business'. Rather, it addresses the integral value of every citizen to his or her community, and the need for society as a whole to protect the life and health of each individual. Hill (1997) makes a similar point, referring to an elderly woman in Papua New Guinea:

> On the surface she consumed rather than produced resources; thus there was little incentive to spend still more on maintaining her health. But what of the value of her knowledge and wisdom in the resolution of family conflicts? What of her value in the education of the children through myths, storytelling and personal history? What of her knowledge of herbal and household remedies for common illnesses? How to assess in monetary terms the fact that she can call upon the support of other community members in times of hardship, just as she has assisted them in times past? These are vital contributions to the continued health of her community, but we have a long way to go before we can cost them.

Traditional health providers practising in rural areas may decide to waive fees for the poorest members of the community, to negotiate instalments, or to accept payments in kind. Such payments are often at the discretion of the consumer, and may include livestock, palm wine, token gifts or even services. Some TCAM practitioners provide treatments free of charge in return for prestige and special privileges within the community (Lantum, 2005). Others, particularly spiritual healers, view their skills as a gift from God and refuse to accept any recompense (El-Gendy, 2005). The flexibility of payment methods in the traditional sector translates into a significant improvement in affordability for patients with restricted access to cash. It often reduces the need for households to borrow money, sell productive assets or sacrifice basic needs such as education (Bodeker, 2002).

2.3. Provision of TCAM in Public Sector Hospitals and Clinics

Traditional health care forms an integral part of the national health service, provided free of charge or at a nominal cost in public sector hospitals and clinics, in a number of countries. Viet Nam, for example, has three national research institutes with beds for inpatients; 52 provincial hospitals of TCAM; over 250 departments of TCAM in general hospitals; and TCAM providers in public health centres at the district and community levels. The national budget for TCAM is approximately 2.7% of the total national health budget (Hien & Truong, 2005). Similarly, in Pakistan, about 360 *tibb* dispensaries and clinics provide free medication to the public under the control of the health departments of provincial governments (Gilani & Hassan, 2005).

Within the Region of the Americas, two countries have dedicated public-sector hospitals for TCAM. In Peru, there are currently 12 Complementary Medicine Centres at the national level, serving over 40,000 patients in total. A study has shown the overall cost-effectiveness of TCAM to be 53–63% higher than that of allopathic treatment for eight selected pathologies. In Cuba, the Ministry of Health supports a Traditional and Natural Medicine (TNM) Program, consisting of a system of Provincial and Municipal TNM Centres providing facilities for treatment, education, research and administration (Pan American Health Organization/WHO Regional Office for the Americas, personal communication, 2005). In Argentina, homeopathy and acupuncture are provided in two standard public hospitals (Zacchino, 2005).

In Europe, only the United Kingdom has dedicated TCAM hospitals in the public sector. There are four specialist homeopathic hospitals (Ong *et al.*, 2005a). Five other European Region countries — Croatia, Georgia, Israel, Malta and Romania — offer one or two TCAM therapies free of charge in public general hospitals, while Luxembourg has publicly funded acupuncture clinics (Ong *et al.*, 2005b). In the Russian Federation, allopathic physicians may provide herbal medicine, nutritional therapy, manipulation, light treatment and hydrotherapy as standard hospital treatments, at public expense (Ullman, 1991).

2.4. Public Health Insurance

Public health insurance is widely used as a financing mechanism for TCAM service provision in the European Region and in a few other countries, mainly within the industrialised world. Table 2.1 gives details of the therapies reimbursed by public health insurance, and the circumstances under which reimbursement is permitted, in 21 countries within the European Region.

In the United States, there are two publicly funded health insurance programmes — Medicare and Medicaid — which, in certain cases, reimburse TCAM treatments. Medicare, which serves primarily people over 65, may cover chiropractic, massage therapy and 'other scientifically proven alternative therapies'. Over 75% of state Medicaid programmes, providing medical assistance to low-income families, reimburse at least one TCAM therapy, most commonly chiropractic or acupuncture (Brixey *et al.*, 2005). Private health insurers in the US also offer coverage for certain CAM modalities. None of the countries of Latin America have provisions for health insurance coverage for TCAM treatment and products (Gupta, 2005).

Traditional health care and herbal medicines are reimbursed in some countries of the Western Pacific Region (Roh, 2005). Since 1976, the Ministry of Health and Welfare of Japan has approved 147 Kampo formulations, as well as their individual herbal components, to be covered by the national health insurance system (Yamada, 2005). In the Republic of Korea, national health insurance has covered traditional medicine since 1987. This move was initially resisted by Korean herbalists, as the profit margin of herbal medicines when paid out-of-pocket has been estimated to be between 100% and 500% (Cho, 2000). New Zealand allows for the reimbursement of services provided by over 600 registered Maori traditional healers (Scrimgeour, 1996).

The Chinese system, which combines public health insurance and direct subsidies, is unique. In 1995, there were over 2500 dedicated traditional medicine hospitals in China, and 95% of general hospitals had departments of traditional medicine (State Administration of Traditional Chinese Medicine, 1997). Traditional health services are covered by health insurance, but the proportion of uninsured people may be as high as 50%. In hospital settings, insured patients are more likely to receive traditional Chinese

Table 2.1. Reimbursement of TCAM by Public Health Insurance in the European Region.

Country	Therapies Reimbursed	Details	Refs.
Austria	Balneotherapy, electrotherapy, homeopathy, massage	Reimbursed only when provided by allopathic physicians.	WHO, 2001
Belgium	Various therapies	At least partial reimbursement when provided by allopathic physicians.	WHO, 2001
Czech Republic	Acupuncture and spa treatment	Partial reimbursement of acupuncture (legally restricted to physicians). Spa treatment is reimbursed only if the patient's physician makes a referral.	Fisher & Ward, 1994; Thorne, 1995
Denmark	Chiropractic	Fully reimbursed, as practitioners are legally recognised.	Høg, 2005
Finland	Various therapies	All TCAM is reimbursed when provided by allopathic physicians during normal sessions. Treatments provided by registered chiropractors, naprapaths and osteopaths are reimbursed if referred by allopathic physician, and TCAM provider works in institution led by an allopathic physician or a registered physiotherapist. Medications are not covered.	WHO, 2001
France	Homeopathy and acupuncture	Reimbursed when provided by allopathic physicians. 65% of expenses for homeopathic medicines are refunded, provided they are not in Korsakovian dilutions or LM potencies. Other consultations (e.g. physicians providing herbal medicine or osteopathy) may be reimbursed, but no refund is available for herbal products purchased over the counter.	WHO, 2001; Bouchayer, 1990; Finne & Viksveen, 1999

                                      G. Burford et al.

Table 2.1. *(Continued)*

Country	Therapies Reimbursed	Details	Refs.
Germany	Homeopathy, anthroposophical medicine, herbal medicine; usually acupuncture	Only prescription herbal drugs reimbursed. TCAM treatment by physicians or *Heilpraktiker* (healing practitioners) may be reimbursed if the aetiology of the illness is unknown; if no allopathic treatment is available, or previous allopathic treatment has failed; if allopathic treatment has side-effects or causes a risk to the patient; or if TCAM is more cost-effective than allopathic treatment.	Bornhöft, 2005
Greece	Acupuncture	Partial reimbursement only.	Fisher & Ward, 1994
Hungary	Acupuncture	Partial reimbursement only.	Fisher & Ward, 1994
Iceland	Acupuncture, massage, hydrotherapy, relaxation, aromatherapy, lifestyle classes, mud treatments, nutritional therapy	Acupuncture is reimbursed when provided by a trained nurse or physiotherapist, but not by a lay acupuncturist. All other therapies are part of residential health care programmes, reimbursed only if patients are referred by their own doctor.	Veal, 1997; Veal, 2001
Ireland	Various therapies, excluding homeopathy	Only when provided by registered allopathic physicians.	WHO, 2001
Italy	Various therapies	Depends on region, but part payment is usual. Purchase of homeopathic medications may be reimbursed.	WHO, 2001; Jütte, 1999
Latvia	Acupuncture, homeopathy, electro-acupuncture, iridology, bio-resonance therapy	Full reimbursement. Officially, only allopathic physicians are entitled to practise.	Monckton *et al.*, 1999

Table 2.1. (*Continued*)

Country	Therapies Reimbursed	Details	Refs.
Luxembourg	Homeopathy	Reimbursed at 80% of fees when provided by a registered allopathic physician. Other treatments may be unofficially reimbursed in the context of normal medical consultations.	WHO, 2001
Netherlands	Homeopathy, anthroposophic medicine, chiropractic	Homeopaths must belong to nationally recognised professional organisations to qualify for reimbursement. National health insurance for 10 visits to chiropractor per year (average US$45).	WHO, 2001; Finne & Viksveen, 1999; Kadel, 1991
Norway	Chiropractic	Partial reimbursement if referred by allopathic physician.	Pedersen, 1990
Poland	Acupuncture	Full reimbursement. Practice is limited to allopathic physicians.	Fisher & Ward, 1994
Portugal	Not known	No details given.	Monckton *et al.*, 1999
Slovak Republic	Acupuncture	Partial reimbursement only.	Fisher & Ward, 1994
Sweden	Chiropractic	Legally recognised chiropractors can try to negotiate reimbursement agreements with local county councils, for part payment only; about two-thirds of them have succeeded in doing so.	Leboeuf-Yde *et al.*, 1997
Switzerland	Various therapies	Mandatory reimbursement for TCAM services provided by physicians, for a test phase of 6 years (1999–2005)	Heusser, 2000

medicine, as one of the primary sources of a hospital ward's profit is the 15–25% mark-up for prescribed medications. Even with this mark-up, it is hard to cover operational costs, and government subsidies currently ensure survival (Phillips *et al.*, 1997).

2.5. Financing TCAM Research and Development

Both India and China have large national departments of traditional medicine research. China's Scientific, Technical and Educational Department, within the State Administration of Traditional Chinese Medicine, directs construction of scientific research institutes and laboratories; organises research, development, appraisal and academic exchanges, etc; and directs protection of intellectual property rights. It also administers examinations in TCM. China has recently established six dedicated universities of traditional medicine, each with substantial research programmes funded by the Government (State Administration of Traditional Chinese Medicine, 1997). India's Central Council for Research in Ayurveda and Siddha, the Central Council for Research in Unani Medicines and the Council for Research in Yoga and Naturopathy conduct research at units, institutes and centres throughout India. This research includes clinical studies, drug research, survey and cultivation of medicinal plants, pharmacognosy, phytochemistry, pharmacology, toxicology, drug standardisation, family welfare research, and literary research on the revival of classical medical literature (Lavekar & Sharma, 2005).

Every country in the South-East Asia Region provides some degree of public funding for TCAM research and development within the national health budget, although the amount of money involved may be relatively small — as in Bangladesh, where total spending on TCAM is only 2% of the allopathic health care budget. In addition to the funding, a number of these countries have received grants from international organisations such as WHO, UNDP and the European Union to improve their TCAM infrastructure (Gaitonde & Kurup, 2005). In Bhutan, for example, a new Pharmaceutical and Research Unit was commissioned in 1997 through a project funded by the European Community. Small-scale mechanised production began in 1982, with support from WHO, and since 1998 all TCAM products are have been produced mechanically according to good manufacturing practice (GMP) regulations. Eight products have been introduced for commercial sale in the local market (Wangchuk, 2005).

The United States has a national governmental centre dedicated to TCAM research. This is the National Center for Complementary and Alternative Medicine (NCCAM) at the National Institutes of Health, Department of Health and Human Services. It was established by Congress in 1992, originally as the Office of Alternative Medicine, and mandated to support rigorous scientific research, train researchers and disseminate its findings (Brixey *et al.*, 2005). Currently the budget for NCCAM is in excess of US$100 million. In addition there is growing support from the non-profit sector, with health-oriented private foundations and medial insurers providing research funding for CAM studies. No other country in the Region of the Americas provides public finance for TCAM research or development on a regular basis (Gupta, 2005), although in Argentina, exceptional grants are provided by the Agency for Promoting Science and Technology (Zacchino, 2005). In Suriname, there is no public financing system, but two non-governmental organisations work together on a project to promote collaboration between allopathic and traditional systems of medicine (Pan American Health Organization/WHO Regional Office for the Americas, personal communication, 2004).

Only two European Region countries are known to have provided public funding for TCAM research. The Government of Norway has undertaken to fund collaborative projects between allopathic physicians and a variety of TCAM providers (Dr. Vegard Nore, personal communication, 2003). In Germany, the Federal Ministry of Education and Research funded a number of TCAM research projects between 1981 and 1999, providing a total of US$17 million, although since then there has been no further government support, and ongoing research is supported by the private sector (Bornhöft, 2005).

Funding for TCAM research and development in Africa is mainly provided by international donor organisations, although individual projects may be executed by national government agencies. It often reflects the unspoken aim of increasing industrialisation and raising national GDP, rather than understanding and improving traditional health care as it is utilised at the local level. For example, in Nigeria, the UN Development Program is funding a pilot project to develop a medicinal and aromatic plant industry. The project is implemented by the National Institute of Pharmaceutical Research and Development, and has already developed two commercial phytomedicines, for treating sickle-cell anaemia and malaria, respectively (Gamaniel *et al.*, 2005). Likewise, in Tanzania, the WHO Regional Office for Africa is providing technical support for the commercial production of dihydroartemisinin-based anti-malarial medications from *Artemisia annua* (WHO-AFRO, 2003).

In the context of the high utilisation of TCAM worldwide, it is perhaps surprising that no national government or intergovernmental organisation has yet provided funding for comparative research into the relative cost-effectiveness of traditional and biomedical systems of health care, and of integrating the two approaches. Such research might focus either on the costs of achieving specified public health outcomes, or on the potential benefits obtainable per dollar (or other currency unit). Retrospective analysis of insurance records may be one possible approach to evaluating cost-effectiveness, especially in terms of interventions intended to improve general health or prevent disease. Herron & Hillis (2000) (see also Bodeker *et al.*, Chapter 1 of this volume) have demonstrated the value of such analysis, showing that the use of the Transcendental Meditation technique in Canada resulted in cost savings of up to $300 million per year in health insurance payments.

2.6. Discussion

In countries where traditional health care systems have not yet been formalised or officially recognised, they are closely bound to specific social and cultural contexts. Payments for service provision are made out-of-pocket, but there is often a personal understanding between patient and practitioner to overcome problems of affordability. As steps are taken towards incorporating these systems of medicine into national health services, they are almost inevitably taken out of context and adapted to resemble allopathic health systems more closely. 'Traditional health care' undergoes the same transformations as 'indigenous agricultural knowledge' (c.f. Fairhead, 1993) when incorporated into national and international development programmes: political and personal aspects are omitted, together with any beliefs and practices that do not conform to the explanatory models of biomedical science. Herbalism may be separated from ritual practices such as divination, and transplanted into clinical settings, in order to present a more 'modern' image and avoid allegations of witchcraft or superstition.

In this process of formalisation, there is a real risk of losing the flexibility that characterises traditional health systems, as their practitioners begin to follow allopathic professionals in demanding immediate cash payment. Unless service provision is directly funded by national governments, user fees may also rise, to compensate for higher overheads and the expense of processed herbal products. Incorporation of improved traditional health care services into medical insurance programmes will benefit only those with enough disposable income to afford the premiums, thereby excluding a considerable proportion of society: 'The poor may be relegated to purchasing unregulated drugs from unlicensed street vendors, as already happens in so many poor countries. This would stand in contrast to the customary role of traditional medicine serving as the first and last resort for available health care for the poor' (Bodeker, 2002).

Some TCAM therapies — such as Chinese phytotherapy and acupuncture — appear to be undergoing a transition from 'traditional medicine', accessible to the poorest in low-income countries, to 'complementary and alternative medicine', favoured by urban elites in the industrialised world (Bodeker *et al.*, 2005). A similar trend may soon be evident for Ayurveda, which is already gaining popularity in Europe and the Middle East. This shift in the global socio-demographic profile of users increases the likelihood that the cost of TCAM services will rise worldwide. At the national level, this could be viewed as advantageous, in terms of raising the GDP of developing countries and increasing commercial opportunities. However, care must be taken to avoid a further widening of the gap between rich and poor within these countries. Public sector investment will be needed to prevent disenfranchisement of poor and marginalised groups from access to safe and effective traditional health care, as the 'improved' TCAM increasingly becomes the domain of those with greater levels of disposable income.

2.7. Conclusions

At a global level, a large proportion of the cost of TCAM is still paid out-of-pocket, often in the context of customary mechanisms to ensure affordability for all patients. Public financing systems exist in a number of countries, but some of these are health insurance programmes that cover only certain approved TCAM therapies, and may provide only partial reimbursement of treatment costs.

In an ideal situation, the most equitable financing model would incorporate TCAM into a national health service, free of charge to all members of the population. More commonly, where this is not possible due to national budget restrictions, economic policies on traditional medicine should aim to keep user fees affordable, perhaps also providing backing for various payment instruments, including payments in kind and instalments.

International organisations such as WHO have an important role to play in raising the profile of economic research on TCAM and thereby working to ensure that TCAM remains accessible to the poorest members of society, throughout the world. There is an urgent need for comparative research on the relative cost-effectiveness of traditional and biomedical systems of health care, and of integrated systems that combine aspects of both, in order for governments to make informed decisions about the best use of scarce resources to improve public health.

References

African Development Bank/UNICEF. *Les Strategies d'Adaptation Sociales des Populations Vulnerables d'Abidjan facé à la Developpement et à ses Effets [Strategies of Social Adaptation to Development and Its Effects Among Vulnerable Populations in Abidjan]*. Abidjan, 1995.

Ahorlu CK *et al.* Malaria-related beliefs and behaviour in southern Ghana: implications for treatment, prevention and control. *Trop Med Int Health* 1997;2: 488–499.

Astin JA. Why patients use alternative medicine: results of a national study. *JAMA* 1998;279:1548–1553.

Betti JL. Medicinal plants sold in Yaoundé markets, Cameroon. *Afr Study Monogr* 2002;23:47–64.

Bodeker G. A framework for cost benefit analysis of traditional medicine and conventional medicine. In: Chaudhury RR (ed). *Traditional Medicine in Asia*. Delhi: World Health Organization Regional Office for South East Asia, 2002.

Bodeker G, Ong, C-K, Grundy C, Burford G, Maehira Y (eds.) *WHO Global Atlas of Traditional Complementary and Alternative Medicine*. Kobe, Japan: WHO Centre for Health Development, 2005.

Bornhöft G. Federal Republic of Germany. In: Bodeker G, Ong C-K, Grundy C, Burford G, Maehira Y (eds.) *WHO Global Atlas of Traditional,*

Complementary and Alternative Medicine. Kobe, Japan: WHO Centre for Health Development, 2005, pp. 125–134.

Bouchayer F. Alternative medicines: a general approach to the French situation. *Complement Med Res* 1990;4:4–8.

Brixey RJD, Kun KE, Killen J. United States of America. In: Bodeker G, Ong C-K, Grundy C, Burford G, Maehira Y (eds.) *WHO Global Atlas of Traditional, Complementary and Alternative Medicine*. Kobe, Japan: WHO Centre for Health Development, 2005, pp. 63–74.

Cho HJ. Traditional medicine, professional monopoly and structural interests: a Korean case. *Social Sci Med* 2000;50:123–135.

El-Gendy AR. Regional Overview: Eastern Mediterranean Region. In: Bodeker G, Ong C-K, Grundy C, Burford G, Maehira Y (eds.) *WHO Global Atlas of Traditional, Complementary and Alternative Medicine*. Kobe, Japan: WHO Centre for Health Development, 2005, pp. 153–158.

Fairhead J. Representing knowledge: the 'new farmer' in research fashions. In: Pottier J (ed.) *Practising Development: Social Science Perspectives*. London: Routledge, 1993, pp. 187–204.

Finne B, Viksveen P. *A Survey of Ten Countries Where Homeopathy is Being Practised*. Oslo: Norwegian Homeopathic Association, 1999.

Fisher P, Ward A. Complementary medicine in Europe. *Br Med J* 1994;309: 107–110.

Gaitonde BB, Kurup PNV. Regional Overview: South-East Asia. In: Bodeker G, Ong C-K, Grundy C, Burford G, Maehira Y (eds.) *WHO Global Atlas of Traditional, Complementary and Alternative Medicine*. Kobe, Japan: WHO Centre for Health Development, 2005, pp. 75–82.

Gamaniel KS, Fakeye T, Sofowora A. Federal Republic of Nigeria. In: Bodeker G, Ong C-K, Grundy C, Burford G, Maehira Y (eds.) *WHO Global Atlas of Traditional, Complementary and Alternative Medicine*. Kobe, Japan: WHO Centre for Health Development, 2005, pp. 27–32.

Gilani AH, Hannan A, Islamic Republic of Pakistan. In: Bodeker G, Ong C-K, Grundy C, Burford G, Maehira Y (eds.) *WHO Global Atlas of Traditional, Complementary and Alternative Medicine*. Kobe, Japan: WHO Centre for Health Development, 2005, pp. 165–170.

Gupta MP. Regional Overview: Region of the Americas. In: Bodeker G, Ong C-K, Grundy C, Burford G, Maehira Y (eds.) *WHO Global Atlas of Traditional, Complementary and Alternative Medicine*. Kobe, Japan: WHO Centre for Health Development, 2005, pp. 41–50.

Hayatie Amal M, Hardaningsih MHA. Republic of Indonesia. In: Bodeker G, Ong C-K, Grundy C, Burford G, Maehira Y (eds.) *WHO Global Atlas of*

Traditional, Complementary and Alternative Medicine. Kobe, Japan: WHO Centre for Health Development, 2005, pp. 97–102.

Health Canada. *Perspectives on Complementary and Alternative Health Care. A Collection of Papers Proposed for Health Canada*. Ottawa, 2001.

Herron RE, Hillis SL. The impact of the transcendental meditation program on government payments to physicians in Quebec: an update. *Am J Health Promot* 2005;14:284–291.

Heusser P. Commentary on Sommer *et al*. A randomized experiment of the effects of including alternative medicine in the mandatory benefit package of health insurance. *Complement Ther Med* 2000;8:50–53.

Hien TV, Truong CQ. Socialist Republic of Viet Nam. In: Bodeker G, Ong C-K, Grundy C, Burford G, Maehira Y (eds.) *WHO Global Atlas on Traditional, Complementary and Alternative Medicine*. Kobe, Japan: WHO Centre for Health Development, 2005, pp. 205–211.

Hill E. Over the edge: health care provision, development, and marginalisation. In: Hill E (ed.) *Development for Health*, Oxford: Oxfam Publications, 1997:6–13.

Høg E. Kingdom of Denmark. In: Bodeker G, Ong C-K, Grundy C, Burford G, Maehira Y (eds.) *WHO Global Atlas of Traditional, Complementary and Alternative Medicine*. Kobe, Japan: WHO Centre for Health Development, 2005, pp. 117–124.

Jütte R. Homöopathie im europäischen Trend [European trends in homeopathy]. *Biol Med* 1999;28:242–247.

Kadel RE. Chiropractic in the Netherlands. *Digest Chiropr Econ* 1991; 33:64–67.

Kale R. Traditional healers in South Africa: a parallel health care system. *Br Med J* 1995;310:1182–1185.

Lantum DN. Republic of Cameroon. In: Bodeker G, Ong C-K, Grundy C, Burford G, Maehira Y (eds.) *WHO Global Atlas of Traditional, Complementary and Alternative Medicine*. Kobe, Japan: WHO Centre for Health Development, 2005, pp. 13–18.

Lavekar GS, Sharma SK. Republic of India. In: Bodeker G, Ong C-K, Grundy C, Burford G, Maehira Y (eds.) *WHO Global Atlas of Traditional, Complementary and Alternative Medicine*. Kobe, Japan: WHO Centre for Health Development, 2005, pp. 89–96.

Leboeuf-Yde C *et al*. Chiropractic in Sweden: a short description of patients and treatment. *J Manipulative Physiol Ther* 1997;20:507–510.

MacLennan AH, Wilson DW, Taylor AW. Prevalence and cost of alternative medicine in Australia. *Lancet* 1996;347:569–572.

Menges LJ. Regular and alternative medicine: the state of affairs in The Netherlands. *Social Sci Med* 1994;39:871–873.

Monckton J *et al. COST Action B4: Unconventional Medicine in Europe. Final Report of the Management Committee, 1993–1998.* Brussels, European Commission Directorate-General for Science, Research and Development, 1999.

Ong CK, Banks B. *Complementary and Alternative Medicine: The Consumer Perspective.* London: The Prince of Wales's Foundation for Integrated Health, 2003.

Ong CK, Bodeker G, Burford G. United Kingdom. In: Bodeker G, Ong C-K, Grundy C, Burford G, Maehira Y (eds.) *WHO Global Atlas on Traditional, Complementary and Alternative Medicine.* Geneva: WHO, 2005a, pp. 143–152.

Ong CK, Høg E, Bodeker G, Burford G. Regional Overview: European Region. In: Bodeker G, Ong C-K, Grundy C, Burford G, Maehira Y (eds.) *WHO Global Atlas on Traditional, Complementary and Alternative Medicine.* Geneva: WHO, 2005b, pp. 109–116.

Ong CK *et al.* Health status of people using complementary and alternative medical practitioner services in four English counties. *Am J Public Health* 2002;92:1653–1656.

Pedersen P. The identity of chiropractic practice with special reference to Western Europe: a literature review. *Eur J Chiropr* 1990;38:41–55.

Phillips MR, Lu S, Wang R. Economics reform and the acute inpatient care of patients with schizophrenia: the Chinese experience. *Am J Psychiatry* 1997;154:1228–1234.

Roh P-U. Regional Overview: Western Pacific Region. In: Bodeker G, Ong C-K, Grundy C, Burford G, Maehira Y (eds.) *WHO Global Atlas of Traditional, Complementary and Alternative Medicine.* Kobe, Japan: WHO Centre for Health Development, 2005, pp. 183–186.

Scrimgeour D. Funding for community control of indigenous health services. *Aust N Z J Public Health* 1996;20:17–18.

State Administration of Traditional Chinese Medicine of the People's Republic of China. *Anthology of Policies, Laws and Regulations of the People's Republic of China on Traditional Chinese Medicine.* Shangdong University, 1997.

Thomas KJ, Nicholl JP, Coleman P. Use and expenditure on complementary medicine in England: a population-based survey. *Complement Ther Med* 2001;9:2–11.

Thorne S. Spas accepted part of health care in Czech Republic. *Can Med Assoc J* 1995;153:94–95.

Ullman D. The international homeopathic Renaissance. *Berlin J Res Homeopath* 1991;1:118–120.

Veal L. Complementary therapies in Iceland. *Complement Ther Nurs Midwifery* 1997;3:12–15.

Veal L. A comparison of the use of complementary therapies in Australia and Iceland. *Complement Ther Nurs Midwifery* 2001;7:72–77.

Wangchuk D. Kingdom of Bhutan. In: Bodeker G, Ong C-K, Grundy C, Burford G, Maehira Y (eds.) *WHO Global Atlas of Traditional, Complementary and Alternative Medicine.* Kobe, Japan: WHO Centre for Health Development, 2005, pp. 83–88.

World Health Organization (2001) *Legal Status of Traditional Medicine and Complementary/Alternative Medicine: A Worldwide Review.* Geneva: World Health Organization, 2001 (WHO/EDM/TRM/2001.2).

World Health Organization, Regional Office for Africa (WHO/AFRO) Press Release, 25 April 2003. *WHO to Support Production of Indigenous Anti-Malarial Medicine in Africa.* Brazzaville: WHO/AFRO. http://www. afro.who.int/press/2003/pr2003042502.html (2003).

Yamada H. Japan. In: Bodeker G, Ong C-K, Grundy C, Burford G, Maehira Y (eds.) *WHO Global Atlas of Traditional, Complementary and Alternative Medicine.* Kobe, Japan: WHO Centre for Health Development, 2005, pp. 193–198.

Zacchino SA. Argentine Republic. In: Bodeker G, Ong C-K, Grundy C, Burford G, Maehira Y (eds.) *WHO Global Atlas of Traditional, Complementary and Alternative Medicine.* Kobe, Japan: WHO Centre for Health Development, 2005.

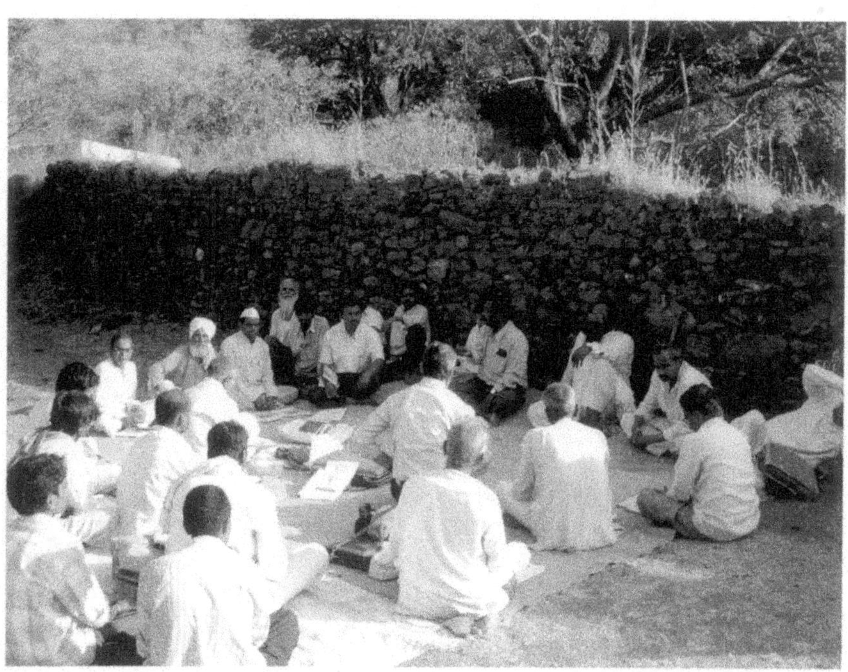

Rural herbalists in Karnataka, South India, participate in a training session focused on the documentation and assessment of local health traditions. [*Source*: Foundation for Revitalization of Local Health Traditions, Bangalore, India (www.frlht.org.in).]

TRAINING

Gerard Bodeker, Cora Neumann, Chi-Keong Ong
and Gemma Burford

3.1. Informal Training Trends

As described in a number of country chapters and regional overviews in this volume, indigenous health systems and informal training programmes can be found throughout the world. Informal overview systems for TCAM training also exist in many communities, through networks of master practitioners, local TCAM associations and self-regulation by community members.

Informally trained traditional health practitioners (THPs) include bonesetters, herbalists, masseurs, snake/insect bite healers, spiritual practitioners, traditional birth attendants and midwives, as well as 'master practitioners' offering a variety of treatments. Danish medical law also allows that 'anyone may care for the ill', within certain limitations (Høg, 2005).

The informal training process can be characterised by two current trends. The first is informal training and registration that allows THPs to move relatively easily into an 'official' TCAM system, or one that is accepted by the community. Such training and registration can take place at either the local or the national level. The second is the emerging practice of training THPs in public health methods such as HIV/AIDS education and safe childbirth practices, which allows them registration and a degree of acceptance into the allopathic sector.

3.1.1. *Informal Training and Registration in the TCAM Sector*

3.1.1.1. Local level

Local training and registration processes can be seen in Afghanistan, Cameroon, Ghana, Indonesia, Latin America and several countries in the Western Pacific Region. In Afghanistan, most of the professional practitioners (*hakim* and *tabib*) of Unani medicine receive instruction from local *tabibs*. Some, however, study in Pakistan or India. TCAM education may be passed from one generation to the next at home, through experienced elderly women; through 'quasi-professional' specialists; or through apprenticeships under master practitioners (*ustâ, xalifa*) (El-Gendy, 2005a).

In Cameroon, compounds of master practitioners constitute informal schools for inculcation by apprenticeship or participant-observation. Initiation is often done by these masters or community leaders, as community recognition is an important part of the 'certification' process (Lantum, 2005). In Ghana (Oppong-Boachie, 2005) and Nigeria (Gamaniel *et al.*, 2005), traditional medicine practitioners (TMP) are defined as persons who are recognised and accepted for healthcare based on indigenous theories, beliefs and experiences handed down through generations.

Latin American countries, in particular Bolivia, Guatemala, Peru and Ecuador, have high percentages of native Amerindian populations who depend heavily on their indigenous medicines. Due to lack of educational infrastructure in rural areas, informal local training is provided for herbalists, masseurs, bonesetters and spiritualists. The services of traditional midwives (*partera empírica* or *comadrona*) are heavily used throughout these countries (Gupta, 2005).

All countries of the South-East Asia Region report the existence of unregistered, informally trained practitioners. In Indonesia, for example, non-standardised local training is available in Jamu medicine and supernatural healing (Gaitonde & Kurup, 2005).

In the Western Pacific Region, informally-trained THPs are those with neither institutional training nor qualifications, who are allowed to practice after several years of apprenticeship under an established local traditional health practitioner (Roh, 2005).

3.1.1.2. National Level

Informal training and registration regulated at the national level can be seen throughout the South East Asia Region. The majority of South East Asian countries have adopted national legislation to mainstream TCAM practice and education, with an increasing focus on registration and licensing (Gaitonde & Kurup, 2005). Compulsory registration of trained as well as untrained practitioners has been introduced in most countries of the Region. Traditional healers and other TCAM practitioners are currently required to register with the ministry of health in all countries, with the exception of Indonesia and the Maldives. In Thailand, master-apprentice training ends with a licensing examination through the Division of Medical Registration in the Ministry of Health. Though this training is informal, the standardised examination indicates some level of self-regulation.

3.1.2. *Public Health Training for Traditional Health Care Providers*

3.1.2.1. Traditional Birth Attendants (TBAs)

A significant trend in the informal training sector is the growing number of public health training programmes available to THPs. According to a recent WHO report, over 500,000 women die every year from childbirth-related complications, including haemorrhage, infection and obstructed labour. In many developing countries, traditional midwives are the primary care-givers during the childbirth process, and though many midwives are highly trained and experienced, the overwhelming majority of maternal deaths occur in these regions. In light of these vital health concerns, a 2004 meeting of the WHO Regional Office for Africa called for widespread training of traditional midwives and birth attendants in safe delivery and safe motherhood practices, including sanitation, nutrition and timely referral to allopathic clinics during emergencies (WHO/AFRO, 2004).

Today, training programmes for traditional birth attendants (TBAs) can be found in at least some countries of every WHO region. Across the African and Eastern Mediterranean Regions, various national authorities and international agencies, such as the WHO Safe Motherhood Initiative, provide training in allopathic primary health care to traditional midwives and birth attendants. Seventeen of the 36 countries in the WHO African Region have such programmes (Kasilo *et al.*, 2005). In Malawi, for example, the training and control of TBAs has been an aspect of Ministry of Health policy since the late 1970s. Development of a national training programme began in 1978 and was expanded by the whole country by 1982. The four-week course involves lectures, observation, discussions, role play, demonstrations, practice, evaluation exercises, field trips, tours of health centres, and social activities specific to health issues such as personal hygiene and sanitation (Smit, 1994). In Djibouti, it is reported that traditional birth attendants, trained by health ministry staff, work within the primary health structure and receive supplies from UNICEF. A long period of breastfeeding is encouraged to promote birth spacing and nutrition (Hatem, 1996). In Sudan, TBAs are trained and utilised in family planning programmes, where they succeed in increasing contraception use (El-Gendy, 2005a).

Training programmes for TBAs have sometimes been criticised, both for over-simplifying complex situations and neglecting the realities of rural homebirth, thus effacing or excluding much of what local people actually believe and do (Pigg, 1995; Davis-Floyd, 2000) and for failing to bring about any significant change in TBA practice (Anderson, 2004). In Mexico, UNICEF has now discontinued funding for TBA training courses, in the absence of any noticeable decrease in maternal mortality over 20 years of training (Davis-Floyd, 2000).

Sibley *et al.* (2004) have conducted a critical review of 16 studies to determine whether TBA training improves the rate of referral of women with obstetric complications to health facilities. They found a medium, positive, non-significant association between training and TBA knowledge of risk factors and conditions requiring referral; and small, positive, significant associations between TBA referral behavior and maternal service use. These results cannot be causally attributed to TBA training because of the overall quality of studies, and the fact that in several of the studies, TBA training was a component of integrated intervention packages. The authors concluded that it is difficult to justify the effort and expense of more rigorous research focusing on TBA training, if the goal is to improve access to emergency obstetric care, due to the complexity of the referral process. They further assert that the real effects of TBA training on TBA and maternal behaviour are likely to be small.

Anderson *et al.* (2004) identify two key issues in the debate: logistical barriers to reaching biomedical health services in a timely manner, and differences in cognitive frameworks between biomedical and traditional practitioners. One potential solution suggested by Davis-Floyd (2000) is the development of a 'partnership paradigm' between TBAs and biomedically trained midwives, based on mutual respect and learning from one another's successes, in contrast to the current system of 'training' that implies the imposition of the biomedical model of birth. She cites a model developed by Dr. Galba Araujo, the former Head of Obstetrics and Gynaecology at a tertiary care centre in Fortaleza, north-east Brazil:

> *'Concerned about high mortality rates in the rural regions his hospital served, he went out to the rural communities and asked the midwives what was needed. Their answer was that women needed a clean and safe place to give birth; most of their houses had dirt floors, and cleanliness was almost impossible to maintain. So he created a system of maternity care clinics in numerous rural villages... Each centre was equipped with the hammocks in which local women preferred to give birth, and with the drugs and equipment that Dr. Araujo felt the midwives should have. He also created an efficient ambulance system, so that transport was readily available should the midwives call for it. Outcomes in these maternity centres were so good that Dr. Araujo began to study what the traditional midwives did, and ended up incorporating hammocks, more patience, and upright positions for birth into the hospital'* (Davis-Floyd, 2000).

There is increasing evidence that many of the 'standard' obstetric interventions widely utilised in global biomedical practice, such as amniotomy (rupture of the amniotic membrane), imposition of a prone position, epidural anaesthesia and episiotomy, may in fact be counterproductive and even harmful in certain circumstances. Bright lights, noise and mother-infant separation, all of which are characteristic of childbirth in biomedical settings, have also been associated with poorer postpartum outcomes and even psychiatric problems in later life (Odent, 2002). In the light of this research, it might be advisable to reconsider the concept of 'training TBAs', and to promote partnership-based models as described above — in which TBAs participate in the 'training' of obstetricians and hospital-based midwives, as well as the reverse. The issue of TCAM training for allopathic health care providers is discussed in Section 3.2.2 below.

3.1.2.2. Other Traditional Health Practitioners (THPs)

Another important move in the training of traditional practitioners in allopathic approaches is found in the management of global epidemics such as HIV/AIDS and tuberculosis. Up to 80% of populations in many African countries rely on traditional medicine for their primary health care, not only out of choice but also due to the lack of allopathic facilities and providers. In Ghana, for example, the three northern regions have only 68 doctors, or 6% of the national total. It has been recommended that public health facilities staff another 268 doctors and over 15,000 other health care professionals to reach optimum operational standards (Ministry of Health, Ghana, 2001).

In the light of the current HIV/AIDS crisis in the African Region, the training of THPs in necessary allopathic approaches has been encouraged. Information sharing and educational programmes in South Africa have resulted in THPs providing correct HIV/AIDS advice as well as demonstrations of condom use. One such programme trained 1510 THPs, and it was calculated that during the first ten months of the programme, some 845,600 of their clients may have been reached with AIDS/STD prevention messages. In similar programmes in Mozambique, traditional healers learned that AIDS is transmitted by sexual contact, by blood and unsterile razor blades used in traditional practice. In a follow-up evaluation, 81% of those trained reported that they had promoted condom use with at least their STD patients (Green, 1997).

King and Homsy (1997) have reviewed the initial outcomes and challenges of programmes aiming to train traditional healers as HIV/AIDS educators and counsellors in Zambia, Uganda, Botswana, Malawi, Mozambique, South Africa, and Central African Republic. At the time of the review, none of the projects had completed a comprehensive evaluation of the different approaches used, or of their real impact on the population served. Overall, however, the authors concluded that traditional healers are capable of performing at least as well as their biomedical counterparts in this arena. They identified the lack of systematic follow-up, after initial training, as an area of concern for many projects.

Similar training programmes have also been implemented outside Africa, notably in Brazil (Nations & de Souza, 1997) and Nepal (Poudel *et al.*, 2005). In the Brazilian programme, which involved 126 Afro-Brazilian healers working in urban slums, significant increases (P < 0.001) in AIDS awareness, knowledge about risky HIV behaviour, information about correct condom use, and acceptance of lower-risk, alternative ritual blood practices, and significant decreases (P < 0.001) in prejudicial attitudes related to HIV transmission were found among mobilized healers as compared to 100 untrained controls. Likewise, in western Nepal, training was found to lead to significant improvements in healers' knowledge of HIV transmission, misconceptions and preventative measures.

Public health training programmes with a non-HIV focus appear to be less common, but a few examples have been identified from published literature. In Ghana, for example, the Danfa Project has been established to decrease the verbal dissemination of inaccurate and dangerous information about traditional remedies; reduce opportunities for unskilled and unrecognised practitioners to operate within the health system; and educate villagers about 'improved' traditional health care, including the safe preparation of home remedies (Yeboah, 2000). In Chikwaka District, Malawi, an interactive training programme was conducted with traditional healers to reduce the incidence of corneal disease and vision loss among patients using traditional eye medicines (TEM) (Courtright *et al.*, 1996). The authors reported that blindness among patients reporting the use of TEM decreased from 44% to 21%, while bilateral corneal disease in patients using TEM decreased from 31% to 10%.

As discussed in Section 3.4.2 below, 'training' is often used as a synonym for the medicalisation of traditional health care. In Nepal, for example, the expressed objective of one training programme (Poudyal *et al.*, 2003) was to improve healers' knowledge of allopathic medicine — i.e. the causes, prevention and treatment of common illnesses according to the biomedical model, as well as the use of first aid kits — and their relationship with government health workers. The authors stated that 'up-scaling this model is a challenge for improving community health care in Nepal in the future'.

3.2. Formal Training and Regulation

The term 'formal training' can be loosely defined as those programmes recognised by national authorities, granting nationally recognised degrees and certifications. Formal training in TCAM can be found in both public and private colleges and universities, technical schools, continuing education courses, short certification programmes, and TCAM association-run courses and degree programmes.

As many formal training programmes are run either solely or through collaborations between government departments, private institutions and national TCAM associations, these same bodies are often involved in the regulation of TCAM programme content, practitioner licensing and curriculum standardisation. This overlap may enhance or hinder quality control and objective standardisation of the TCAM sector. Licensing and practitioner 'registration' often coincide with training regulations, and are regulated by both training institutions and national authorities.

3.2.1. *Formal Training for TCAM Providers*

Formal education programmes leading to TCAM degrees, which exist outside conventional medical school settings, offer courses of varying levels and durations. Some of these courses are also available to allopathic medical students, though the majority specialises in training for TCAM-only practitioners.

Within the WHO African Region, Ghana offers a Bachelor of Science degree in herbal medicines; Kenya has established a Karati Rural Service and School of Alternative Medicine and Technology; Zimbabwe has established a School of Traditional Medicine and a Bachelor of Science in Natural Medicine; and Nigeria has a formalised diploma course for traditional herbalists (Kasilo *et al.*, 2005).

TCAM training courses are offered by various associations and private institutions in many countries of the Region of the Americas: for example, through societies and schools in Argentina, Bolivia, Canada, Chile, Colombia, Mexico and the United States. In Cuba, national state-run universities offer formal TCAM degree programmes. In Argentina, various TCAM associations provide training in chiropractic, natural medicine, medicinal plants, acupuncture, homeopathy, Ayurveda and phytomedicine. In the United States, TCAM accrediting boards and councils currently run 70 acupuncture schools, 16 chiropractic colleges, 63 massage therapy schools, three naturopathic programmes and 20 osteopathic colleges. Association-run training courses in chiropractic, massage therapy, naturopathy, acupuncture and Traditional Chinese Medicine are available in Canada (Gupta, 2005).

TCAM associations in the Americas are involved to varying degrees in regulation and practitioner licensure. In Argentina, Canada and the United States, national councils oversee TCAM generally, and regional or state accreditation bodies regulate training and licensure. In the United States, TCAM professional licensure is regulated at the state level: acupuncture is currently licensed in 42 states; chiropractic in all states; homeopathy in three states; massage therapy is in 33 states; and naturopathy in 12 states. In Canada, chiropractic is regulated in all provinces, massage therapy in three provinces, naturopathy in four, and acupuncture and Traditional Chinese Medicine in three (Gupta, 2005).

In the Eastern Mediterranean Region, TCAM training varies greatly from one country to another. In Pakistan, the Ministry of Health oversees the qualifications of practitioners in Unani, Ayurvedic and Homeopathic medicine, as well as the subject of the 'old system' of medicine. The Board of Homeopathic Systems of Medicine registers practitioners who have completed a four-year course at recognised teaching institutions, or who are deemed as 'possessing the requisite knowledge and skill'. In order to practice legally in the United Arab Emirates, TCAM practitioners (including homeopaths, herbalists, acupuncturists, chiropractors and Ayurveda, Traditional Chinese Medicine and Unani practitioners) must possess a degree from an accredited TCAM institution, and must also pass the national TCAM qualifying examinations administered by the Ministry of Health (El-Gendy, 2005b).

As in the Americas, TCAM associations are largely responsible for TCAM training in the European region. In Germany, TCAM associations offer training in osteopathy, Ayurvedic medicine, electroacupuncture, bioresonance, Bach-flower therapy and other therapies (Bornhöft, 2005). In the United Kingdom, the European Herbal Practitioners' Association plans to develop a core curriculum for herbal medicine, together with specific curricula for the Western, Chinese and Ayurvedic herbal traditions, and has established an accreditation board to assess training standards (Lampert, 2001).

In many South and South East Asian countries, national legislation to mainstream TCAM practitioners has either preceded or followed the establishment of facilities for formal TCAM training. Ministries of Health oversee most of these programmes, and in India, 30% of Ayurveda, Yoga, Unani, Siddha or Homeopathy (AYUSH) colleges are government or state-run (Gaitonde & Kurup, 2005).

Several countries of the Western Pacific Region have formal training for TCAM providers. There are more than 30 universities or colleges for traditional medicine in China, and examinations are overseen by the National Scientific, Technical and Educational Department. Traditional Chinese Medicine (TCM) and integrated TCM–allopathic care are offered for ambulatory emergency care in 52.2% of urban health centres and 48.3% of rural clinics in China (Baoyan, 2005). In Japan, providers of acupuncture, moxibustion and Judo-seifuku therapy are trained in technical schools and universities, and all TCAM practitioners must pass national qualifying examinations for licensing by the Ministry of Health, Labor and Welfare (MHLW). In Vietnam, most formal TRM training is organised by the government and is provided by Hanoi University, four provincial medical colleges, the Military Academy of Medicine, three Ministry of Health secondary schools, and one private Training Bureau (Roh, 2005).

3.2.2. TCAM Training for Allopathic Practitioners

TCAM courses for allopathic health professionals are increasingly being offered in all of the WHO regions. These courses vary in length and level from short courses, through certification programmes lasting one or two years, to Masters and Doctoral level courses.

In the African Region, Burkina Faso, Cameroon, Congo, Equatorial Guinea, Gambia, Ghana, Guinea, Kenya, Lesotho, Liberia, Madagascar, Malawi, Mali, Rwanda, Senegal, Sierra Leone, South Africa, Uganda and the United Republic of Tanzania provide formal training in traditional medicine for pharmacists, doctors and/or nurses. In Tanzania, short traditional medicine exposure courses for medical, pharmacy, dental and nurse undergraduate students are in place at two colleges (Kasilo *et al.*, 2005).

Table 3.1. TCAM Educational Programmes in South East Asia Region.

Country	Programme(s)	Curriculum
Bangladesh	9 Unani and Ayurveda institutes under Ministry of Health (MOH) regulation	4–5 year courses + 1 year clinical internship
Bhutan	1 programme under MOH National Institute of Traditional Medicine	5½ year graduate course, 3½ year assistant course + 6 month internship. Includes some allopathic medicine methods
DPRK	TRM programme within each medical school (one per province)	7 year course. 30% of curriculum focused on allopathic medicine
India	259 undergraduate colleges; 69 postgraduate institutes	Bachelor, MD and PhD degrees of various lengths in Ayurveda, Siddha, Unani, Homeopathy, Naturopathy and Yoga (AYUSH)
Myanmar	1 national institute (Mandalay); various local	4 years + 1 year internship for diploma; 10-month qualification and 2-month refresher courses for TCAM practitioners
Nepal	1 programme (Tribhuvan University)	Bachelors degree (BAMS) in Ayurveda
Sri Lanka	Various indigenous and Ayurveda programmes	Basic medical and PhD degrees
Thailand	Various public and private, formal and informal	National Institute and national NGO offer 3 year courses in pharmacy, Thai TRM, Ayurveda, massage, reflexology; primary and secondary school programmes (non-formal)

Adapted from Gaitonde & Kurup (2005).

Similarly, in Zimbabwe, all medical students spend part of their training in rural areas in order to gain first-hand experience in traditional medicine (Barrett, 1996).

In the Region of the Americas, Argentina, Canada and the United States offer TCAM programmes for allopathic practitioners. In Argentina, programmes in various TCAM disciplines are offered at the University of Buenos Aires, two schools of pharmacy and one regional medical school (Gupta, 2005). In the United States and Canada, a growing number of universities offer continuing education and elective courses on different TCAM therapies, and 98 of the 126 medical schools in the U.S. currently include CAM instruction as part of their required curriculum, as well as a range of TCAM electives (Brixey *et al.*, 2005).

Within the Eastern Mediterranean Region, medical students in both Somalia and the United Arab Emirates attend short courses on TCAM. Allopathic doctors in the United Arab Emirates may earn additional TCAM qualifications through a diploma or postgraduate certificate in any of the MOH recognised TCAM specialties, but must also pass the national TCAM qualifying examinations administered by the Ministry of Health. Pharmacy schools in the Syrian Arab Republic and the Islamic Republic of Iran include curricula on herbal medicines. In Saudi Arabia, the Ministry of Health restricts acupuncture licenses to those persons who have at least 200 hours of training; are anaesthetists, rheumatologists, or orthopaedists; and comply with hygienic standards (El-Gendy *et al.* 2005b).

Within the European Region, Georgia, Germany, Hungary and the United Kingdom offer TCAM training for medical students. In Georgia, all medical students study the pharmacology and pharmacognosy of certain officially recognised herbal medicines. In Germany, the study of naturopathy (including phytotherapy) during medical training became mandatory in October 2003, and state licensing examinations for pharmacists include a compulsory paper on herbal medicines and other 'natural healing substances'. Postgraduate medical specialisations in TCAM can be obtained in naturopathy (including phytotherapy), balneotherapy, chiropractic, homeopathy and acupuncture. The German Federal Chamber of Physicians regulates postgraduate TCAM education of physicians, and TCAM medical associations have developed an internationally standardised postgraduate education. In Hungary, where the practice of 'higher-level' therapies such as homeopathy, Ayurveda and traditional Tibetan medicine is restricted to allopathic physicians, these subjects are taught in medical universities. In the United Kingdom, short courses on TCAM are offered as part of the undergraduate curriculum in many medical schools, and the Faculty of Homeopathy has accredited training centres for registered healthcare professionals (Ong *et al.*, 2005).

Various countries of the South East Asia Region offer continuing education for allopathic practitioners, and in Indonesia, doctors and nurses may train in acupuncture (Gaitonde & Kurup, 2005).

The Western Pacific Region countries in which TCAM is offered within formal education systems are Australia, China, Hong Kong, Japan, Korea, Macao, Malaysia, Mongolia, Singapore and Vietnam. In Japan, Kampo medicine is included in the curriculum of 93% of Japan's medical schools and 91% of pharmacy schools (Roh, 2005).

3.3. Allopathic Medicine and TCAM

As can be seen from the examples given above, there is enormous variation in the nature of TCAM training programmes for allopathic health care providers, with a corresponding diversity of objectives. Clearly, in the light of the high utilisation of TCAM worldwide (Bodeker *et al.*, Chapter 1 of this volume), it is vital for all health care professionals to understand the nature of the TCAM therapies that their patients may be using, and the implications for conventional treatment, such as the possibility of drug-herb interactions. However, some of the longer courses are clearly not aimed at providing 'exposure' alone; rather, they are intended to develop practical skills, and to encourage allopathic health care providers to incorporate TCAM therapies into their regular practice. It is unclear to what extent the distinctive features of TCAM therapies are incorporated into any of these programmes — encouraging conventional physicians, for example, to take a more holistic and socially situated view of health care — and, conversely, to what extent individual healing modalities are isolated from their social and cultural contexts in order to make them more acceptable within biomedical settings. As discussed in Chapter 1, the emerging global discipline of 'medical acupuncture' represents one such example of recontextualisation (see also Barnes, 2003).

More worrying than the content and nature of training programmes is the trend, observed in a number of countries, for allopathic health care professionals with *no* specific TCAM training to be permitted to provide these therapies in biomedical contexts. In the *WHO Global Atlas of Traditional, Complementary and Alternative Medicine* (Bodeker *et al.*, 2005), the maps detailing the extent to which allopathic health care professionals are entitled to provide TCAM have revealed rather surprising patterns.

                    G. Bodeker et al.

3.3.1. *Conventional Physicians*

Only eight countries, which include Bolivia, Indonesia and Portugal, have structures that expressly forbid conventional physicians from practicing TCAM. Thirty-eight countries allow physicians with no recognisable TCAM training to provide TCAM. This list includes countries such as Australia, Belgium, Denmark, France, Japan, the Netherlands, Qatar, the United Kingdom and the United States.

Another 42 countries allow physicians with TCAM training to provide TCAM. India, Pakistan, China, Brazil, Singapore, Vietnam, Saudi Arabia, the United Arab Emirates, Hungary and Iceland are among the countries that allow physicians to provide TCAM only after recognised TCAM training (Bodeker *et al*, 2005).

3.3.2. *Nursing Profession*

More stringent standards appear to apply to nursing and the other allied health professions. Forty-six countries, including the USA, Brazil, France, Japan, Indonesia and Venezuela, disallow nurses from providing TCAM. Clearly, two sets of standards apply. In certain nations such as the USA, Japan, Denmark and France, where physicians are allowed to provide TCAM with little or no training, nurses are excluded. Only 14 countries, including China, Cyprus, Hungary, Iceland, India and the United Arab Emirates, allow nurses to provide TCAM if they have obtained recognised training. Eight countries, including the United Kingdom, Australia, Germany, the Netherlands and Norway, allow nurses to provide TCAM without any formally recognised training (Bodeker *et al.*, 2005).

3.3.3. *Other Allied Health Professions: Physiotherapists, Pharmacists and Midwives*

Forty-six countries do not permit physiotherapists to provide TCAM, while ten countries allow the practice of TCAM by physiotherapists without recognised training. Australia, Belgium, the Netherlands, Norway, Switzerland and the United Kingdom fall into the latter category. Eight countries, including India, Hungary and Iceland, allow physiotherapists to practice TCAM if they have the requisite training.

Forty-six countries prevent midwives from providing TCAM, with nine allowing practice if recognised training has been obtained. Eight countries allow the practice of TCAM without formally recognised training.

Although sparse data was available for pharmacists, 29 countries were found to prevent pharmacists from providing TCAM, with 11 allowing practice if recognised training has been obtained, and another 11 countries allowing the practice of TCAM without formally recognised training.

Five countries allowed all of the listed categories of allopathic health care providers — physicians, nurses, midwives, physiotherapist and pharmacists — to provide TCAM without formally recognised training. These countries are Ireland, Malta, the United Kingdom, Norway and the Netherlands (Bodeker *et al.*, 2005). Clearly, this raises issues of patient safety, and these countries might well be advised to tighten regulation and control of who is allowed to practice TCAM within their borders.

3.4. Emerging Trends in TCAM Training and Policy

3.4.1. *Regional Policy Trends*

Policy commitment to the development and regulation of TCAM education and training is widespread in all WHO Regions. While many ministries of health acknowledge progress towards fulfilling their policies, substantial gaps remain, implying a need for increased funding for TCAM.

In the African Region, 16 countries (44%) have a national expert committee on TCAM; 14 countries (39%) have a national programme on TCAM; and 31 countries (86%) have established a national office of TCAM in the Ministry of Health (Kasilo *et al.*, 2005). Gaps between legislation and practice continue to exist in some of these areas, however. For example, although legislation in the United Republic of Tanzania (Government of the United Republic of Tanzania, 2002) mandates TCAM training for both allopathic and TCAM providers, and the Tanzania Traditional and Alternative Medicine Council plans to develop and oversee education and training, these policies have not yet been implemented.

TCAM policies in the Region of the Americas are, on the whole, less developed than those in Africa, despite the fact that many of the indigenous populations rely on TCAM for their primary care. Argentina is focused only on CAM, perhaps because of its relatively small indigenous population. The United States allows CAM associations and accrediting bodies to run the majority of TCAM education and regulation. Although policy calls for formalisation, this process remains divided between private and national organisations (Gupta, 2005).

In Europe, the 1999 European Commission final report on TCAM under the Cooperation in Science and Technology (COST) framework (Monckton *et al.*, 1999) recommended that TCAM organisations set up boards for licensing and accreditation purposes, and it was hoped that these organisations would oversee guidelines for training, practice and research within their respective fields. Despite these recommendations, training and licensing vary greatly across European countries. The Russian Federation is another example of a country with significant gaps between policy and practice: a certification system for folk healers was first introduced in 1993, but to date, only three of the 89 regions making up the Russian Federation have enforced the law (A. Goryunov, personal communication, 2003).

With the exception of the Democratic People's Republic of Korea, where TCAM is integrated by law, countries of the South-East Asia Region are focused equally on THP registration and education (Gaitonde & Kurup, 2005). In the Western Pacific Region, some countries allow only conventional doctors to provide TCAM, although in others, traditional practitioners are recognised and in part registered (Roh, 2005). In the Eastern Mediterranean Region, renewed interest in TCAM is seen in Kuwait and the Islamic Republic of Iran, but policy has not yet been enacted. Pakistan and Afghanistan follow the South East Asian trends of recognising and registering THPs (El-Gendy, 2005b).

3.4.2. *Medicalisation of TCAM*

As discussed above, there are global trends towards providing both public health training for TCAM practitioners, and TCAM training for conventional health care professionals. The net result is a growing medicalisation of TCAM therapies, as they are integrated into formal health systems. Contributing factors include fears about the safety and efficacy of TCAM, particularly with regard to the absence of standardised dosages; power and economic dynamics, including the legacy of colonialism and the general global dominance of the 'West' (Burford *et al.*, Chapter 2 of this volume; Davis-Floyd, 2000); and the familiar nature of institutionalised allopathic medicine to policy-makers in many countries, due to the nature of the respective education systems in those countries.

Possible implications of medicalisation include a decreased emphasis on the value of local knowledge and THPs; endangering the therapeutic qualities of TCAM-only practice (Bornhöft, 2005); and a continued marginalisation of TCAM-only practitioners. These outcomes, in turn, could contribute towards the disappearance of beneficial traditional practices that might otherwise — in a more supportive policy environment — have enhanced the provision of care in formal health facilities, as in the example given by Davis-Floyd (2000) and cited in Section 3.1.2.1 above.

3.5. Conclusions

In countries with long histories of formal TCAM development and standardised knowledge, such as India and China, and regions with large indigenous populations, such as Africa and South East Asia, strong policies and practical commitments exist for developing education and recognising THPs. Training courses in HIV/AIDS and safe motherhood in the two latter regions are also helping to consolidate the valuable contribution of THPs to public health, although care must be taken to ensure that the content and delivery of these courses remains culturally relevant and appropriate.

Throughout the world, gaps in the provision of TCAM training remain, due to a lack of funding and/or political will. There is a general trend towards greater government commitments to standardising and regulating TCAM education, particularly in industrialised countries, driven by increasing consumer demand and commercial interest. Nonetheless, in many cases these policy commitments have yet to be translated into practice. The integration of TCAM into national education systems in Europe, the United States, Canada and Japan may increase as scientific evidence for its efficacy and safety becomes available. In the meantime, however, TCAM remains 'the other mainstream' in these countries.

Countries with long traditions of TCAM, as well as those with significant financial resources, may become the leaders in shaping future trends. The South East Asia Region, in particular, can lead the way through continued registration and integration of THPs into the formal sector. Registration and licensing systems potentially encompass both those THPs who have been apprenticed to an acknowledged master, and those who have gained a nationally recognised qualification, thereby offering a meeting point between formal and informal systems of training.

One caveat to this approach, however, is that it may result in an increasing medicalisation of TCAM without full integration into the 'modern' infrastructure. This could potentially lead to further marginalisation and a perception of THPs as under-qualified doctors for the poor, rather than providers of distinct and separate forms of treatment. It is important for policy-makers, allopathic practitioners and traditional health care providers themselves to be alert to the issue of the medicalisation of TCAM, and consciously seek partnership models in which the advantages of both health care systems are maintained.

Training should not be construed merely as something that is given *by* doctors and hospital-based midwives, *to* traditional healers and birth attendants, respectively. Rather, it can be framed as an ongoing process of dialogue between different paradigms of health care, with the shared aim of optimising the services provided to patients and their families within their specific socio-cultural contexts. In this two-directional model, registered and licensed providers of TCAM — having already passed through training programmes recognised by their own communities, governments or the respective leaders of their professions — should be accepted by allopathic health care providers as equals, and as potential teachers. Such a model is contigent on the acceptance of non-biomedical health care modalities as 'complementary', rather than 'alternative', ways of understanding well-being and managing illness.

Carefully targeted programmes of national funding for appropriate training, research and development can help to ensure that TCAM retains its distinctive nature and continues to serve the needs of the poorest in society, while also offering greater health care choices to those with the ability to pay. International agencies such as WHO, and private foundations involved in funding health care research and development, also have important roles to play in this process.

References

Anderson BA, Anderson EN, Franklin T, Dzib-Xihum de Cen A. Pathways of decision making among Yucatan Mayan traditional birth attendants. *J Midwifery Womens Health* 2004;49(4):312–319.

Baoyan L. People's Republic of China. In: Bodeker G, Ong C-K, Grundy C, Burford G, Maehira Y (eds.) *WHO Global Atlas of Traditional, Complementary and Alternative Medicine: Text Volume*. Kobe, Japan: WHO Centre for Health Development, 2005, pp. 187–192.

Barnes LL. The acupuncture wars: the professionalizing of American acupuncture — a view from Massachusetts. *Med Anthropol* 2003 (Jul–Sep) 22(3): 261–301.

Barrett S. Zimbabwe uses all medical resources to find solutions. *AIDS Anal Afr* 1996;6(1):13.

Bodeker G, Ong C-K, Grundy C, Burford G, Maehira Y (eds.) *WHO Global Atlas of Traditional, Complementary and Alternative Medicine: Map Volume*. Kobe, Japan: WHO Centre for Health Development, 2005.

Bornhöft G. Federal Republic of Germany. In: Bodeker G, Ong C-K, Grundy C, Burford G, Maehira Y (eds.) *WHO Global Atlas of Traditional, Complementary and Alternative Medicine: Text Volume*. Kobe, Japan: WHO Centre for Health Development, 2005, pp. 125–134.

Brixey RJD *et al.* United States of America. In: Bodeker G, Ong C-K, Grundy C, Burford G, Maehira Y (eds.) *WHO Global Atlas of Traditional, Complementary and Alternative Medicine: Text Volume*. Kobe, Japan: WHO Centre for Health Development, 2005.

Courtright P, Lewallen S, Kanjaloti S. Changing patterns of corneal disease and associated vision loss at a rural African hospital following a training programme for traditional healers. *Br J Ophthalmol* 1996;80(8):694–697.

Davis-Floyd R. Anthropological perspectives on global issues in midwifery. *Midwifery Today* 2000; 53.

El-Gendy AR. *Status of Traditional Medicine/Complementary and Alternative Medicine in the Eastern Mediterranean Region*. Cairo: World Health Organization Regional Office for the Eastern Mediterranean, 2004 (unpublished internal document). Cited in abridged form as El-Gendy AR, Regional Overview: Eastern Mediterranean Region. In: Bodeker G, Ong C-K, Grundy C, Burford G, Maehira Y (eds.) *WHO Global Atlas of Traditional, Complementary and Alternative Medicine, Text Volume*. Kobe, Japan: WHO Centre for Health Development, 2005a, pp. 153–158.

El-Gendy AR. Regional Overview: Eastern Mediterranean. In: Bodeker G, Ong C-K, Grundy C, Burford G, Maehira Y (eds.) *WHO Global Atlas of Traditional, Complementary and Alternative Medicine: Text Volume.* Kobe, Japan: WHO Centre for Health Development, 2005b, pp. 153–158.

Gaitonde BB, Kurup PNV. Regional Overview: South-East Asia. In: Bodeker G, Ong C-K, Grundy C, Burford G, Maehira Y (eds.) *WHO Global Atlas of Traditional, Complementary and Alternative Medicine: Text Volume.* Kobe, Japan: WHO Centre for Health Development, 2005.

Gamaniel KS, Fakeye T, Sofowora A. Nigeria. In: Bodeker G, Ong C-K, Grundy C, Burford G, Maehira Y (eds.) *WHO Global Atlas of Traditional, Complementary and Alternative Medicine: Text Volume.* Kobe, Japan: WHO Centre for Health Development, 2005.

Government of the United Republic of Tanzania. *The Traditional and Alternative Medicine Act No. 23 of 2002.* Dar es Salaam: Government Printer, 2002.

Green EC. Participation of traditional healers in AIDS prevention programs. *Trop Doct* 1997;27(Suppl 1):56–59.

Gupta MP. Regional Overview: Region of the Americas. In: Bodeker G, Ong C-K, Grundy C, Burford G, Maehira Y (eds.) *WHO Global Atlas of Traditional, Complementary and Alternative Medicine: Text Volume.* Kobe, Japan: WHO Centre for Health Development, 2005.

Hatem MM. Health development in Djibouti. *World Health Forum* 1996;17: 390–391.

Høg E. Denmark. In: Bodeker G, Ong C-K, Grundy C, Burford G, Maehira Y (eds.) *WHO Global Atlas of Traditional, Complementary and Alternative Medicine, Text Volume.* Kobe, Japan: WHO Centre for Health Development, 2005.

Kasilo OMJ *et al.* Regional Overview: African Region. In: Bodeker G, Ong C-K, Grundy C, Burford G, Maehira Y (eds.) *WHO Global Atlas of Traditional, Complementary and Alternative Medicine: Text Volume.* Kobe, Japan: WHO Centre for Health Development, 2005.

King R, Homsy J. Involving traditional healers in AIDS education and counselling in sub-Saharan Africa: a review. *AIDS* 1997;11(Suppl A):S217–S225.

Lampert N. *Briefing Document on Statutory Self-regulation for Herbal Medicine in the UK.* London: European Herbal Practitioners Association, 2001.

Lantum DN. Cameroon. In: Bodeker G, Ong C-K, Grundy C, Burford G, Maehira Y (eds.) *WHO Global Atlas of Traditional, Complementary and Alternative Medicine: Text Volume.* Kobe, Japan: WHO Centre for Health Development, 2005.

Ministry of Health, Government of Ghana. *The Health of the Nation: Reflections on the First Five Year Health Sector Programme of Work.* Accra, 2001; 1–68.

Monckton J *et al. COST Action B4: Unconventional Medicine in Europe. Final Report of the Management Committee*, 1993–1998. Brussels: European Commission Directorate-General for Science, Research and Development, 1999.

Nations MK, de Souza MA. Umbanda healers as effective AIDS educators: case-control study in Brazilian urban slums (*favelas*). *Trop Doct* 1997; 27(Suppl 1):60–66.

Odent M. *The Farmer and the Obstetrician*. London: Free Association Books Ltd, 2002.

Ong C-K *et al.* United Kingdom. In: Bodeker G, Ong C-K, Grundy C, Burford G, Maehira Y (eds.) *WHO Global Atlas of Traditional, Complementary and Alternative Medicine: Text Volume*. Kobe, Japan: WHO Centre for Health Development, 2005.

Oppong-Boachie FK. Ghana. In: Bodeker G, Ong C-K, Grundy C, Burford G, Maehira Y (eds.) *WHO Global Atlas of Traditional, Complementary and Alternative Medicine: Text Volume*. Kobe, Japan: WHO Centre for Health Development, 2005.

Pigg SL. Acronyms and effacement: traditional medical practitioners (TMP) in international health development. *Soc Sci Med* 1995;41(1):47–68.

Poudel KC, Jimba M, Joshi AB, Poudel-Tandukar K, Sharma M, Wakai S. Retention and effectiveness of HIV/AIDS training of traditional healers in far western Nepal. *Trop Med Int Health* 2005;10(7):640–646.

Poudyal AK, Jima M, Murakami I, Silwal RC, Wakai S, Kuratsuji T. A traditional healers' training model in rural Nepal: strengthening their roles in community health. *Trop Med Int Health* 2003;8(10):956–960.

Roh P-U. Regional Overview: Western Pacific. In: Bodeker G, Ong C-K, Grundy C, Burford G, Maehira Y (eds.) *WHO Global Atlas of Traditional, Complementary and Alternative Medicine: Text Volume*. Kobe, Japan: WHO Centre for Health Development, 2005.

Sibley L, Sipe TA, Koblinsky M. Does traditional birth attendant training improve referral of women with obstetric complications: a review of the evidence. *Soc Sci Med* 2004;59(8):1757–1768.

Smit JJ. Traditional birth attendants in Malawi. *Curationis* 1994;17(2): 25–28.

World Health Organization Regional Office for Africa (WHO/AFRO). Press Release, 17 February 2004, *Meeting on Reducing Maternal and Newborn Mortality Opens in Harare*. http://www.afro.who.int/press/2004/pr2004021702.html. Accessed 25 April 2004 at 12:02.

Yeboah T. Improving the provision of traditional health knowledge for rural communities in Ghana. *Health Libr Rev* 2000;17(4):203–208.

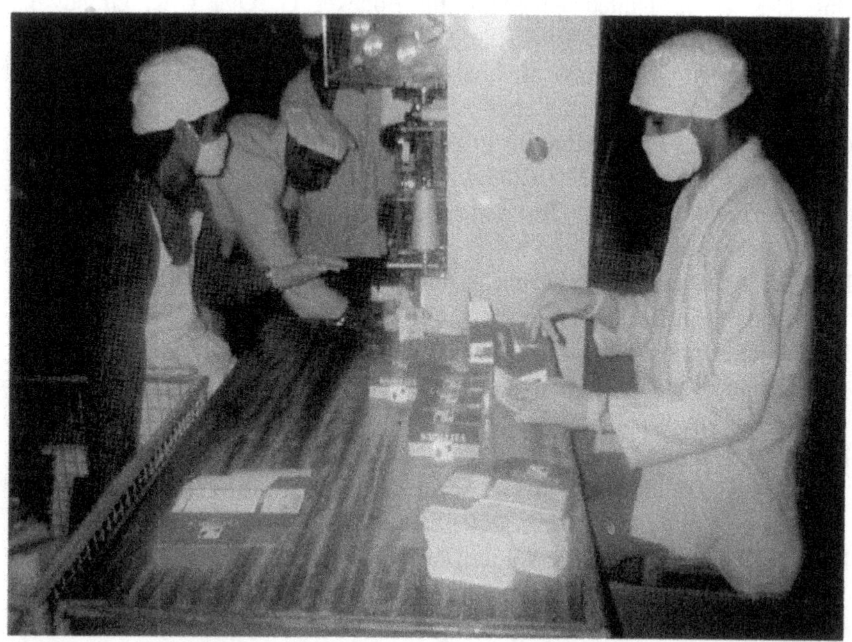

Adherence to international standards of good manufacturing practice is a key factor in ensuring the safety of herbal products. Ayurvedic teas being packaged at the Maharishi Ayurveda Products factory in Noida, India. (*Photo courtesy of G. Bodeker.*)

CHAPTER 4

SAFETY: ISSUES AND POLICY

Gilbert Shia, Barry Noller and Gemma Burford

4.1. Introduction

The global growth in the popularity of traditional, complementary and alternative medicine (TCAM) has been well reviewed (Bodeker *et al.*, Chapter 1 of this volume). This growth is evident both in countries with a long history of traditional medicine use and those in which certain forms of treatment, such as acupuncture and herbal medicine, are alternative or complementary to the dominant allopathic health care system. In spite of this, there is still a serious lack of data on the safety of TCAM methodologies around the world.

Evidence of traditional use of a given plant or formula, or of a particular technique, is often regarded as equivalent to proof of safety, but this assumption may not always hold. The globalisation of TCAM has important implications for both the quality control of medications, and the training and competence of practitioners. Furthermore, when traditional health care approaches are taken out of their original contexts and incorporated into 'alternative and complementary' health care in industrialised countries — as in the case of acupuncture, traditional Chinese herbalism and Ayurveda — there is an increased need for vigilance (c.f. Burford *et al.*, Chapter 2 of this volume; Barnes, Chapter 5 of this volume). It cannot necessarily be assumed that a known technique will produce the desired effects, and no others, in a physiologically different population. Unexpected side effects can also result from modification of formulations, techniques, or methods of preparation and storage, as well as the inevitable human error factor.

The World Health Organization has issued a number of documents relevant to the safety of traditional health care approaches, as reviewed in Section 4.2 below. In this chapter, we have also reviewed the national policies of a number of individual WHO Member States in respect of this issue (Section 4.4), with the aim of drawing parallels between countries and districts, and highlighting policies adopted by particular states that could be useful to others.

4.2. Relevant WHO Guidelines on Safety of Traditional Medicine

The World Health Organization (WHO) has a long-standing interest in traditional medicine. In 1978, at the International Conference on Primary Health Care, the Declaration of Alma-Ata was made. One of its recommendations was the inclusion of proven traditional remedies into national drug policies and regulatory measures (WHO, 1978). In 1989, the World Health Assembly urged Member States to make a comprehensive evaluation of their traditional systems of medicine, and to identify medicinal plants with a satisfactory efficacy/side-effect ratio (Resolution WHA42.43). It also recommended introducing regulation to maintain the standard of medicinal plant products. The policy of WHO with respect to traditional medicine was presented in the Director-General's Report on Traditional Medicine and Modern Health Care to the 44th World Health Assembly 1991. The report stated that 'WHO collaborated with its Member States in the review of national policies, legislation and decisions on the nature and extent of the use of traditional medicine in their health systems'. The major objectives of the Traditional Medicine Programme were derived from the relevant resolutions.

Guidelines for the Assessment of Herbal Medicines were drafted at a WHO Consultation in Munich, Germany in June 1991, and adopted for general use by the Sixth International Conference on Drug Regulatory Authorities in Ottawa later that year (WHO, 1991). These guidelines define basic criteria for the evaluation of quality, safety and efficacy of herbal medicines, to assist national regulatory authorities. As a general rule, such assessment should take into account the medical, historical, and ethnological background of herbal products, and traditional experience of their use. Detailed descriptions of the products from medical or pharmaceutical literature, or other written accounts of their application, must be provided. Safety assessment should incorporate documented experience of safety (in traditional use) and toxicological studies, where indicated. The Guidelines for the Assessment of Herbal Medicines also set out important requirements for product labelling, and for package inserts providing information to consumers.

In 1994, the WHO Regional Office for the Eastern Mediterranean published Guidelines for Formulation of National Policy on Herbal Medicines (WHO/EMRO, 1994). The WHO Traditional Medicine Strategy 2002–2005 stated that the World Health Organization would promote the safety of traditional medicine by expanding evidence-based information. It would also monitor the safety of herbal medicines and related products, and provide technical guidelines and methodology for evaluating their safety (WHO, 2002).

In 2001, the World Health Organization Traditional Medicine Programme Team published an informal document entitled 'Legal Status of Traditional Medicine and Complementary/Alternative Medicine: A Worldwide Review' (WHO, 2001). This constituted an updated and expanded version of the 1998 document 'Regulatory Situation of Herbal Medicines: A Worldwide Review' (WHO, 1998). These two documents describe the policy of Member States individually.

4.3. Global Forum on Safety of Herbal and Traditional Medicine

In July 2001 a conference entitled the Global Forum on Safety of Herbal and Traditional Medicine was held at the Gold Coast, Australia (Noller *et al.*, 2001). The inputs of various groups covered the status of complementary medicine in Australia and comparative examples from Africa and Bangladesh, the status of databases and needs for a focus on safety outcomes as a point of direction from the forum. Safety evaluation, which incorporates quality procedures, was identified as another point of focus. The issues identified were incorporated into a statement, the 'Gold Coast Declaration on Safety of Herbal and Traditional Medicine', which was prepared and endorsed by the forum (Noller *et al.*, 2001). It was recommended that an international centre be established within the Commonwealth to implement the needs and knowledge gaps in the good manufacture and safe use of herbal and traditional medicine. Steps have been taken to create such a centre in Bangladesh, following a series of planning meetings during 2003–2005. A symposium on safety and quality issues and challenges of the herbal medicine industry was also held at Brisbane, Australia in 2002.

4.4. National Policies and Regulation

While traditional medicine is used in a large majority of WHO Member States (123 of 191 countries) (WHO, 2001), there are considerable differences in utilisation spectra. Countries such as China and Viet Nam use almost exclusively indigenous forms of medicine, which have been their main health care systems for many centuries. Their practice is well accepted in everyday life, and their benefits are recognised by the public. Traditional medicine is part of their culture, and regulations were developed with this pretext. Furthermore, policies have been developed around one or a small number of traditional therapies, and laws have been evolving over centuries. Many countries, on the other hand, have recognised the use of traditional medicine relatively recently, and a wide selection of different health care traditions have become popular in a short period of time. Therapies identified during a survey in the United States included relaxation techniques, herbal medicines, massage, chiropractic, spiritual healing, megavitamins, imagery, diets, energy healing, homeopathy, hypnosis, biofeedback, and acupuncture (Eisenberg *et al.*, 1998). In Australia, traditional therapies are considered to include Traditional Chinese Medicine, Ayurveda, traditional European herbal medicine, homeopathy, aromatherapy, and a number of other traditional systems of health care. Many of the users from these countries have little cultural identification to these alternative medicines, and accept them on their holistic and naturalistic credentials. Regulations have been developed to protect both consumer rights and public health (WHO, 2001). These regulations must be equally applicable to medicine from all traditions, and many are in the early days of being exercised. All these factors influence the attitude of policy makers towards the issue of safety.

4.4.1. *Regulation of Herbal Products*

Some countries have accepted the experience from historical use, and have regulated herbal medicine separately from allopathic medicine. In Japan, for example, some herbal medicines are included in the Japanese Pharmacopoeia. Herbal medicines that are in frequent use, but not included in the Pharmacopoeia, are examined according to specific criteria and officially recognised by inclusion in *The Japanese Herbal Medicine Codex*.

In Jamaica, the Food and Drug Regulations were revised by Parliament in 2001. The new law states that herbal products must be approved, although the requirements are not as strict as those for pharmaceuticals. The onus is on manufacturers to demonstrate quality, efficacy and safety (Ministry of Health of the Government of Jamaica, 1999).

The European Parliament is seeking to adopt a simplified registration procedure, the 'traditional use registration', for herbal medicinal products. The registration requirement accepts bibliographic data and historical experience as evidence to support safety and efficacy claims (Commission of the European Communities, 2002; see also Barnes, Chapter 5 of this volume).

Australia has explicitly accepted that traditional experience can be used as evidence to support medical claims. The Complementary Medicines Evaluation Committee recognises two types of evidence to support claims on therapeutic goods: scientific evidence and traditional use. The extent of required evidence depends on the claims made for the product. For the Committee, traditional use refers to written or orally recorded evidence that a substance has been used for three or more generations for specific health-related or medicinal purposes (Therapeutic Goods Administration of Australia, 1999). Similarly, in the Republic of Korea, the Ministry of Public Health and Welfare published a notification in 1969 permitting pharmaceutical companies to produce herbal preparations whose formula is described in the 11 classic books on traditional Korean and Chinese medicine, without first having to submit clinical or toxicological data (WHO, 2001).

In Estonia, only plants included in an official list may legally be used in TCAM treatments. The 1998 Rules for Categorisation of Semi-Medicinal

Products classified such plants into three groups: 'proprietary medicinal products' (prescription only), 'semi-medicinal products' (sold in pharmacies over the counter) and non-medicines (natural products or food additives — no restrictions on sale). The classification of a plant is dependent largely on its perceived potential to cause harm. Semi-medicinal products are subject to the same licensing requirements as proprietary medicinal products, with the proviso that a scientific bibliography detailing 'medicinal background and traditional spheres of use' for each plant drogue — based on approved literature — may be substituted for pre-clinical and clinical testing (Estonia State Agency of Medicines, undated).

As well as relying on historical experience to assure safety, certain countries have established schemes to carry out post-marketing surveillance of herbal medicine. In the United Kingdom, the Medicines and Health care Products Regulatory Agency has extended its Yellow Card scheme for reporting suspected adverse drug reactions (CSM/MHRA, 2004a) to include herbal medicine. The topic of pharmacovigilance of herbal medicines in the UK context is covered in more detail by Barnes (Chapter 5 of this volume). In China, the Centre for Drug Re-evaluation is establishing a nationwide network of monitoring centres to collect adverse effect reports for licensed proprietary herbal medicines (China Concept Consulting and The Information Centre of the State Drug Agency, 2000).

Safety data, whether historical or contemporary, do not necessary have an equal influence on policy in all countries. Countries with their own indigenous systems of health care are more likely to measure risks against benefits, even when the evidence for efficacy is empirical rather than pharmacological. The fate of their traditional practice is never in question. Policies are tailored to enable it to continue in the safest environment. For example, the Health Law Act of Indonesia classifies traditional medicines (*jamu*) into two groups: The first group consists of traditional medicines produced by individual persons or by home industries. The second group consists of traditional medicines produced and packed on a commercial scale, whether large or small. The first group of medicines do not require registration. They are made by traditional medicine practitioners for use by their own patients. They may not be labelled or marked except with the vernacular name. The Minister of Health permits the use of only 54 species of plants in these medicines. The safety of these species is known through traditional experience. Herbal medicines of the second group, on the other hand, must be registered and licensed before they may be sold. In order to be registered, the product must undergo scientific studies to ensure the safety and efficacy, composition and rationality of the composition, dosage form, and claimed indications for the medicines (WHO, 2001).

India has developed a classification for herbal medicines depending on their market availability, and the nature of the herbs themselves. Herbs that have already been used for more than five years are classified as Category 1; those in use for less than five years as Category 2; and new medicines as Category 3. The classification of herbal medicines also depends on whether they contain processed or unprocessed parts of plants, and whether they contain potentially poisonous plants. Requirements for safety and efficacy vary according to the classification and market availability of the product (Chakravarty, 1993). In South Africa, issues of safety and quality take precedence over demonstrations of efficacy. The aim is to regulate, and not to prevent access to, systems of health care that are often used in preference to allopathic medicine (Gray, 1998).

In countries where TCAM has become popular only in recent years, safety is often considered by itself. The regulations in the United States of America, for example, emphasise safety rather than efficacy. They aim to safeguard consumers against fraud, and against dangerous practices and practitioners (WHO, 2001). In the United Kingdom, a list of restricted herbal ingredients has been compiled by considering only adverse effect profiles (CSM/MHRA, 2004b). The German Federal Health Office has set up several commissions of experts to evaluate scientific data on herbal, anthroposophic and homeopathic medications, and to prepare indications for use (Steinhoff, 1993). Evidence of traditional use may be accepted in place of clinical proof of efficacy, but manufacturers of all such products are required to present pharmacological, toxicological and clinical data as proof of safety, with no exemptions given on the basis of long-term utilisation (Steinhoff, 1994; Kraft, 2001).

Quality control of herbs is vital for ensuring safety. A 1993 incident in which a large number of patients in Belgium suffered kidney damage, due to aristolochic acid present in a Chinese herbal medicine, highlighted this issue (Vanherweghem *et al.*, 1993; Vanhaelen *et al.*, 1994). Several incidents of poisoning were believed to be due to the inadvertent confusion of two ingredients with similar names (Vanhaelen *et al.*, 1994). In both Norway and Indonesia, medicinal plants have to be described using several systems of nomenclature, including Latin, local and foreign names, at the same time (WHO, 1998). In Malaysia, there is a legal requirement for registered traditional medicines to be free from dangerous or hazardous ingredients. Incorporation of chemical drugs or scheduled poisons is forbidden. The content of heavy metals such as lead, mercury and arsenic, and also pesticides, should be below the acceptable limits. Likewise, in Germany, Chinese herbs must have a certificate of identification and must demonstrate that heavy metals, pesticides and fungicides are all within permitted limits (Grandjean, 2000).

Labels for TCAM products must give adequate information, which is clear enough for the consumers to use the product properly and safely (WHO, 1998). In Japan, importers of herbal medicine and manufacturers of herbal-based pharmaceutical products have to comply with the provisions laid down in the Japanese Standards for Herbal Medicines (Government of Japan, 1993). In China, all herbal medicine manufacturers must comply with Good Manufacturing Practice (GMP) requirements by the end of 2004 (State Administration of Traditional Chinese Medicine of the People's Republic of China, undated).

4.4.2. *Regulation of TCAM Practitioners*

At present, most countries impose their safety requirements on locally manufactured products and on importers. This leaves out practitioners who are importing small amounts of their own medicine privately. In Australia, medicines can be imported by individuals to bypass normal regulatory controls. In a number of incidents in Queensland, formulated Traditional Chinese Medicines on sale to the public were found to contain excessive quantities of arsenic, lead and mercury (Cooper *et al.*, 2003; Rutherford *et al.*, 2003). Some of these products had not been registered by the Therapeutic Goods Administration, but were removed from sale. Similarly, certain herbal preparations on sale in the United Kingdom were found to contain 'prescription only' medications, and topical skin preparations compounded by individual practitioners were found to contain steroids (Keane *et al.*, 1999).

These examples illustrate that ensuring safety requires the regulation of practitioners, as well as the products they use. The Chinese Medicine Regulation Act (2000) in Victoria, Australia, emphasises an interconnected system of policy controls incorporating both products and practitioners as part of the regulatory framework. In Japan, the Society of Japanese Oriental Medicine has started a system that requires its members to renew their registration every five years. The Japan Pharmacists' Education Centre issues a certificate for pharmacists specialising in Kampo medicines and herbal materials, in accordance with its own qualification criteria. Renewal of this certificate is required every three years (WHO, 2001).

In a number of European countries, legislation to promote safe TCAM practice requires the involvement of a licensed allopathic physician. In Denmark, for example, acupuncturists can practice only under medical supervision, and chiropractors — while not supervised directly — are required to inform the patient's physician of their diagnosis and treatment (WHO, 2001). Conversely, in Italy, chiropractors are regarded as equivalent to medical auxiliaries, and do require a physician's direct supervision (Forieri, 1992). In Hungary, any 'unconventional' treatment must be preceded by a conventional medical diagnosis, and all TCAM providers without medical training must follow the guidance of a licensed physician (Monckton *et al.*, 1999). In Norway, providers of TCAM may treat 'serious diseases' only if there is no objection from the patient's physician (Dr. Vegard Nore, personal communication, 2003).

Some countries in Europe have implemented legislation to prevent TCAM practitioners from carrying out specific medical procedures that have the potential to cause harm if performed incorrectly, such as X-rays, anaesthesia and surgery, and from dispensing prescription-only medications. Others have banned TCAM providers from treating particular conditions that are regarded as especially dangerous to public health, or assumed to be unresponsive to non-allopathic treatment, e.g. venereal diseases, cancer, diabetes, psychiatric conditions or epilepsy. In all of these cases, a licensed physician must be consulted. In the United Kingdom, while TCAM practitioners are permitted to treat cancer, diabetes, epilepsy, glaucoma, tuberculosis and venereal diseases, they may not advertise their treatments or make any claims with respect to these conditions (Walker & Budd, 2002). An overview of restricted medical procedures (other than the use of prescription medicines), and health conditions that may be treated only by allopathic physicians, in various European countries is given in Table 4.1.

Supervision by the allopathic medical establishment is not, however, the only way of promoting the safety of TCAM practice. In a number of countries, voluntary self-regulation has been established, with professional associations of practitioners responsible for devising their own training programmes, setting their own examinations, admitting members, issuing ethical guidelines and monitoring standards. Professional organisations operating as voluntary self-regulatory bodies in Europe include the Danish Chiropractic Association (Launsø, 1995); the French Academy of Osteopathy (Stubbe, personal communication, 2003); the Israeli Association for Classical Homeopathy (Shemmer, 1997); the European Herbal Practitioners' Association, based in the UK (Lampert, 2001); and the Professional Register of Traditional Chinese Medicine (PRTCM), the associated professional body of the Irish College of Traditional Chinese Medicine. The PRTCM has a strictly imposed Code of Ethics and Code of Practice, closely modelled on those accepted by the UK Department of Health, and only fully qualified practitioners who have passed the Licentiate examination may be admitted to the Register. There is also a separate Professional Register of Chinese Herbal Medicine for those who successfully complete the Irish College of Traditional Chinese Medicine's postgraduate course in herbalism (T. Shanahan, personal communication, 2003; PRTCM website, undated).

In the Netherlands, where there are a great many professional organisations representing TCAM practitioners, the Health Inspectorate has been working with patient organisations and health insurers to develop a quality framework. The current framework has 36 criteria, which include recognised training programmes and continuing education, a register of qualified members, codes of conduct, disciplinary rules, complaints procedures and relationships with other health care providers. An independent research organisation is monitoring the progress that is being made in implementing the quality policy, and found, for example, that 82% of the TCAM practitioner organisations had a register of qualified members in 2000, compared to only 63% in 1996 (Sluijs & de Bakker, 2001).

Statutory, rather than voluntary, self-regulation of TCAM professions is another legislative option that has been utilised effectively in some countries. The Norwegian Chiropractors' Association has the status of a

Table 4.1. Medical Procedures and Health Conditions Restricted to Licensed Allopathic Physicians in Europe.

Country	Medical Procedures	Health Conditions	References
Denmark	Anaesthesia Electrical devices Obstetrics Surgery X-rays	Tuberculosis Venereal diseases	WHO, 2001
Germany	Anaesthesia Gynaecology Obstetrics Vaccination X-rays	Infectious diseases Venereal diseases	WHO, 2001; Bornhöft & Matthiessen, pers. comm., 2003
Ireland	Anaesthesia Obstetrics	Venereal diseases	WHO, 2001
Liechtenstein	Surgery	Infectious diseases	WHO, 2001
Netherlands	Anaesthesia (general) Artificial insemination Cardioversion Catherisation Defibrillation Endoscopy Electroconvulsive therapy Injections Lithotripsy Narcosis Obstetrics Surgery X-rays	None stated	WHO, 2001
Norway	Anaesthesia Injections Surgery	Cancer* Infectious diseases	Nore, pers. comm., 2003; WHO, 2001
Russian Federation	None stated	Cancer Infectious diseases Psychiatric conditions Tuberculosis	ECCH, 2002
Sweden	Acupuncture Anaesthesia Obstetrics X-rays	Cancer Diabetes Epilepsy Notifiable diseases	WHO, 2001
Ukraine	None stated	Cancer Infectious diseases Psychiatric conditions	ECCH, 2002

*Non-medical TCAM providers in Norway may not treat cancer-affected tissue directly.

statutory self-regulatory body (Langworthy & Birkelid, 2001), while in the United Kingdom, statutory self-regulation for osteopathy and chiropractic has been in place since 1993 and 1994 respectively, overseen by the General Osteopaths' Council and General Chiropractors' Council (Ong *et al.*, 2002).

In 1999, a Select Subcommittee of the House of Lords in the UK commenced an enquiry into TCAM, and a report was published in 2000, which classified therapies into three groups. These were: (1) professionally organised alternative therapies (acupuncture, chiropractic, herbal medicine, homeopathy and osteopathy); (2) complementary therapies, which included aromatherapy, counselling, healing, hypnotherapy, massage, shiatsu and yoga; and (3) alternative disciplines, such as Ayurvedic, Chinese, naturopathic and anthroposophical medicine. The report's strongest recommendation was for statutory regulation of Group 1 therapies, particularly herbal medicine, in order to ensure patient safety (Thomas *et al.*, 2001). In 2001, the UK Government responded by recommending that practitioners of both herbal medicine and acupuncture should seek statutory regulation as soon as possible, and in 2002, this was followed by the establishment of two independent committees, the Herbal Medicine Regulatory Working Group (HMRWG) and the Acupuncture Regulatory Working Group (ARWG), whose mandate was to consider how such regulation could best be achieved. On the basis of their reports, the Department of Health published a public consultation document in March 2004 that proposed the establishment of a shared CAM Council, which could potentially be extended to other unregulated professions. The consultation document requested feedback, within a three-month period, on a number of questions, such as legal protection of professional titles (e.g. 'herbal practitioner' and 'acupuncturist') and the composition and functions of the Council. After considering the responses, the Government plans to publish a formal proposal for statutory regulation, together with draft legislation, and it has been suggested that both professions could be regulated by 2006 (McIntyre, 2004).

4.5. Conclusions

In summary, most countries have taken account of the popularity of TCAM, and WHO has taken initiatives to issue guidelines on regulation. While safety is a common goal for all policy-makers, their perspectives on risk assessment differ. Some countries assess risk by itself, while others measure it against benefit. The quality of processing can add to the inherent risk of herbal products. Regulating the standard of practitioners is also important in ensuring the safe use of traditional, complementary and alternative medicine by the public. Different methods of achieving this include supervision by the medical profession, voluntary self-regulation, and statutory regulation.

References

Chakravarty BK. *Regul Aff J* 1993;4:699–701.

China Concept Consulting and the Information Centre of the State Drug Agency. *China Pharmaceuticals Guide: New Policy and Regulation*. London: Urch Publishing, 2000.

Commission of the European Communities. *Proposal for a Directive of the European Parliament and of the Council, Amending the Directive 2001/83/EC As Regards Traditional Herbal Medicinal Products*. Brussels: Commission of the European Communities, 2002. Available at: http://europa.eu.int/eur-lex/en/com/pdf/2002/en_502PC0001.pdf (Accessed 24 February 2004 at 00:28).

Cooper KJ, Noller B, Connell D, Yu J, Sadler R, Olszowy H, Golding G, Tinggi U, Moore MR, Myers S. Development of a probabilistic risk assessment approach to assess public health risks associated with heavy metals and metalloids of traditional Chinese medicines. *Abstracts First World Congress on Chinese Medicine*. Melbourne: Melbourne Town Hall, 21–24 November 2003.

ECCH. *European Council for Classical Homeopathy, Report on the Status of Homeopathy in Europe*. Published on the Internet: http://www.homeopathy-ecch.org (2002).

Eisenberg DM *et al*. Trends in alternative medicine use in the United States, 1990–1997. *JAMA* 1998;280:1569–1575.

Estonia State Medicines Agency (undated). Home page: http://www.sam.ee

Forieri DC. Chiropractic education: a critical view from Italy. *Dig Chiropr Econ* 1992;35(2):40–43.

Government of Japan. *The Japanese Standards for Herbal Medicines*. Tokyo: Yakuji Nippo Ltd., 1993.

Grandjean M. Traditionelle chinesische Phytotherapie in Deutschland: sinnvoll oder gefährlich? [Traditional Chinese phytotherapy in Germany: sensible or dangerous?] *Natura Med* 2000;15(4):17–19.

Gray A. *Health Sys Trust Update* 1998;37:9–10.

Keane FM *et al.* Analysis of Chinese herbal creams prescribed for dermatological conditions. *Br Med J* 1999;318:563–564.

Kraft K. History of herbal medicinal use in Germany, with a treatise on present day practice. *J Herbal Pharmacother* 2001;1(2):43–49.

Lampert N. *Briefing Document on Statutory Self-Regulation for Herbal Medicine in the UK.* London: European Herbal Practitioners' Association, 2001.

Langworthy JM, Birkelid J. General practice and chiropractic in Norway: how well do they communicate and what do GPs want to know? *J Manipulative Physiol Ther* 2001;24(9):576–581.

Launsø L. People choose alternative therapies! Consequences for future pharmacy practice. *J Soc Admin Pharm* 1995;12(1):43–52.

McIntyre M. British Government calls for regulation of herbal and acupuncture practitioners in UK. *HerbalGram* 2004;62:66–67.

Ministry of Health of the Government of Jamaica. *Amendments to the Food and Drugs Act and Food and Drugs Regulations to Include Herbal Products: Draft Cabinet Submission, 2 March 1999.* Kingston: Ministry of Health of the Government of Jamaica, 1999.

Monckton J, Belicza B, Betz W, Engelbart H, van Wassenhoven M. *COST Action B4: Unconventional Medicine in Europe. Final Report of the Management Committee, 1993–1998.* Brussels: European Commission Directorate-General for Science, Research and Development, 1999. Published on the Internet in the website of the Research Council for Complementary Medicine, http://www.rccm.org (accessed 27.06.05 at 12:24).

Noller BN, Myers S, Abegaz B, Mohinder Singh M, Kronenberg F, Bodeker G. Global forum on safety of herbal and traditional medicine, 7 July 2001, Gold Coast, Australia. *J Altern Complement Med* 2001;7(5):583–601.

Ong CK, Petersen S, Bodeker G, Stewart-Brown S. Use of complementary and alternative medical services in England: a population survey. *Am J Public Health* 2002;92(10):1653–1656.

PRTCM (undated). *Professional Register of Traditional Chinese Medicine, Ireland.* Published on the Internet: http://www.chinesemedicine.ie

Rutherford S, Marshall I, Loan A, Tempany G, Golding G, Holling N. A pilot survey of the presence of undeclared drugs and health risk associated with metal contamination of complementary medications offered for sale in Queensland. *Aust J Environ Health* 2003;3(4):21–28 .

Shemmer Y. Homoeopathy in Israel. *Homeopath Links* 1997;10(2):63.

Sluijs E, de Bakker D. *Quality Policy of Alternative Practitioners in The Netherlands, Paper Commissioned by Department of Health and Children.* Dublin: Department of Health and Children, 2001 (unpublished paper). Cited in: O'Sullivan T., *Report on the Regulation of Practitioners of Complementary and Alternative Medicine in Ireland*. Dublin: Institute of Public Administration, Health Services Development Unit, 2002.

State Administration of Traditional Chinese Medicine of the People's Republic of China, 未取得ＧＭＰ证书的药厂明年７月１日起一律停产. [Requirements for Good Manufacturing Practice]. http://www.satcm.gov.cn/lanmu/zhongyao/tcm031104gmp.htm (accessed 25 February 2004 at 12:20).

Steinhoff B. The legal situation of phytomedicines in Germany. *Br J Phytother* 1993;3(2):76–80.

Steinhoff B. New developments regarding phytomedicines in Germany. *Br J Phytother* 1994;3(4):190–193.

Therapeutic Goods Administration of Australia. *Overview of the Regulatory Requirements for the Manufacture and Supply of Medicine in Australia and for Export*. Woden: Therapeutic Goods Administration of Australia, 1999.

Thomas KJ, Nicholl JP, Coleman P. Use and expenditure on complementary medicine in England: a population-based survey. *Complement Ther Med* 2001;9:2–11.

United Kingdom Committee on Safety of Medicines (CSM)/Medicines and Healthcare Products Regulatory Agency (MHRA). *Monitoring the Safety and Quality of Medicines: The Yellow Card Scheme*. London: CSM/MRSA, 2004a. http://www.mca.gov.uk/aboutagency/regframework/csm/csmhome.htm (accessed 25 February 2004 at 12:11).

United Kingdom Medicines and Healthcare Products Regulatory Agency. *List of Herbal Ingredients Which are Prohibited or Restricted in Medicines*. Medicines and Healthcare Products Regulatory Agency, 2004b. http://www. mca.gov.uk/ourwork/licensingmeds/herbalmeds/prohibit2.pdf (accessed 25 February 2004 at 12:05).

Vanhaelen M *et al. Lancet* 1994;343:174.

Vanherweghem JL *et al. Lancet* 1993;341:387–391.

Walker LA, Budd S. UK: the current state of regulation of complementary and alternative medicine. *Complement Ther Med* 2002;10:8–13.

World Health Organization. *International Conference on Primary Health Care*, Alma-Ata, USSR, 6–12 Spetember 1978. Available at: http://www.who.int/ hpr/NPH/docs/declaration_almaata.pdf (accessed 9 April 2006 at 01:20).

World Health Organization. *Traditional Medicine Strategy 2002–2005*. Geneva: World Health Organization, 2002. Available at: http://www.who.int/ medicines/organization/trm/orgtrmmain.shtml (accessed 24 February 2004 at 00:04).

World Health Organization. *Legal Status of Traditional Medicine and Complementary/Alternative Medicine: A Worldwide Review*. Geneva: World Health Organization, 2001. Available at: http://www.who.int/medicines/library/trm/who-edm-trm-2001-2/legalstatus.pdf (accessed 24 February 2004 at 00:23).

World Health Organization. *Regulatory Situation of Herbal Medicines: A Worldwide Review*. Geneva: World Health Organization, 1998. Available at: http://www.who.int/medicines/library/trm/who-trm-98-1/who-trm-98-1.pdf (accessed 24 February 2004 at 00:05).

World Health Organization. *Guidelines for the Assessment of Herbal Medicines, WHO/TRM/91.4*. Geneva: World Health Organization, 1991.

World Health Organization Regional Office for the Eastern Mediterranean. *Guidelines for Formulation of National Policy on Herbal Medicines*. Alexandria: WHO Regional Office for the Eastern Mediterranean, 1994.

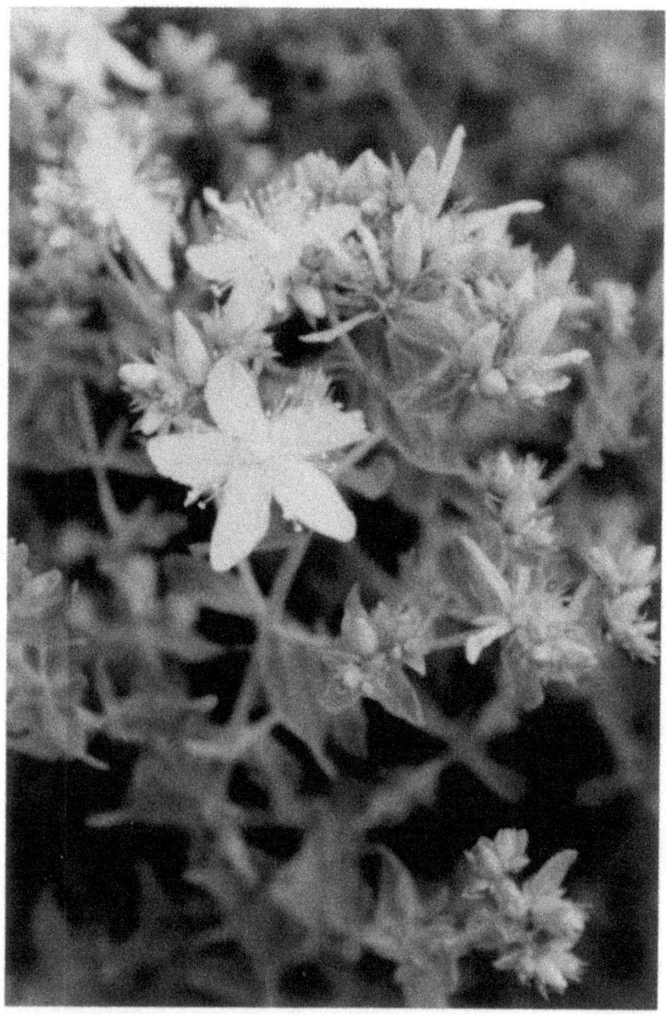

Hypericum perforatum (St. John's Wort) is a popular antidepressant in Europe. Pharmacovigilance has revealed important interactions with several modern medications. (*Photo courtesy of M. L. Willcox.*)

CHAPTER 5

PHARMACOVIGILANCE OF HERBAL MEDICINES: A UNITED KINGDOM PERSPECTIVE[1]

Joanne Barnes

5.1. Introduction

Pharmacovigilance has been defined as '*the study of the safety of marketed drugs under the practical conditions of clinical usage in large communities*' (Mann & Andrews, 2002). It involves monitoring drug safety and identifying adverse drug reactions (ADRs) in humans, assessing risks and benefits, and responding to and communicating drug safety concerns; recently, it has been suggested that there could be more emphasis on extending knowledge of safety rather than focusing on demonstrating harm (Waller & Evans, 2003).

---

[1] This chapter was first published as Barnes J. Pharmacovigilance of herbal medicines: a United Kingdom perspective. *Drug Safety* 2003;26(12):829–851, and is reprinted here by kind permission of Adis International. Footnotes have been added (2005) to update the original text.

                                    J. Barnes

The above definition makes no distinction between pharmacovigilance of conventional and herbal medicines.[2] Indeed, there is no need, nor is it desirable, to separate the two; pharmacovigilance should embrace all preparations used medicinally regardless of their regulatory status, pharmaceutical composition, cultural use and philosophical framework. Hence, the same aims and activities of pharmacovigilance apply to herbal medicines. However, pharmacovigilance activities largely have been focused on conventional medicines, and the current model of pharmacovigilance and its science and processes have developed in relation to synthetic drugs. Applying the existing model and its tools to monitoring the safety of herbal medicines presents unique challenges in addition to those described for conventional medicines, and it is important that these are understood by all stakeholders.

There is an increasing awareness at several levels of the need to develop pharmacovigilance practices for herbal medicines; the WHO, for example, has produced draft guidelines on this (WHO, 2003). Awareness has arisen not only because of the extensive use of herbal medicines, but also because in recent years there have been several high-profile herbal safety concerns which have had an impact on public health. Against this background, this paper aims to provide a critical overview of the current state of pharmacovigilance of herbal medicines in the UK, and to discuss the particular challenges that this area presents. The paper is written from a UK perspective, but also has wider international relevance, particularly to those countries with spontaneous reporting schemes and a health care system similar to those of the UK.

5.2. Herbal Medicines: Challenges for Pharmacovigilance

The unique characteristics of herbal medicines, and the ways in which herbal medicines are named, perceived, sourced, utilised and regulated raise important issues and challenges for pharmacovigilance.

---

[2]For simplicity, the term 'conventional medicines' is used here to describe licensed medicinal products typically comprising a single characterised chemical entity, but also includes more complex products such as vaccines. It is recognised there are licensed herbal medicinal products, and that in the UK some of these are considered conventional medicines, for example, formulations of ispaghula husk licensed for use as bulk-forming laxatives and in hypercholesterolaemia, and standardised formulations of sennosides, licensed for use as stimulant laxatives.

Some issues arise because most herbal medicines can be obtained without a prescription from various outlets, not only pharmacies. Thus, the problems that apply to pharmacovigilance of conventional non-prescription medicines, for example, that generally their use does not involve a prescriber and is not recorded or monitored through the National Health Service (NHS), also apply to herbal medicines. Other problems are specific to herbal medicines and present difficulties over and above those described for conventional prescription and non-prescription medicines.

5.2.1. *Characteristics of Herbal Medicines*

Herbal medicinal products (also known as phytomedicines or phytotherapeutic preparations) are '*medicinal products containing as active substances exclusively herbal drugs or herbal drug preparations*' (European Agency for the Evaluation of Medicinal Products, 2001): i.e. they contain as active ingredients only crude and/or processed plants and/or plant parts; an isolated chemical constituent which originates from plant material is not a herbal medicine. The term 'herbal medicines' is also used generally to describe both relatively crude preparations, such as herbal tinctures, usually supplied by herbal-medicine practitioners (medical herbalists), and manufactured or finished herbal medicinal products, usually formulated as tablets or capsules and available for purchase without a prescription. Legal definitions relating to herbal medicines and explanations of other terms used are given in Table 5.1.

In contrast with conventional medicines, herbal medicines are chemically rich complex mixtures comprising several hundreds of constituents, often more. For many herbal medicines, the chemical constituents are unknown, and even for those with well-documented phytochemistry, there are few for which the specific constituents responsible for pharmacological activity are fully understood.

The profile of constituents is not uniform throughout a plant, and for many plants, only a specific plant part, or parts, such as roots or leaves, is (or should be) used medicinally. Moreover, the precise profile of constituents is likely to vary both qualitatively and quantitatively between different batches of herbal starting materials because of one or more of the following factors

 J. Barnes

Table 5.1. Formal Definitions and Other Terms Used in Relation to Herbal Medicines.

Term	Definition
Herbal remedy	'A medicinal product consisting of a substance produced by subjecting a plant or plants to drying, crushing or any other process, or of a mixture whose sole ingredients are two or more substances so produced, or of a mixture whose sole ingredients are one or more substances so produced and water or some other inert substances' (The Medicines Act, London, 1968).
Herbal substance (herbal drug)	'All mainly whole, fragmented or cut plants, plant parts, algae, fungi, lichen in an unprocessed, usually dried form but sometimes fresh. Certain exudates that have not been subjected to a specific treatment are also considered to be herbal substances. Herbal substances are precisely defined by the plant part used and the botanical name according to the binomial system (genus, species, variety and author)' (Commission of the European Communities, 2002).
Herbal preparation (herbal drug preparation)	'Preparations obtained by subjecting herbal substances to treatments such as extraction, distillation, expression, fractionation, purification, concentration and fermentation. These include comminuted or powdered herbal substances, tinctures, extracts, essential oils, expressed juices and processed exudates' (Commission of the European Communities, 2002).
Herbal medicinal product	'Any medicinal product, containing as active ingredients one or more herbal substances or one or more herbal preparations, or one or more such herbal substances in combination with one or more such herbal preparations; **in addition, the product may contain vitamins or minerals or other non-biological substances for which there is well-documented evidence for its safety; the action of the non-herbal substances must be ancillary to that of the herbal active ingredients**' (Commission of the European Communities, 2003).
Herbal constituent	A specific chemical compound found in a herbal ingredient, e.g. hyperforin found in the aerial parts (herb) of St John's wort.
Herbal ingredient	A specific individual medicinal plant and the plant part, present in a herbal medicine, e.g. St John's wort herb present in St John's wort tablets.

Note that the text in bold type is a recent amendment, the wording of which is still to be confirmed at a European level.

These definitions have now been formally approved in Directive 2004/24/EC (see also footnote 4), with two changes: (1) the definition of a herbal preparation should read 'concentration *or* fermentation'; (2) the section in bold type has now been included in a later section of the Directive, namely Article 16a(2), and slightly modified (Commission of the European Communities, 2004).

(Barnes *et al.*, 2002):

- inter- or intraspecies variation in constituents
- environmental factors, such as climate, and growing conditions
- time of harvesting — the profile of constituents can vary even over the course of a day
- post-harvesting factors, such as storage conditions and drying.

The method of processing crude herbal material, for example, the type of extraction, can also influence the precise chemical composition of a herbal preparation or product. Many herbal medicinal products contain several herbal ingredients, and medical herbalists usually prescribe combinations of herbal tinctures often supplied as a mixture, in both cases, further adding to the chemical complexity of the herbal medicine taken by the patient. The chemical complexity of herbal medicines creates difficulties in determining their clinical pharmacokinetics, pharmacodynamics and toxicology and, equally, where a safety concern has been identified in association with a particular herbal medicine, establishing which constituent(s), even which herbal ingredient(s) with combination herbal medicines, are implicated is problematic.

For the reasons given above, it is likely that there will be variations in the chemical composition of herbal medicines containing the same herbal ingredient but produced by different manufacturers; this will apply to both licensed herbal medicinal products and unlicensed herbal medicines. Several studies have found important differences in the pharmaceutical quality of different products on the US market. For example variations in the content of major constituents in St John's wort (*Hypericum perforatum*) products (which in several cases also differed markedly from the concentrations stated on the label) (De Los Reyes & Koda, 2002), and variations in and unacceptably high concentrations (in several cases, over 25,000 parts per million) of ginkgolic acids, which potentially are allergenic, in ginkgo products (Kressman *et al.*, 2002). Standardisation on content of certain constituents is an approach used by some manufacturers to achieve more consistent pharmaceutical composition, but its usefulness is limited at present since the specific active constituents are known only for a few herbal medicines.

Because of the variations that can exist between different manufacturers' products and preparations of the same herbal ingredient, evidence of safety (and efficacy) should be considered in this light; strictly speaking, evidence is product- or extract-specific, and should be extrapolated only to those products or extracts which have been shown to be pharmaceutically equivalent and bioequivalent (Loew & Kaszkin, 2002). This is largely impractical at present, given the limited data available for herbal medicines; nevertheless, the differences between different preparations of a herbal ingredient should not be ignored. In many cases, because of the nature of herbal medicines, a group of related constituents, rather than a single constituent, is likely to be responsible for an observed adverse effect. In this case, it may be appropriate to group together different preparations and products containing the same herbal ingredient or group of constituents in order to detect signals. In some ways, this is similar to investigating 'class effects' with conventional medicines.

The names that are used for herbal medicines present a further problem (see also the section on 'ADR Reporting Form'). Often, common or vernacular names are used to describe herbal medicines, but these vary widely, and may be used to describe more than one species, and cannot be precise.

Contrary to popular belief, herbal medicines are not 'safe' because they originate from natural sources; some plants are highly poisonous, and many others have inherently toxic constituents. For example, metabolites of 'unsaturated' pyrrolizidine alkaloids, such as senecionine, are hepatotoxic in humans, and carcinogenic and mutagenic in animals (Barnes *et al.*, 2002). Senecionine is found in liferoot (*Senecio aureus*) and in other *Senecio* species, such as *Senecio scandens*, which has been reported as an ingredient in a traditional Chinese medicine product *Qianbai Biyan Pian* found in the UK (Woodfield, 2002; MHRA, 2003a). Other known intrinsically toxic groups of constituents, their effects and examples of plant sources include aristolochic acids (nephrotoxic and carcinogenic), found in *Aristolochia* species throughout the plant, sesquiterpene lactones (allergenic), found in feverfew (*Tanacetum parthenium*) and other species in the Asteraceae family, and furanocoumarins (phototoxic), found in angelica (*Angelica archangelica*) and other species belonging to the Apiaceae family (Barnes *et al.*, 2002).

5.2.2. *Utilisation of Herbal Medicines and Related Issues*

The use of herbal medicines is a popular health care approach among patients and consumers in the UK, although there are few reliable estimates of the prevalence of use. Estimates of herbal medicine use among adults in England come from a cross-sectional survey (n = 5010; response rate: 59%) carried out in 1998 which found that 19.8% (95% CI 18.3–21.3) had purchased an over-the-counter herbal medicinal product and that 0.9% (95% CI 0.6–1.3) had consulted a medical herbalist in the previous year (Thomas *et al.*, 2001). There are no longitudinal data for prevalence of use of herbal medicines for the UK at present, although market research data indicate increasing sales — sales of licensed and unlicensed herbal medicinal products were worth £75 million in 2002, an increase of 57% over the previous five years (Mintel International Group Ltd, 2003). Studies carried out in other developed countries, such as Australia and the US, also suggest increasing prevalence of use of herbal medicines among the general adult population (Eisenberg *et al.*, 1998; MacLennan *et al.*, 2002). Extrapolating estimates of herbal medicine use from such studies suggests that large numbers of people are being exposed to herbal medicines; this in itself is of concern for the public health.

In the UK, herbal medicines are used by a wide range of individuals for both acute and chronic conditions. Many herbal medicinal products are purchased for maintenance of general health and well-being, and for use in the prevention and treatment of minor, common ailments. Use is not necessarily based on evidence, nor limited to symptoms and conditions suitable for self-treatment. Herbal medicinal products are also used by individuals with serious chronic diseases, including cancer, AIDS, multiple sclerosis, and asthma, and many other conditions, by older patients, and pregnant or breast-feeding women, and are administered by parents/guardians to children (Barnes, 2002). Similarly, medical herbalists use herbal medicines to treat a variety of conditions (Barnes & Ernst, 1999). Some patient groups, such as children and older people, are at increased risk of adverse drug effects, and there is no reason why this should not also apply where they use herbal medicines. Other groups, for example, pregnant women, may use herbal medicines in preference to conventional medicines because they are perceived to be safer, without realising that little is known about the effects of herbal medicines taken during pregnancy.

Typically, users of herbal medicinal products do not seek professional advice in selecting herbal medicines, but rather rely on friends' or relatives' recommendations, and information in the popular media (Barnes *et al.*, 1998; Gulian *et al.*, 2002). Herbal medicines are widely available for purchase over the internet and from retail outlets in which there is no trained health care professional available (Vickers *et al.*, 1998; see Section 5.3.1). Even where herbal medicinal products are purchased from pharmacies, a consumer or patient may not have any interaction with a pharmacist or trained pharmacy counter assistant, or if a consultation does occur, pharmacy staff may not have sufficient knowledge to feel confident about providing information and advice on herbal medicines (Quinn & Waterman, 1997). A small proportion of users of herbal medicines seeks treatment from a herbal medicine practitioner, but at present, there is no legal requirement for such practitioners to have undertaken training in herbal medicine or to belong to a professional organisation for herbal medicine practitioners, and while many herbal medicine practitioners will have taken these steps, some will not.

A related issue is that some users of herbal medicines may not disclose this use to a health care professional (Gulian *et al.*, 2002); equally, health care professionals do not ask their patients routinely whether they are using herbal medicines, even when receiving reports from patients of suspected ADRs associated with conventional medicines, and rarely record information on herbal medicine use on patient records (Barnes & Abbot, 1999; Barnes, 2001). It is possible, therefore, that undisclosed herbal medicine use could be an alternative explanation for reports of suspected ADRs associated with conventional medicines.

Disclosure of herbal medicine use to health care professionals is particularly important where patients start, stop, or are already receiving treatment with conventional medicines and, equally, individuals consulting medical herbalists should disclose their current use of conventional medicines, because there may be a potential for drug-herb interactions. Information on the extent to which concurrent use of herbal and conventional medicines occurs is limited, although preliminary data suggest that it may be extensive. In a cross-sectional survey of complementary therapy use among adults in the United States (n = 2055 respondents; 60% weighted overall response rate), 44% were regular users of prescription medicines and, of these, 18.4% were using concurrently a herbal or high-dose vitamin preparation (Eisenberg *et al.*, 1998). In a small study conducted in the UK, 59% of herbal-medicine users identified in pharmacies and health-food stores claimed that they had used herbal medicines concurrently with conventional medicines, mostly prescription medicines, in the previous year (Gulian *et al.*, 2002).

In summary, the ways in which herbal medicines are described (named), perceived and obtained, together with users' behaviour towards herbal medicines and issues relating to health care professionals' and herbal practitioners' practice present opportunities for herbal medicines to be used inappropriately, even unsafely, and for suspected ADRs to go undetected and unreported.

5.3. Regulation of Herbal Medicines

5.3.1. *Current Regulatory Framework*

As with all medicines, the origins of regulation and pharmacovigilance for herbal medicines lie in the thalidomide tragedy of the 1950s and 1960s. This was the milestone which led, of course, to the establishment of the Committee on Safety of Drugs (now the Committee on Safety of Medicines, CSM), an 'early-warning system' (the 'yellow card' scheme) for doctors to report their suspicions on adverse effects of drugs, and legislation in the form of the Medicines Act 1968 requiring pharmaceutical companies to satisfy the competent authority (now the Medicines and Health care Products Regulatory Agency, MHRA) of the quality, safety and efficacy of their new medicines before marketing.

There are around 600 licensed herbal medicinal products on the UK market, although most of these are not 'new' marketing authorisations, but are products which initially were granted product licences of right (PLRs) as they were on the market when the medicines licensing system was set up in 1971. When PLRs for herbal medicinal products were reviewed by the competent authority, manufacturers of those intended for use in minor self-limiting conditions were permitted to rely on bibliographic evidence to support efficacy and safety, rather than being required to carry out new tests and controlled clinical trials (Barnes *et al.*, 2002). So, although many herbal medicinal products have product licences, the products have not necessarily undergone the stringent testing required to obtain a full marketing authorisation today, but rather have relied on evidence from long-standing use.

Other herbal medicines available in the UK are sold either as herbal remedies exempt from licensing under section 12 of the Medicines Act 1968, or as unlicensed food supplements without making medical claims and regulated under food, not medicines, legislation (Barnes *et al.*, 2002). Herbal medicines meeting the definition of a herbal remedy (Table 5.1) and compounded and supplied by 'herbal practitioners' on their own recommendation currently are exempted from licensing requirements under Section 12 (1) (Medicines Act, 1968). This exemption was initially intended to give 'herbal practitioners' the flexibility to prepare remedies for their patients, although the term is not defined and, at present, there is no statutory regulation of herbalists in the UK. A Herbal Medicine Regulatory Working Group has been established to consider appropriate legislation and reform of Section 12 (1) and is expected to report during 2003 (Department of Health, undated).[3]

Many herbal medicinal products are sold under the Section 12 (2) exemption, which exempts from licensing requirements those herbal remedies consisting solely of dried, crushed or comminuted (fragmented) plants sold under the plant or botanical name and with no written recommendations as to their use (Medicines Act, 1968). In other words, such products must not contain any non-herbal 'active' ingredients, must not use proprietary names and must not make medical claims. Some manufacturers are unaware of, or ignore, these conditions and illegal unlicensed herbal products can be found for sale, as currently there is no requirement for manufacturers to consult the competent authority before placing an unlicensed herbal medicinal product on the market. MHRA does have the statutory power to decide whether a particular marketed unlicensed product satisfies the definition of a relevant 'medicinal product' and, therefore, is subject to the usual provisions of regulations relating to Medicines for Human Use, unless it meets criteria for exemption (i.e. as provided in Section 12 of the

---

[3]The Department of Health consultation on statutory regulation of herbal medicine and acupuncture closed on 7 June 2004, and an analysis of the responses was published on 14 February 2005. The Department of Health plans to publish draft legislation for further comment by the autumn of 2005 (Department of Health, 2005, website). See also Shia *et al.*, Chapter 4 of this volume.

Medicines Act). Herbal medicines available in the UK include some traditional Chinese medicines (TCM) and Ayurvedic medicines (both of which often also contain non-herbal substances), and these are subject to the same legislation as are 'Western' herbal medicines (Medicines Control Agency, 2001). There are further restrictions on certain toxic herbal ingredients, such as *Aristolochia* species, found in some TCM products, and on other herbal ingredients that may be confused with toxic herbal ingredients (The Medicines (Aristolochia and Mu Tong) (Prohibition) Order 2001). However, unlicensed herbal products containing these banned species continue to be found (MHRA, undated).

In the UK, licensed medicinal products, including licensed herbal medicinal products, are classified as prescription-only medicines (POMs; generally may only be sold or supplied from a registered pharmacy in accordance with a prescription given by an appropriate practitioner), pharmacy medicines (P; may only be sold or supplied from a registered pharmacy and by or under the supervision of a pharmacist), and general sales list medicines (GSL; may be sold or supplied at registered pharmacies or other businesses which can be closed to exclude the public) (Medicines Act, 1968). Most licensed herbal medicinal products are GSL medicines. Potentially hazardous herbal substances (e.g. *Digitalis* leaf) are controlled as POMs; certain other plants or plant parts (e.g. yohimbe bark; *Pausinystalia yohimbe*) are controlled as P medicines, but some of these (e.g. belladonna herb; *Atropa belladonna*) can be sold or supplied by 'herbal practitioners' (see earlier in this section) if certain conditions are met (e.g. limits on maximum dose, maximum daily dose and/or strength). In practice, these restricted herbal substances are rarely, if ever, sold or supplied by pharmacists, but some, such as *Ephedra* species, where permitted, are utilised by herbal practitioners in their practice.

The current regulatory framework presents several major problems for pharmacovigilance of herbal medicines. Whereas manufacturers of licensed herbal medicinal products are required to comply with regulatory provisions on pharmacovigilance as set out in Directive 2001/83/EC (Commission of the European Communities, 2001), manufacturers of unlicensed herbal products and those sold under exemptions from licensing are not required to do so, i.e. for these products, which comprise the majority of herbal medicines on the UK market, manufacturers have no

                                    J. Barnes

obligation to keep records of suspected ADRs associated with these products, nor to report these suspected ADRs to the competent authority. This is also the case where herbal medicines are supplied to patients by medical herbalists.

In addition, the range of possible regulatory actions that the competent authority can take in response to a herbal safety concern is limited for unlicensed herbal medicinal products and, for some responses, requires the voluntary cooperation of herbal medicines manufacturers. For example, after important interactions between St John's wort and certain prescription medicines emerged around 1999/2000, MHRA took the decision that provision of warnings on St John's wort products was an appropriate part of the regulatory response, but this required the cooperation of manufacturers of unlicensed St John's wort products. At the same time, marketing authorisation holders of conventional medicines believed to interact with St John's wort products were obliged to make variations to product information for their relevant products. Similarly, when an association between use of kava-kava (*Piper methysticum*) preparations and liver toxicity was being investigated by the CSM, the herbal sector agreed to withdraw kava-kava products from sale. Voluntary withdrawal worked reasonably well initially, but as the period of evaluation drew on, some retail outlets began selling kava-kava products again. Community pharmacists, however, had a professional and ethical responsibility not to do so (Adcock, 2002; Royal Pharmaceutical Society, 2003).

Other issues relevant to pharmacovigilance arise because manufacturers of unlicensed herbal medicinal products are not required to demonstrate to MHRA the quality, safety and efficacy of their products before marketing. The importance of pharmaceutical quality for the safety (and efficacy) of herbal medicinal products is well-recognised (Barnes *et al.*, 2002; De Smet *et al.*, 1992; Busse, 2000), but manufacturers are required only to demonstrate pharmaceutical quality standards for their licensed herbal medicinal products. Some manufacturers of unlicensed herbal medicinal products may have appropriate quality control and quality assurance procedures for their products, but others do not, and the pharmaceutical quality of many unlicensed herbal medicinal products is of real concern. In addition to difficulties with assuring pharmaceutical quality due to the variation in chemical composition, quality problems with unlicensed herbal products include intentional or accidental substitution of species, contamination with restricted or toxic substances, including prescription medicines, and differences between labelled and actual contents (Barnes *et al.*, 2002; MHRA, undated). It is essential, therefore, when assessing reports of suspected ADRs associated with a particular unlicensed herbal medicine to establish whether the herbal ingredient(s) implicated are what the product actually contains, and whether the product could be adulterated or contaminated. Ideally, a sample of the suspected herbal medicine should be retained for pharmaceutical analysis if necessary.

There is a general lack of objective information on the safety of many herbal medicines. This has arisen in part because under the current regulatory framework there is little incentive for manufacturers to carry out pre-clinical tests and clinical trials. Post-marketing surveillance studies involving certain herbal medicinal products have been conducted by some manufacturers (usually those based in Germany) but this is the exception. Generally speaking, there is a lack of information on the types and frequency of adverse effects, including interactions with other medicines, foods, alcohol, disease and so forth, and other aspects relevant to safety for herbal medicines, such as their active constituents, pharmacokinetics, pharmacology, use in special patient groups (e.g. children, older people, individuals with renal or hepatic disease, pregnant or breast-feeding women), effects of long-term use, and so on. It is often argued that herbal medicines have a long history of traditional use and that this provides evidence for their safety (and efficacy). However, while the 'test of time' may have identified inherently toxic plants, it cannot, for example, identify delayed adverse effects, effects that may arise from use in patients with 'modern' illnesses, such as HIV/AIDS, and safety issues arising from how herbal medicines are utilised today, for example, concurrently with conventional medicines (Ernst *et al.*, 1998). Certainly, there are examples of type A reactions (those that typically are dose dependent and related to the pharmacological effects of the medicine) and type B reactions (typically unrelated to dose, idiosyncratic) and other types of ADRs (e.g. delayed effects in the user or offspring remote from medicine use in the user) associated with the use of certain herbal medicines (De Smet, 1995).

In addition, the efficacy of many herbal medicines has not been evaluated in randomised clinical trials. Even for well-tested herbal medicines, such as certain extracts of St John's wort herb which have been assessed in around 30 randomised clinical trials in depression, only a small number of clinical trial participants has been exposed to a specific manufacturer's product. Furthermore, there are few long-term clinical trials of herbal medicines intended for long-term use. For comparison, conventional medicines have been tested in around 1500 patients before they reach the market. The lack of information on the safety and efficacy of herbal medicines makes it difficult to carry out benefit-risk assessments.

In summary, in the UK, the current regulatory framework allows unlicensed herbal medicines, which may be of inadequate pharmaceutical quality and for which there is a lack of information on safety aspects, to be placed on the market and obtained by consumers and patients from a range of retail outlets without a prescription or other involvement of a health care professional. Manufacturers are under no obligation to carry out pharmacovigilance of such products. By contrast, conventional P or GSL medicines are permitted to be sold or supplied without a prescription because they have a history of relative safety.

5.3.2. *Proposed New Regulatory Framework*

The need for a new regulatory framework for herbal medicinal products was first discussed in the late 1980s and, for several reasons, today it is recognised widely that the existing regulatory framework does not adequately protect the public health. In particular, the current system does not give consumers and patients adequate protection against poor-quality and unsafe unlicensed herbal medicinal products. It also discriminates against manufacturers of licensed herbal medicinal products, as their costs are likely to be higher because of the need to comply with the principles of good manufacturing practice and other regulatory provisions.

Against this background, a draft European Union (EU) directive (2002/0008, which amends 2001/83/EC) has been produced which aims to establish a harmonised legislative framework for authorising the marketing of traditional herbal medicinal products (Commission of the European Communities, 2002). The directive will require EU member states to set up a simplified national registration scheme for traditional herbal medicinal products meeting defined criteria. The key features

Table 5.2. Key Features of Proposed European Union (EU) Directive 2002/0008 (Amends 2001/83/EC) on Traditional Herbal Medicinal Products (Commission of the European Communities, 2002 and 2003).

Establishes a Committee on Herbal Medicinal Products which will be part of the EMEA and will take over the tasks of the CPMP with regard to authorisations or registrations of herbal medicinal products by member states. Other tasks will include producing EC herbal monographs, and establishing a 'positive list' of herbal substances (to include indication, route of administration, strength, and so on) allowed under the directive.
Requires EU member states to set up a specified simplified national registration procedure for traditional herbal medicinal products that could not fulfil medicines licensing criteria.
Main features of requirements for registration include: • products for oral, external or inhalation use only • minor indications only (suitable for self-diagnosis and self-treatment) • evidence that the herb has been used traditionally for at least 30 years, including at least 15 years within the EC; period of traditional use can include the transition period • reliable identification of raw materials and use of appropriate quality herbal ingredients, i.e. compliance with Ph Eur standards where they exist and with manufacturer's own specification otherwise • systematic quality assurance and quality control throughout the manufacturing process: compliance with principles of GMP and other relevant European guidelines; qualified person responsible for release of batches onto the market; manufacturer's licence or wholesale dealer's licence where appropriate; inspection of premises • provision of bibliographic data on safety with an expert report • labelling, information and advertising requirements in accordance with 2001/83/EC and relevant national regulations • compliance with pharmacovigilance requirements in accordance with 2001/83/EC • transition period of at least five years, probably seven years, once the directive comes into force.

CPMP = Committee on Proprietary Medicinal Products; EC = European Community; EMEA = European Agency for the Evaluation of Medicinal Products; GMP = good manufacturing practice; Ph Eur = European Pharmacopoeia.

of the directive at the time of writing are summarised in Table 5.2, although the directive is still under discussion and amendments may yet be made.[4]

---

[4]The directive has now been agreed by the European Parliament as 2004/24/EC; see also footnote 5.

In essence, the proposed directive will require manufacturers wishing to obtain registrations for their traditional herbal medicinal products under a national scheme to demonstrate the quality and, to some extent, the safety of their products, whereas the usual efficacy and, to some extent, safety requirements will be replaced by evidence of traditional use. Another major change is that manufacturers of products registered under the directive will be required to comply with information and labelling requirements. Currently there is no requirement for manufacturers of unlicensed herbal medicinal products to provide systematic information with their products.

The proposed directive will have an important impact on pharmacovigilance of herbal medicines, once it comes into force. Manufacturers of traditional herbal medicinal products registered under the UK national scheme established under the directive will be required to comply with relevant existing pharmaceutical legislation, including the provisions on pharmacovigilance (Commission of the European Communities, 2001). Several of these may pose problems for manufacturers with little or no experience in this area. For example, the requirement to have constant access to an appropriately qualified and experienced person responsible for pharmacovigilance, implementation of the use of Medical Dictionary for Regulatory Activities (MedDRA) and connection to and compliance with EudraVigilance. There has been some discussion about the possibility of making some allowances for manufacturers with regard to the qualified person responsible for product quality; it is not clear whether any similar allowances will be made with respect to the qualified person responsible for pharmacovigilance. According to the current time-scale, the directive is expected to come into force around the end of 2004; following this, there will be a transition period of at least five years (the precise duration is currently under discussion but probably will be seven years) (Woodfield, 2003).[5]

---

[5]The directive has now been agreed by the European Parliament and has to be tranposed into national legislation (in all 25 member states, including the UK) by the end of October 2005. The correct title is now: Directive 2004/24/EC on Traditional Herbal Medicinal Products. This directive amends Directive 2001/83/EC (the European Community code on medicinal products for human use) to introduce the Traditional Herbal Medicines Registration Scheme. Many of the existing requirements in Directive 2001/83/EC will apply to traditional herbal medicinal products, e.g. regulatory provisions on pharmacovigilance. However, Directive 2001/83/EC is to be separately amended by Directive 2004/27/EC (after a review of pharmaceutical legislation). This comes into effect at the same time as the traditional herbal registration scheme comes into effect, so manufacturers wishing to register their traditional herbal medicinal products under the Traditional Herbal Medicines Registration Scheme will need to be aware of the requirements of both Directives 2001/83/EC and 2004/27/EC as well, of course, as those in Directive 2004/24/EC.

Other developments at the European level are concerned, at least in part, with pharmacovigilance of herbal medicines. The European Agency for the Evaluation of Medicinal Products' Herbal Medicinal Products Working Party (previously the *ad hoc* Herbal Medicinal Products Working Group, set up in 1997) has several pharmacovigilance issues on its agenda (EMEA, 2003).

5.4. Methods for Pharmacovigilance of Herbal Medicines

Some standard methods used in pharmacovigilance, particularly spontaneous reporting schemes, are used to monitor the safety of herbal medicines, although these methods are less well established than for conventional medicines. Other methods, such as prescription-event monitoring, have not yet been applied to exploring the safety of herbal medicines. All available pharmacovigilance tools have important limitations with regard to their use in investigating the safety of herbal medicines, in addition to those already recognised, and it is likely that modified, even novel, methods are required. This section discusses the available methods, with a focus on spontaneous reporting schemes, and the particular challenges that herbal medicines present for each.

5.4.1. *Spontaneous Reporting Schemes*

The future of spontaneous reporting schemes in pharmacovigilance has been questioned (Waller & Evans, 2003), although it is likely that this point was raised in relation to conventional medicines for which other well-established tools, such as computerised health-record databases, can be used for pharmacovigilance purposes. By contrast, spontaneous reporting for herbal medicines is in the early stages of its development and, at present, in the absence of other tools and/or resources, is the main method of generating and detecting signals of potential safety concerns associated with herbal medicines. Spontaneous reporting schemes appear to function reasonably effectively as a pharmacovigilance tool for herbal medicines in countries such as Germany where herbal medicinal products are regulated as medicines, frequently prescribed by physicians and well known to other health care professionals, particularly pharmacists (De Smet, 1997). However, spontaneous reporting is likely to be far less effective in countries such as the UK where herbal medicines are marketed mainly as unlicensed products with no obligation for manufacturers to report suspected ADRs to the competent authority, and where herbal medicines are used mostly in self-treatment without any supervision from a health care professional.

5.4.1.1. UK National Spontaneous Reporting Scheme

The CSM/MHRA's national spontaneous reporting scheme for suspected ADR reporting by health care professionals (also known as the 'yellow card' scheme because of the form used to report suspected ADRs to the CSM/MHRA) has applied to licensed medicines, including licensed herbal medicines, since its inception in 1964. However, the inclusion of licensed herbal medicines in the scheme was not well-publicised until October 1996, over 30 years later, when the scheme was extended to include reporting for unlicensed herbal medicines (Anonymous, 1996). This move followed a five-year study of traditional remedies and food supplements, carried out by a UK Medical Toxicology Unit (Shaw *et al.*, 1997), which identified suspected ADRs associated with these types of products. The extension allowed those with official reporter status — at the time, doctors, dentists and coroners only — to submit reports for unlicensed herbal medicines, but did not (and could not) place any statutory obligation on manufacturers to report suspected ADRs associated with their unlicensed herbal products.

In April 1997 and November 1999, the scheme underwent further extensions to allow reporting of suspected ADRs by all hospital and community pharmacists, respectively. Community pharmacists were encouraged by the CSM and MHRA to concentrate on areas of limited reporting by doctors, namely licensed and unlicensed herbal products, and other non-prescription medicines (Anonymous, 1997a). This extension followed a one-year pilot scheme for community pharmacist ADR reporting, carried out in the four CSM regions during 1997–98 and involving around 3200 pharmacies, which showed that community pharmacists, compared with general practitioners (GPs), submitted a greater proportion of reports of suspected ADRs associated with herbal medicines (the numbers of herbal ADR reports as a proportion of the total number of reports submitted by pharmacists and GPs were 4/96 (4.2%) and 8/1975 (0.4%), respectively; $p < 0.001$) (Davis & Coulson, 1999). However, numbers of herbal ADR reports submitted by both groups of reporters were very low and represented an average of only one and two reports per CSM region for pharmacists and GPs, respectively.

Despite these initiatives to stimulate reporting of suspected ADRs associated with both licensed and unlicensed herbal medicines, numbers of herbal ADR reports submitted to the CSM/MHRA remain very low. From 1964 until the end of 1995, 832 reports were received (MHRA, 2003b). For the period 1996 (when the yellow card scheme was extended to unlicensed herbal medicines and when its inclusion of herbal medicines was first well publicised) to 2002 inclusive, 467 reports of suspected ADRs associated with herbal medicines were received (see Fig. 5.1). Most frequently, these reports related to products containing the herbal ingredients St John's wort (*Hypericum perforatum*), ginkgo (*Ginkgo biloba*), peppermint (*Mentha piperita*), *Echinacea* species, senna and valerian (*Valeriana officinalis*). It is not known whether the low numbers of reports of suspected ADRs associated with herbal medicines simply reflect a low frequency of

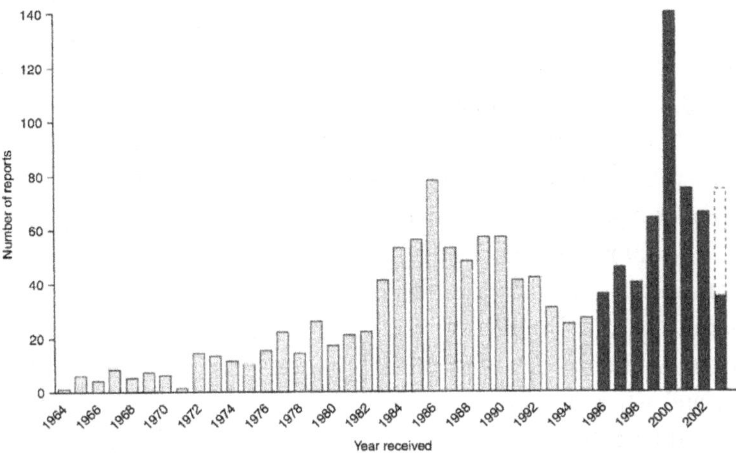

Fig. 5.1. Numbers of reports of suspected adverse drug reactions associated with herbal medicines received by the UK Committee on Safety of Medicines/Medicines and Health care Products Regulatory Agency's yellow card scheme for the period 1964 to 25 July 2003. Gray bars (i.e. pre-1996) represent licensed herbal medicines; black bars (1996 onwards) represent reports for both licensed and unlicensed herbal medicines following extension of the scheme to unlicensed herbal medicines in October 1996; the dotted line above the 2003 bar represents an estimate of the total number of reports for the full year. Source: Adverse Drug Reactions On-line Information Tracking (MHRA, 2003b).

adverse effects with herbal medicines, or whether there are other explanations, for example, substantial under-reporting.

The number of herbal ADR reports received increased over the period 1999–2002, with a peak in the year 2000 around the time that reports emerged of suspected interactions between St John's wort and certain prescription medicines. In part, this simply reflected an increase in numbers of reports of suspected ADRs associated with St John's wort — 60% (82/140) of herbal reports for the year 2000 (42% for 1999 and 13% for 1998) and 40% (138/345) of all herbal reports received during this period related to St John's wort, with around 40 reports in total describing drug interactions with St John's wort — but there was also a (small) general increase in numbers of herbal ADR reports submitted during this period (MHRA, 2003b).

It is not yet clear whether this just reflects year-to-year variation, or whether it has been sustained. Typically, a year-on-year increase in the number of herbal suspected ADR reports submitted could be expected, with further increases with the addition of new recognised reporters and initiatives aimed at stimulating herbal ADR reporting. However, the inclusion of pharmacists does not yet appear to have had a marked impact in this regard, since the additional reports of suspected ADRs associated with herbal medicines submitted during 1999–2002 were not submitted solely by pharmacists but also by other recognised reporters (MHRA, 2003b; Major, 2002). For comparison, in 1964 when the yellow card scheme began, there were 1414 submitted reports of suspected ADRs associated with conventional medicines. This increased steadily until 1977 when there was a surge in reporting (10,921 reports for the year) around the time practolol was associated with oculomucocutaneous syndrome and withdrawn from the market, and when initiatives to encourage reporting of suspected ADRs were introduced, for example, the introduction of the newsletter *Current Problems in Pharmacovigilance* (Davis & Raine, 2002). Annual reporting rates have since increased, with some fluctuations, currently to around 20,000 reports per year (which includes the small number of herbal ADR reports), giving a total of over 450,000 reports to the end of 2002.

Further extensions to the reporter base for the yellow card scheme occurred in October 2002 when all nurses, midwives and health visitors became recognised reporters (MHRA, 2002). At the same time, electronic reporting of suspected ADRs over the internet was launched in an attempt to facilitate reporting (Anonymous, 2002a), and in April 2003, a pilot scheme was introduced to allow patient reporting of suspected ADRs via one of the NHS's 22 NHS Direct telephone call centres (Anonymous, 2003). The impact that these new reporter groups and initiatives will have on the reporting of suspected ADRs associated with herbal medicines is not yet known. The results of the pilot scheme for patient ADR reporting via NHS Direct will be relevant for herbal medicines, given that many users of herbal medicines select and self-treat with such preparations without the advice or supervision of a health care professional, and that some users may not report suspected ADRs associated with herbal medicines to their doctor or a pharmacist (Barnes *et al.*, 1998). Evaluations of pilot schemes have indicated that the completeness of all reports submitted by community pharmacists and GPs was similar (Davis & Coulson, 1999), although in the pilot scheme for ADR reporting by nurses there was some evidence that completeness of doctors' reports was slightly better than that of nurses (Morrison-Griffiths *et al.*, 2003).

ADR Reporting Form

The minimum information required for a report of a suspected ADR is the same for both conventional and herbal medicines, and a standard yellow card is used to collect data, regardless of the type of preparation implicated. In the year 2000, a modified yellow card was introduced which included in the section for '*Other drugs*' the prompt '*(including self-medication and herbal remedies)*' (Anonymous, 2000). Apart from this, the yellow card does not mention herbal medicines specifically, and its current design has several deficiencies with regard to prompting for and collecting information on herbal medicines.

The section '*Suspected drug*' presents several problems. First, the reporter is asked to provide the brand (proprietary) name of the suspected drug(s). While licensed herbal medicinal products are likely to have brand names, unlicensed herbal products legally are not permitted to use them — only the vernacular and/or botanical name, such as St John's wort or *Hypericum perforatum* should be used, although this is ignored by some manufacturers. For unlicensed herbal medicines it would be more appropriate to request the name of the herbal ingredient(s) and the name of the manufacturer/supplier. Identifying the manufacturer is particularly important for reasons mentioned earlier, namely because the composition of products containing the same herbal ingredient can vary both qualitatively and quantitatively between manufacturers. Also, there may be other problems with the pharmaceutical quality (e.g. contamination) of unlicensed herbal products, which should be considered when assessing ADR reports. Ideally, the form should also include space to indicate whether a sample of the suspected product(s) is available.

To identify specifically the herbal ingredient(s) implicated, the binomial botanical name (genus and species) should be given. For example, 'echinacea' is insufficient, since three different *Echinacea* species (*E. purpurea*, *E. pallida* and *E. angustifolia*) are used medicinally and these differ in their phytochemical composition. In addition, the specific plant part used should also be stated, since one or more plant parts may be used medicinally and, again, the phytochemical composition can vary. For example, both the root and the herb (aerial parts) of *E. purpurea* and nettle (*Urtica dioica*) are used medicinally. However, there is no specific request for these details on the yellow card.

Other relevant information not specifically requested includes the method of processing the crude herbal material (e.g. type of extract), since this can also influence the precise chemical composition and, therefore, the potential toxicity of a herbal preparation (De Smet, 1997), the strength of the preparation (e.g. drug:extract ratio), and the formulation of the product (e.g. tablets, tincture). Also, many herbal medicinal products contain several herbal ingredients, some include non-herbal ingredients such as vitamins and minerals, and herbal practitioners often prescribe several herbal tinctures together supplied as a mixture. With respect to these preparations, one or more herbal ingredient(s) may be the suspected agent(s), yet there is limited space on the current yellow card to provide this level of detail.

Although it is not desirable to introduce different reporting forms for different types of preparations, it could be argued that herbal medicines present a special case and that a more specialised reporting form is required. Alternatively, modifications to the existing reporting card could be made so that important details on herbal medicines can be requested.

Signal Detection and Assessment

At present, because of the relatively small number of reports of suspected ADRs associated with herbal medicines held on the MHRA's ADROIT (Adverse Drug Reaction On-line Information Tracking) database reports, signals are detected simply by numbers of reports. It may be possible to obtain proportional reporting ratios for some suspected ADRs associated with certain herbal medicines, such as St John's wort for which around 150 reports in total have been received since 1996. In this case, the comparison is made against the rest of the database, rather than only against the subset of herbal ADR reports. The assumptions made in proportional analysis, and the importance of considering the effect of selected backgrounds, has been discussed in the context of conventional medicines (Gogolak, 2003). Since there are additional biases and other issues in pharmacovigilance of herbal medicines, what is an appropriate comparator requires consideration. This subject is, however, beyond the scope of this article.

Following confirmation of a signal relating to a herbal safety concern, the next stages in its evaluation are also difficult with respect to herbal medicines. In the UK, quantifying the risk is probably impossible as there is no reliable way of determining the number of individuals exposed to the herbal medicine of interest. Benefit-risk analysis is problematic because of the limited clinical data on safety and efficacy of herbal medicines, and identifying at-risk groups is also difficult because the user profile for herbal medicines is poorly defined. A particular problem is that a specific herbal medicine can have numerous uses and may be taken by healthy individuals for 'general well-being', as well as by patients with chronic disease. These problems are further compounded if the variation in different preparations of the same herbal ingredient is considered.

The concerns regarding kava-kava (*Piper methysticum*) and hepato-toxicity illustrate the process of assessing and responding to safety issues relating to unlicensed herbal medicinal products. A signal concerning kava-kava and liver toxicity was first raised in 2000 following a cluster of cases reported in Switzerland, and was strengthened a year or so later following further spontaneous reports from Switzerland and Germany (MCA, 2002). The UK CSM undertook an initial evaluation, including causality assessment, and found that the risks of kava-kava appeared to outweigh its benefits. No regulatory action was taken at that time, although the herbal sector instigated a voluntary withdrawal of products containing kava-kava while the safety concerns were investigated further.

The next stage involved further data collection and evaluation. The CSM set up a working group to assess the issue and requested additional data on benefits and risks of kava-kava from the herbal sector and regulatory authorities. When the CSM next considered the issue in July 2002, a total of 68 reports originating from several countries had been received, although only three originated in the UK (MCA, 2002). The severity of the liver damage described in the reports varied from abnormal liver function test results to liver failure and death; six patients received liver transplants. Different preparations of kava-kava were available (e.g. different types of extracts) and consideration was given as to whether only certain types of kava-kava preparation might be associated with liver toxicity. However, there appeared to be no relationship between the method of processing/type of extract, strength or dose, and the adverse reactions. Thus, on the basis of the data available, the CSM advised that the possible benefits of preparations containing kava-kava do not outweigh the risks, that kava-kava had the potential to cause hepatotoxicity which could be serious in nature, and that kava-kava should be prohibited in unlicensed medicines. On January 13, 2003, a statutory order came into effect in the UK prohibiting the sale, supply and import of unlicensed medicines containing kava-kava. Product licences for licensed kava-kava products were revoked (The Medicines for Human Use (Kava-Kava) (Prohibition) Order 2002).

Some of the difficulties in assessing safety concerns with unlicensed herbal medicines were evident here. For example, the number of unlicensed herbal products containing kava-kava available in the UK, their extent of use, and the extent of use of kava-kava preparations by patients consulting medical herbalists, were not known; reports involved different types of kava-kava preparations; only a very low number of reports was received in the UK; the quality and completeness of the reports was poor, and some reports were duplicated; there are few clinical trials of kava-kava products and a lack of clear evidence of efficacy; regulatory options in responding to the signal were limited, and alternatives, such as including warning information with products, would have required the voluntary co-operation of manufacturers of unlicensed kava-kava products and MHRA would have had no means of enforcement.

Strengths and Weaknesses

Spontaneous reporting schemes have recognised advantages and limitations, and several of these may be even more important with regard to herbal medicines (see Table 5.3). In particular, under-reporting is a well-recognised, important and inevitable limitation of any spontaneous reporting scheme, but for several reasons it may be an even greater problem for herbal medicines.

Under-reporting of suspected ADRs associated with herbal medicines could occur at several levels. First, because of the perception that herbal medicines are 'safe', users of these preparations may not associate an adverse event with their use of a herbal medicine, particularly if they are taking other (conventional) medicines. If the user does make an association between use of a herbal medicine and an adverse event, they may take steps to resolve the problem themselves (for example, stop taking the preparation) and/or may not inform a health care professional (Barnes *et al.*, 1998). Under-reporting can also occur at the level of the health care professional,

Table 5.3. Summary of Advantages and Limitations of Spontaneous Adverse Drug Reaction (ADR) Reporting Schemes with Respect to Herbal Medicines.

Advantages
Monitor all drugs, including all herbal medicines, all the time and for all consumers and patients.
Provide early warnings of undocumented drug safety concerns; important for herbal medicines as information on safety is limited.
Relatively cheap to run; important as the herbal sector may not have the resources to conduct large-scale post-marketing surveillance studies.
Limitations
Under-reporting; likely to be greater for herbal medicines.
Poor quality of data available to or provided by reporter; yellow card does not cater specifically for recording information on herbal medicines as suspected drugs.
Biases in Reporting
Cannot estimate frequency of an ADR as do not provide accurate information on number of individuals exposed to the drug of interest; probably not possible to obtain denominators for unlicensed herbal medicinal products.
Suspected ADRs may be identified/reported outside the formal system (e.g. to herbalists, health food stores).

since doctors, pharmacists and other recognised reporters could filter out reports of suspected ADRs described by patients (van Grootheest *et al.*, 2003). Reasons for under-reporting among health care professionals are well documented, although studies exploring this area have been carried out in the context of conventional medicines, and it is not known if these same reasons apply to under-reporting for herbal medicines. ·

Several studies involving community pharmacists indicate that many pharmacists are unaware that they should report suspected ADRs associated with herbal medicines. A cross-sectional survey carried out in 1998 of over 1300 community pharmacists (response rate: 67%) not involved in the CSM/MHRA pilot scheme for community pharmacist ADR reporting found that 47% of respondents were not aware that the yellow card scheme applied to herbal medicines at all, 37% were aware it applied to licensed herbal medicines, and only 16% knew it applied to both licensed and unlicensed herbal medicines (Barnes, 2001). This finding is not so surprising, since these pharmacists were not recognised reporters at the time of the study and would not have received training materials on ADR reporting. Of more concern is the fact that studies conducted since all community pharmacists became recognised reporters and were encouraged to focus on reporting suspected ADRs associated with herbal and other non-prescription medicines have continued to find that many community pharmacists are unaware of the need to report suspected ADRs associated with herbal medicines, particularly unlicensed herbal medicines (Wingfield *et al.*, 2002; Green *et al.*, 1999). There may also be biases favouring ADR reporting for herbal medicines. An audit of medicines information pharmacists working in a Medicines Information Centre in Wales found that although they encouraged only 41% of enquirers about ADRs to complete yellow cards, they were more likely to give encouragement where an 'alternative' medicine was involved rather than a conventional medicine (Biscoe *et al.*, 2002). In addition, all these studies revealed deficiencies in community pharmacists' knowledge on other aspects of ADR reporting, such as the level of certainty required regarding a causal relationship.

To date, there are very few studies that provide any information on the extent of under-reporting of suspected ADRs associated with herbal medicines. In one cross-sectional survey of community pharmacists who were not involved in the CSM/MHRA pilot scheme for community pharmacist ADR reporting (see earlier in this section), respondents were asked to describe any reports of suspected ADRs associated with complementary medicines that they had received or identified over the previous 12 months (Barnes & Abbot, 1999; Barnes, 2001). In total, among 818 respondents, 44 reports of suspected ADRs associated with herbal medicines were described, an average of one report per 19 pharmacists. By contrast, the CSM/MHRA pilot scheme, which ran over approximately the same period covered by the survey, and involved around 3200 pharmacies, received only four reports (Davis & Coulson, 1999; Anonymous, 1997b). Conclusions cannot be drawn from these crude comparisons, since these studies used different methodologies, involved pharmacists/pharmacies in different regions of the UK, and so on. They do, however, raise the hypothesis that there is significant under-reporting by pharmacists of suspected ADRs associated with herbal medicines.

It is recognised that pharmacists can make an important contribution to ADR reporting for herbal medicinal products, but it is likely that greater vigilance on the part of the pharmacist and initiatives to encourage herbal ADR reporting by pharmacists are required. Against this background, there have been several recent papers in a journal received by all UK pharmacists (Barnes, 2002; Major, 2002; Cox, 2002), and a factsheet on ADR reporting by pharmacists has been produced by the Science Committee of the Royal Pharmaceutical Society of Great Britain (the professional and regulatory body for all pharmacists in the UK) which provides guidance and reminds pharmacists of their professional and ethical responsibilities in this regard (Moffat, 2003).

A further limitation of spontaneous reporting schemes is that herbal medicines are widely available from a range of outlets without the need for interaction with a health care professional and, therefore, suspected ADRs associated with herbal medicines may be identified by or reported to an individual (e.g. herbalist) who is outside the formal system for ADR reporting. Health food stores are a major outlet for herbal medicinal products, but it is not known whether staff in these outlets receive reports of suspected ADRs associated with such products, and if they do, what action, if any, they take.

 J. Barnes

5.4.1.2. WHO/Uppsala Monitoring Centre Traditional Medicines Project

ADR reports, including herbal ADR reports, from the CSM/MHRA yellow card scheme and (in 2003) those from 70 other countries with national ADR monitoring schemes are fed into the WHO/Uppsala Monitoring Centre (UMC). The UMC recognises the problems inherent in ADR reporting for herbal medicines and has established a Traditional Medicines Project to stimulate reporting in this area and to standardise information on herbal medicines, particularly with regard to nomenclature (Farah *et al.*, 2000). For example, a special set of herbal anatomical-therapeutic-chemical (ATC) codes has been developed which is fully compatible with the regular ATC classification system for conventional medicines (Uppsala Monitoring Centre, 2002).

The UMC database, established in 1968, held over two million reports of suspected ADRs by 1999, of which around 0.5% involve herbal medicines (Uppsala Monitoring Centre, 2002). For the period 1968–1997, almost 9000 reports involving herbal medicines were received by the UMC. The UK is among the top five countries in terms of absolute numbers of herbal suspected ADR reports submitted.

5.4.1.3. Herbal-Sector-Initiated Spontaneous Reporting Schemes

At present, herbal medicine practitioners are not recognised as reporters by the CSM/MHRA yellow card scheme. Several herbal medicine practitioners and other herbal sector organisations have initiated their own ADR reporting schemes for herbal medicines based on the CSM/MHRA scheme. While this is a responsible and potentially useful step forward where these schemes have developed a link with the CSM/MHRA or WHO/UMC, *ad hoc* schemes are not encouraged because there is a risk that reports will be dispersed and signals may be not be detected as early as possible, or may be missed. As with any spontaneous reporting scheme, herbal sector-initiated schemes are also likely to be prone to limitations such as under reporting. It is not known whether reasons for under-reporting of suspected herbal ADRs by the herbal sector are different from those for herbal ADR reporting by conventional health care professionals. It is possible that there may be concerns among the herbal sector that the availability of herbal medicines and their freedom to practise herbal medicine may be threatened if significant numbers of herbal ADR reports are submitted.

The National Institute of Medical Herbalists (NIMH), the major organisation for medical herbalists in the UK, requests from its members reports of suspected ADRs associated with herbal treatments. Reports are submitted on a modified 'yellow card' form, which has some additional data fields relevant to herbalists' prescriptions. The NIMH sends an annual summary of reports received to MHRA. For the period January 1994 – November 2001, 23 reports were received by the NIMH (Broughton, 2001). Most reports described reactions experienced by patients who had received a combination of several herbs, which is typical of medical herbalists' treatment approach. A similar scheme has been set up by the Register of Chinese Herbal Medicine (RCHM), which also uses a modified yellow card form to collect data from its practitioners of Chinese herbal medicine. The RCHM scheme also has a link with MHRA. At the time of writing, nine reports (three in 2000) had been received by the RCHM from its members (Ward, 2002).

Other schemes have been established which are not restricted to herbal medicine practitioners. Phytonet is a password-protected, internet-based system for gathering reports of suspected ADRs associated with herbal medicines that was set up by a UK university on behalf of the European Scientific Co-Operative on Phytotherapy in 1996 (ESCOP, undated). Phytonet uses an electronic form based on the CSM/MHRA yellow card, but differs from the schemes described above in that it accepts reports from health care professionals, herbal practitioners, patients and the public. Submitted reports are assessed by an expert panel and, where appropriate, fed into the WHO/UMC. Few reports have been received, however, and support is needed to revive the system. As there is no obligation for manufacturers to report suspected ADRs associated with their unlicensed herbal products, the British Herbal Medicine Association (BHMA), whose members include many herbal medicines manufacturers, has addressed this in its voluntary code of practice for its members (BHMA, 1997). The code includes the requirement that manufacturers send reports of suspected ADRs associated with their unlicensed herbal products to the BHMA, which may, at its discretion, forward such reports to MHRA. At the time of writing, the BHMA had not received from its members any reports of suspected ADRs associated with unlicensed herbal medicinal products. The University of Westminster, London, UK, in conjunction with a supermarket retailer, is developing an ADR reporting scheme for consumers, nutritional advisers and other health practitioners to report suspected ADRs associated with herbal and 'complementary' medicines (University of Westminster, undated). There is at least one other scheme in the UK, set up by a herbal supplier in Leicester, UK, which is inviting purchasers of its products to submit reports of suspected ADRs. It is not clear what are the aims of this scheme, given that it is stated that the information will be used only by the herbal supplier. This is of concern if, for example, a herbalist submits a report of a suspected ADR associated with a herbal medicine to this scheme alone.

5.4.1.4. Intensive Monitoring Schemes

Extensions to the CSM/MHRA yellow card scheme were launched in 1997 and 1998 to stimulate reporting of suspected ADRs associated with medicines used in the treatment of HIV infection, and of ADRs occurring in children (Davis & Raine, 2002). The HIV reporting scheme, launched in 1997, targets specialist health care professionals working with HIV-infected individuals and encourages reports of suspected ADRs on a modified yellow card form which does not request the patient's name. The paediatric reporting scheme also targeted health care professionals but did not involve a modified yellow card. Numbers of reports increased following the introduction of these schemes, although the underlying reporting rate increased only with the HIV scheme; ongoing promotion of the scheme, for example, through a regular newsletter is stated to be important (Davis & Raine, 2002). To date, CSM/MHRA have not introduced an intensive monitoring scheme for herbal medicines and, given that the impact of initiatives to stimulate reporting of herbal ADRs has so far been limited, it may be an appropriate time to set up such a scheme together with a programme of ongoing promotion aimed at maintaining its effectiveness.

The herbal sector has not yet set up any such schemes for pharmacovigilance purposes, although a pilot study run by the Medicinal Plant Research Group collected detailed data, including outcomes, from around 30 herbalists on all their patients treated for irritable bowel syndrome (Logue *et al.*, 2002).

5.4.2. *Prescription Event Monitoring*

The methodology of prescription event monitoring (PEM)[6] in monitoring the safety of newly marketed prescription drugs is well established (Shakir, 2002). The valuable contribution that PEM has made to pharmacovigilance of conventional medicines is clear, but the existing method is of no use at present for pharmacovigilance of herbal medicines because they are rarely prescribed.

A protocol for modified PEM methodology has been developed by the Drug Safety Research Unit, Southampton, UK, in collaboration with the NIMH, the University of Southampton, the Medical Toxicology Unit at Guy's and St Thomas' Hospital Trust, London, and the School of Pharmacy, University of London. This approach involves using herbalists to provide adverse event data on green forms for patients treated with a specific herbal medicine. Where patients give permission, a green form requesting adverse event data would also be sent to their GP. There are limitations to this method, such as whether sufficient patient numbers could be achieved and, particularly, that the herb of interest is not 'newly marketed' so there may be preconceptions about its safety profile. Nevertheless, the protocol represents a step forward in attempting to develop methods for pharmacovigilance of herbal medicines. Funding is being sought to carry out a pilot study of the modified PEM methodology.

Another potential approach, based on PEM concepts, is to use community pharmacists to recruit a cohort of purchasers (where consent is given) of a specific herbal medicinal product who would then be followed up over time and adverse event data collected. The feasibility of this approach has been demonstrated in a pilot study using a conventional non-prescription medicine (Layton *et al.*, 2002; Sinclair *et al.*, 1999), but needs to be evaluated as a method for pharmacovigilance of herbal medicinal products.

---

[6]PEM is a hypothesis-generating, non-interventional, observational form of monitoring for newly marketed medicines carried out by the Drug Safety Research Unit, Southampton, UK. Current PEM methodology involves sending a 'green form' to GPs who have prescribed the medicine being studied; these data are obtained from the UK Prescription Pricing Authority. The green form comprises a simple questionnaire, which requests data on all health events the patient who was prescribed the drug experienced during treatment. These forms are usually sent to the GPs around six months after the patient was first prescribed the medicine under study.

5.4.3. *Other Pharmacoepidemiological Study Designs*

The methodology for case-control and cohort studies is well established and these study designs can be used to investigate safety concerns with herbal medicines, although few studies have been carried out to date. One study explored the relationship between colorectal cancer and use of preparations containing anthranoid laxatives (De Smet, 1997). The strengths and limitations of case-control and cohort studies are well documented (Strom, 2000), but as with other study designs, some of the problems are compounded when these study designs are applied to herbal medicines. For example, to establish and verify both cases' and controls' exposure to the herbal medicine(s) of interest is particularly problematic since herbal medicines are rarely prescribed; even where herbal medicinal products are purchased from pharmacies, pharmacists do not routinely record use of herbal and other non-prescription medicines on computerised patient medication records (Barnes & Abbot, 1999; Barnes, 2001). In addition, for reasons explained earlier, there are likely to be variations in different manufacturers' products and, therefore, defining exposure precisely will be difficult at best.

Case-control and cohort studies involving conventional prescribed medicines can be carried out using UK computerised health-record databases such as the General Practice Research Database and the Medicines Monitoring Unit database, but such tools currently are of no use for studies involving herbal medicines since herbal medicines are rarely prescribed and information on non-prescription medicines, including herbal medicines, is not recorded on GPs' patient records.

As with case-control and cohort studies, experimental studies can be applied to investigating the safety of herbal medicines. At present, notwithstanding recognised limitations, such as sample size and ethical considerations, well-designed and well-conducted randomised clinical trials (RCTs) overcome some of the difficulties that herbal medicines present for other pharmacoepidemiological studies. For example, precisely establishing exposure is simpler since compliance checks can be carried out, and RCTs are unlikely to use herbal medicinal products (containing the same herbal ingredient) from different manufacturers, so product variation and, usually, batch-to-batch variation in products, is eliminated. There is always the possibility, of course, that clinical-trial participants could take purchased herbal medicines in addition to the study medication.

Systematic reviews and meta-analyses of adverse event data from RCTs of specific herbal medicines have been carried out, but this introduces other problems. Many existing RCTs of herbal medicinal products are of poor or limited methodological quality, and/or published reports of studies do not follow Consolidated Standards of Reporting Trials (CONSORT) guidelines. In addition, clinical trials of a particular herbal ingredient usually will have been carried out using several different manufacturers' products, but systematic reviews and meta-analyses often ignore variations between products.

5.5. Communication of Herbal Safety Concerns

The importance of the timing, content and method of delivery of messages regarding safety concerns has been discussed extensively, and the requirements for successful communication of safety concerns should apply equally to herbal medicines. However, communicating information on herbal safety concerns presents additional difficulties for several reasons. 'Dear Doctor/Pharmacist' letters can be sent, but health care professionals are unlikely to know which of their patients are using herbal medicines and, therefore, will be unable to pass on safety messages to specific individuals. Medical herbalists may keep some records of their patients' treatment, but as there is no statutory regulation for herbal medicine practitioners, lists of all individuals practising herbal medicine are not available (see footnote 5 on p. 116).

Moreover, most users of herbal medicines obtain these medicines from outlets where there is no health care professional present and without seeking professional advice. Methods aimed at reaching the public directly (e.g. the internet) and the popular media are often the only ways of communicating herbal safety information to such individuals. There is a lack of research on how herbal medicine users interpret information on risks associated with herbal medicines. It should not be assumed that users' understanding of risk associated with herbal medicines is the same as that for prescription medicines or conventional non-prescription medicines. It has been shown that individuals may overestimate the risks of adverse effects associated with prescription medicines and conventional non-prescription medicines (Berry *et al.*, 2002 and 2003), but given that herbal medicines are widely perceived to be safe, the hypothesis that users of herbal medicines may underestimate risks needs to be tested.

Furthermore, once the proposed directive on traditional herbal medicinal products comes into force, manufacturers of products registered under the new national scheme will be required to provide systematic information with their products, including information on adverse events and special warnings. The impact of this on users' perceptions of the risks associated with herbal medicines will also require evaluation.

The action taken by MHRA to communicate information on interactions between St John's wort and certain prescription medicines after this issue emerged in the year 2000 provides an example of the process of communicating information on herbal safety concerns. Following its decision that manufacturers should include warning information on product packaging, MHRA used various ways of communicating the message. 'Dear Doctor/Pharmacist' letters were sent, and pharmacists in particular were asked to provide advice to consumers and patients on interactions between St John's wort and conventional medicines. A telephone help-line was set up, and information for patients was posted on the MHRA website. However, it is difficult to assess the effectiveness of these measures. Since February 2000 when the information was made public, the CSM/MHRA yellow card scheme has continued to receive reports of suspected interactions between St John's wort and conventional medicines (more than 30 from February 2000 – April 2003), for example, reports of breakthrough bleeding and unintended pregnancy in women taking St John's wort products concurrently with oral contraceptives (MHRA, 2003b).

It is likely that there is scope for improving communication with the public on herbal safety issues. Recognising this, an area on the MHRA website has been set up which is dedicated to providing early information on herbal safety concerns (MHRA, undated).

5.6. The Future for Pharmacovigilance of Herbal Medicines

The potential for herbal medicines to have a significant negative impact on the public health needs to be kept in perspective. Nevertheless, a parallel can be drawn between the lack of a formal medicines regulatory system before the thalidomide disaster and the current situation in the UK as regards herbal medicinal products, in that the sector is largely unregulated. Most herbal medicinal products, including herbs from China, South America and many other countries, which are new to the UK, are sold without any requirement to demonstrate to the licensing authority evidence of quality, safety and efficacy. Post-thalidomide, new initiatives in drug safety monitoring initially followed further high-profile drug safety problems (Edwards & Olsson, 2002). Likewise, several recent high-profile herbal safety concerns, such as renal failure and urothelial cancer associated with exposure to *Aristolochia* species (Cosyns, 2003), drug interactions with St John's wort (Henderson *et al.*, 2002), and hepatotoxicity associated with kava-kava (Anonymous, 2002b), have contributed to the increasing awareness of the need to monitor the safety of herbal medicines. Against a background of increasing use of herbal medicines, particularly by patients using conventional drugs concurrently and those with serious chronic illness, it is likely that new safety concerns will continue to emerge.

However, improvements in the safety and pharmacovigilance of herbal medicines can be expected, if the proposed EU directive for traditional herbal medicinal products is implemented as planned (Commission of the European Communities, 2002). Manufacturers of traditional herbal medicinal products registered under national schemes established under the directive will be required to adhere to quality standards, to provide bibliographic evidence of the safety of their products, and to comply with regulatory provisions on pharmacovigilance. These improvements may not happen immediately across all manufacturers, since some may take advantage of the transition period (which will be at least five years, probably seven years, from the date the legislation comes into force; see footnote 5 on p. 116) before submitting their dossiers to MHRA in order to apply for product registrations.

Another effect of the directive may be to shift the emphasis of research involving herbal medicines. At present, most research in the herbal medicines area is aimed at discovering the pharmacological activities of medicinal plants and providing evidence of clinical efficacy; rather less effort is focussed on investigating safety. However, since the proposed traditional herbal medicinal products directive does not require manufacturers to demonstrate efficacy (other than by way of traditional use), there may be more interest among manufacturers and researchers in extending knowledge of the safety of herbal medicines. While research into the safety of herbal medicines is to be welcomed, research into efficacy is also needed in order to develop herbal medicinal products with favourable benefit-risk profiles.

Statutory regulation of herbal medicine practitioners, as recommended by The House of Lords' Select Committee on Science and Technology's report (2000) on complementary/alternative medicine, is also expected to be implemented over the next few years.[7] Once this has been achieved, it seems reasonable to expect that the yellow card scheme would be extended to include state-registered herbal medicine practitioners as recognised reporters who would be encouraged to report suspected ADRs associated with herbal medicines.

In the longer term, modified, even novel tools for monitoring the safety of herbal medicines may be developed. Pharmacy-record linkage is used in The Netherlands for pharmacovigilance purposes, but no such tool exists currently in the UK. A Department of Health (2003) report, however, discusses the possibility of community pharmacists being able to access a common electronic health record which will be created for all patients and, presumably, to add community pharmacy data to it.

While such a system probably would apply only to prescription medicines initially, with technological advances it might also be developed into a computerised record-linkage database that could be used to monitor the safety of herbal and other non-prescription medicines. Consideration should also be given as to whether consumers and patients could have a greater role in pharmacovigilance of herbal medicines, possibly by their inclusion as recognised reporters in spontaneous reporting schemes and by collecting data directly from patients in studies based on modified PEM methodology.

The future for ensuring the safety of herbal medicines may lie, at least in part, with pharmacogenetics and pharmacogenomics. The importance of genetic factors in determining an individual's susceptibility to ADRs is well documented (Pirmohamed & Park, 2001), and this applies to herbal medicines as well as to conventional drugs. However, optimising treatment, including reducing the potential for ADRs, on the basis of a patient's genotype has barely been discussed in the context of herbal medicines.

---

[7]See footnote 3.

Acknowledgements

The author thanks Mrs Leigh Henderson, Medicines and Healthcare Products Regulatory Agency (MHRA) for providing data from the ADROIT system, and Dr Linda Anderson, MHRA, and the referees for their comments.

No sources of funding were used to assist in the preparation of this manuscript. The author has no conflicts of interest directly relevant to the contents of this review. The views expressed are those of the author alone and do not necessarily represent the views of the MHRA or the individuals mentioned above.

References

Adcock H. Medicines Control Agency proposes ban for kava-containing products. *Pharm J* 2002;269:128.

Anonymous. Extension of the yellow card scheme to unlicensed herbal remedies. *Curr Prob Pharmacovigilance* 1996;22:10.

Anonymous. Extension of the yellow card scheme to pharmacists. *Curr Prob Pharmacovigilance* 1997;23:3.

Anonymous. Pharmacists' adverse drug reaction reporting to start on April 1. *Pharm J* 1997b;258:330–331.

Anonymous. Updated "yellow card" launched. *Pharm J* 2000;265:387.

Anonymous. MCA launches web version of yellow card scheme. *Pharm J* 2002a;269:631.

Anonymous. Kava-kava and hepatotoxicity [news item]. *Curr Prob Pharmacovigilance* 2002b;28:6.

Anonymous. Patients able to report ADRs via NHS Direct. *Pharm J* 2003;270:608.

Barnes J. *An Examination of the Role of the Pharmacist in the Safe, Effective and Appropriate Use of Complementary Medicines*. PhD thesis, University of London, 2001.

Barnes J. Herbal therapeutics (1): an introduction to herbal medicinal products. *Pharm J* 2002;268:804–806.

Barnes J, Abbot NC. Experiences with complementary medicines: a survey of community pharmacists [abstract]. *Pharm J* 1999;263:R37–R43.

Barnes J, Anderson LA, Phillipson JD. *Herbal Medicines: A Guide for Healthcare Professionals*. London: Pharmaceutical Press, 2002.

Barnes J, Ernst E. Traditional herbalists' prescriptions for common clinical conditions: a survey of members of the UK National Institute of Medical Herbalists. *Phytother Res* 1999;12:369–371.

Barnes J, Mills SY, Abbot NC *et al.* Different standards for reporting ADRs to herbal remedies and conventional OTC medicines: face-to-face interviews with 515 users of herbal remedies. *Br J Clin Pharmacol* 1998;45:496–500.

Berry DC, Knapp PR, Raynor DK. Is 15% very common: informing people about the risks of medication side effects. *Int J Pharm Prac* 2002;10: 145–151.

Berry DC, Raynor DK, Knapp P *et al.* Patients' understanding of risk associated with medication use: impact of European Commission guidelines and other risk scales. *Drug Saf* 2003;26(1):1–11.

BHMA (British Herbal Medicine Association). *Code of Good Practice: Unlicensed Herbal Remedies*. Bournemouth: British Herbal Medicine Association, March 1997.

Biscoe R, Houghton JE, Woods FJ. An audit of the level of encouragement given by medicines information pharmacists to enquirers of suspected adverse drug reactions to complete a yellow card report: perspectives in patient safety [abstract]. *28th UK Medicines Information Conference Proceedings* 19–21 September 2002, Chester, UK.

Broughton A. Yellow card reporting scheme. *Eur J Herb Med* 2001;Dec:3–6.

Busse W. The significance of quality for efficacy and safety of herbal medicinal products. *Drug Inf J* 2000;34:15–23.

Commission of the European Communities. Directive 2001/83/EC. Brussels: European Commission, 2001.

Commission of the European Communities. Proposal for amending the directive 2001/83/EC as regards traditional herbal medicinal products. 2002/0008 (COD). Brussels: European Commission, 2002.

Commission of the European Communities. Amended proposal for a Directive of the European Parliament and of the Council amending the directive 2001/83/EC as regards traditional herbal medicinal products. 2002/0008 (COD). Brussels: European Commission, 2003.

Commission of the European Communities. Directive 2004/24/EC. Brussels: European Commission, 2004.

Cosyns J-P. Aristolochic acid and 'Chinese herbs nephropathy': a review of the evidence to date. *Drug Saf* 2003;26(1):33–48.

Cox A. Embracing ADR reporting could improve pharmacists' standing [letter]. *Pharm J* 2002;269:14.

CSM/MHRA (Committee on Safety of Medicines and Medicines and Health-care Products Regulatory Agency). *The Yellow Card Scheme: Extension of the Yellow Card Scheme to Nurse Reporters* [online]. Available from URL: http://medicines.mhra.gov.uk/aboutagency/regframework/csm/csmhome. htm [Accessed 25 July 2003].

Davis S, Coulson R. Community pharmacist reporting of suspected ADRs: (1) the first year of the yellow card demonstration scheme. *Pharm J* 1999;263: 786–788.

Davis S, Raine JM. Spontaneous reporting: UK. In: Mann RD, Andrews E (eds.) *Pharmacovigilance*. Chicester: Wiley, 2002, pp. 195–207.

De Los Reyes GC, Koda RT. Determining hyperforin and hypericin content in eight brands of St John's wort. *Am J Health Syst Pharm* 2002;59:545–547.

Department of Health. Herbal Medicine Regulatory Working Group [online]. Available from URL: http://www.doh.gov.uk/herbalmedicinerwg [Accessed 29 July 2003].

Department of Health. *A Vision for Pharmacy in the New NHS*. London: Department of Health, July 2003.

De Smet PAGM. Health risks of herbal remedies. *Drug Saf* 1995;13(2):81–93.

De Smet PAGM. An introduction to herbal pharmacovigilance. In: De Smet PAGM, Keller K, Hänsel R *et al.* (eds.) *Adverse Effects of Herbal Drugs*, Vol. 3. Berlin: Springer-Verlag, 1997.

De Smet PAGM, Hänsel R, Keller K *et al.* (eds.) Toxicological outlook on quality assurance of herbal remedies. In: *Adverse Effects of Herbal Drugs*, Vol 1. Berlin: Springer Verlag, 1992.

Edwards IR, Olsson S. WHO programme: global monitoring. In: Mann RD, Andrews EB (eds.) *Pharmacovigilance*. Chicester: Wiley, 2002, pp. 169–182.

Eisenberg DM, Davis RB, Ettner SL *et al.* Trends in alternative medicine use in the United States, 1990–1997: results of a national follow-up survey. *JAMA* 1998;280(18):1569–1575.

EMEA. Press release, revised. Meeting of the Working Party on Herbal Medicinal Products. 24–25 February 2003, European Agency for the Evaluation of Medicinal Products, London. Document reference:EMEA/CPMP/ HMPWP/1090/03Rev.1.

EMEA (European Agency for the Evaluation of Medicinal Products). Committee for Proprietary Medicinal Products (CPMP). Note for guidance on quality of herbal medicinal products. CPMP/QWP/2819/00 (EMEA/CVMP/814/00). London: EMEA, 26 July 2001 [online]. Available from URL: http://www.emea.eu.int/pdfs/human/qwp/281900en.pdf [Accessed 13 August 2003].

Ernst E, De Smet PA, Shaw D *et al.* Traditional remedies and the "test of time". *Eur J Clin Pharmacol* 1998;54(2):99–100.

ESCOP (European Scientific Co-operative on Phytotherapy). PhytoNET [online]. Available from URL: http://www.escop.com [Accessed 29 July 2003].

Farah MH, Edwards R, Lindquist M *et al.* International monitoring of adverse health effects associated with herbal medicines. *Pharmacoepidemiol Drug Saf* 2000;9:105–112.

Gogolak VV. The effect of backgrounds in safety analysis: the impact of comparison cases on what you see. *Pharmacoepidemiol Drug Saf* 2003;12: 249–252.

Green CF, Mottram DR, Raval D *et al.* Community pharmacists' attitudes to adverse drug reaction reporting. *Int J Pharm Prac* 1999;7:92–99.

Gulian C, Barnes J, Francis S-A. Types and preferred sources of information concerning herbal medicinal products: face-to-face interviews with users of herbal medicinal products [abstract]. *Int J Pharm Prac* 2002;10(Suppl):R33.

Henderson L, Yue QY, Bergquist C *et al.* St John's wort: drug interactions and clinical outcomes. *Br J Clin Pharmacol* 2002;54:349–356.

House of Lords Select Committee on Science and Technology, Session 1999–2000, 6th report. *Complementary and Alternative Medicine.* London: The Stationery Office, 2000.

Kressman S, Muller WE, Blume HH. Pharmaceutical quality of different *Ginkgo biloba* brands. *J Pharm Pharmacol* 2002;54:661–669.

Layton D, Sinclair HK, Bond CM *et al.* Pharmacovigilance of over-the-counter products based in community pharmacy: methodological issues from pilot work conducted in Hampshire and Grampian, UK. *Pharmacoepidemiol Drug Saf* 2002;11:503–513.

Loew D, Kaszkin M. Approaching the problem of bioequivalence of herbal medicinal products. *Phytother Res* 2002;16:705–711.

Logue M, Pendry B, Waters E *et al.* Irritable bowel syndrome: herbal research update [abstract]. *Phytotherapy Research Conference*, April 2002, Glasgow.

MacLennan AH, Wilson DH, Taylor AW. The escalating cost and prevalence of alternative medicine. *Prev Med* 2002;35:166–173.

Major E. The yellow card scheme and the role of pharmacists as reporters. *Pharm J* 2002;269:25–26.

Mann RD, Andrews EB (eds.) *Pharmacovigilance.* Chicester: Wiley, 2002.

Medicines Act. London: The Stationery Office, 1968.

Medicines (Aristolochia and Mu Tong) (Prohibition) Order 2001 (SI 2001/1841). London: The Stationery Office, 2001.

Medicines and Healthcare Products Regulatory Agency. Herbal safety news [online]. Available from URL: http://medicines.mhra.gov.uk [Accessed 29 July 2003a].

Medicines and Healthcare Products Regulatory Agency. Adverse drug reaction on-line information tracking (ADROIT) system, 25 July 2003b.

Medicines Control Agency. *Traditional Ethnic Medicines: Public Health and Compliance with Medicines Law*. London: Medicines Control Agency, November 2001.

Medicines Control Agency. *Consultation MLX 286: Proposals to Prohibit the Herbal Ingredient Kava-Kava (Piper methysticum) in Unlicensed Medicines*. London: Medicines Control Agency, 19 July 2000.

Medicines for Human Use (Kava-Kava) (Prohibition) Order 2002 (SI2002/3170). London: The Stationery Office, 2003.

Mintel International Group Ltd. *Complementary Medicines, UK*. London: Mintel International Group Limited, April 2003.

Moffat T. *Adverse Drug Reaction (ADR) Reporting by Pharmacists*. London: Royal Pharmaceutical Society of Great Britain, 2003 (in press).

Morrison-Griffiths S, Walley TJ, Park BK *et al.* Reporting of adverse drug reactions by nurses. *Lancet* 2003;361:1347–1348.

Pirmohamed M, Park BK. Genetic susceptibility to ADRs. *Trends Pharmacol Sci* 2001;22(6):298–305.

Quinn CG, Waterman P. *A Comparison of the Teaching of Herbal Medicine in the United Kingdom and Europe*. University of Strathclyde, 1997.

Royal Pharmaceutical Society of Great Britain. *Medicines, Ethics and Practice: A Guide for Pharmacists*. London: Royal Pharmaceutical Society of Great Britain, July 2003, p. 920.

Shakir SAW. PEM in the UK. In: Mann RD, Andrews EB (eds.) *Pharmacovigilance*. Chicester: Wiley, 2002, pp. 333–344.

Shaw D, Leon C, Kolev S *et al.* Traditional remedies and food supplements: a 5-year toxicological study (1991–1995). *Drug Saf* 1997;17(5):342–356.

Sinclair HK, Bond CM, Hannaford PC. Pharmacovigilance of over-the-counter products based in community pharmacy: a feasible option? *Pharmacoepidemiol Drug Saf* 1999;8:479–491.

Strom BL. How should one perform pharmacoepidemiology studies? Choosing among the available alternatives. In: Strom BL (ed.) *Pharmacoepidemiology*, 3rd edn. Chicester: Wiley, 2000, pp. 401–413.

Thomas KJ, Nicholl JP, Coleman P. Use and expenditure on complementary medicine in England: a population based survey. *Complement Ther Med* 2001;9:2–11.

University of Westminster (undated). Nutraceuticals adverse events database. Executive summary [online]. Available from URL: http://www.wmin. ac.uk/sih/research/proj_nutraceuticals.html [Accessed 25 July].

Uppsala Monitoring Centre (World Health Organisation Collaborating Centre for International Drug Monitoring). *Draft Guidelines for Herbal ATC Classification*. Uppsala: The Uppsala Monitoring Centre, 2002.

van Grootheest K, de Graaf L, de Jong-van den Gerg LTW. Consumer adverse drug reaction reporting: a new step in pharmacovigilance? *Drug Saf* 2003;26(4):211–217.

Vickers AJ, Rees RW, Robin A. Advice given by health food stores: is it clinically safe? *J R Coll Phys Lond* 1998;32(5):426–428.

Waller PC, Evans SJW. A model for the future conduct of pharmacovigilance. *Pharmacoepidemiol Drug Saf* 2003;12:17–29.

Ward T. *Register for Chinese Medical Herbalists*. 18 September 2002.

Wingfield J, Walmsley J, Norman C. What do Boots pharmacists know about yellow card reporting of adverse drug reactions? *Pharm J* 2002;269:109–110.

Woodfield R. Senecio species in unlicensed herbal remedies [letter]. London: Medicines Control Agency, 2002.

Woodfield R. *Proposed Directive on Traditional Herbal Medicinal Products: Progress in European Negotiations [letter]*. London: Medicines and Healthcare Products Regulatory Agency, 2003.

World Health Organization. *Draft WHO Guidelines on Safety Monitoring and Pharmacovigilance of Herbal Medicines*. Geneva: World Health Organization, 2003.

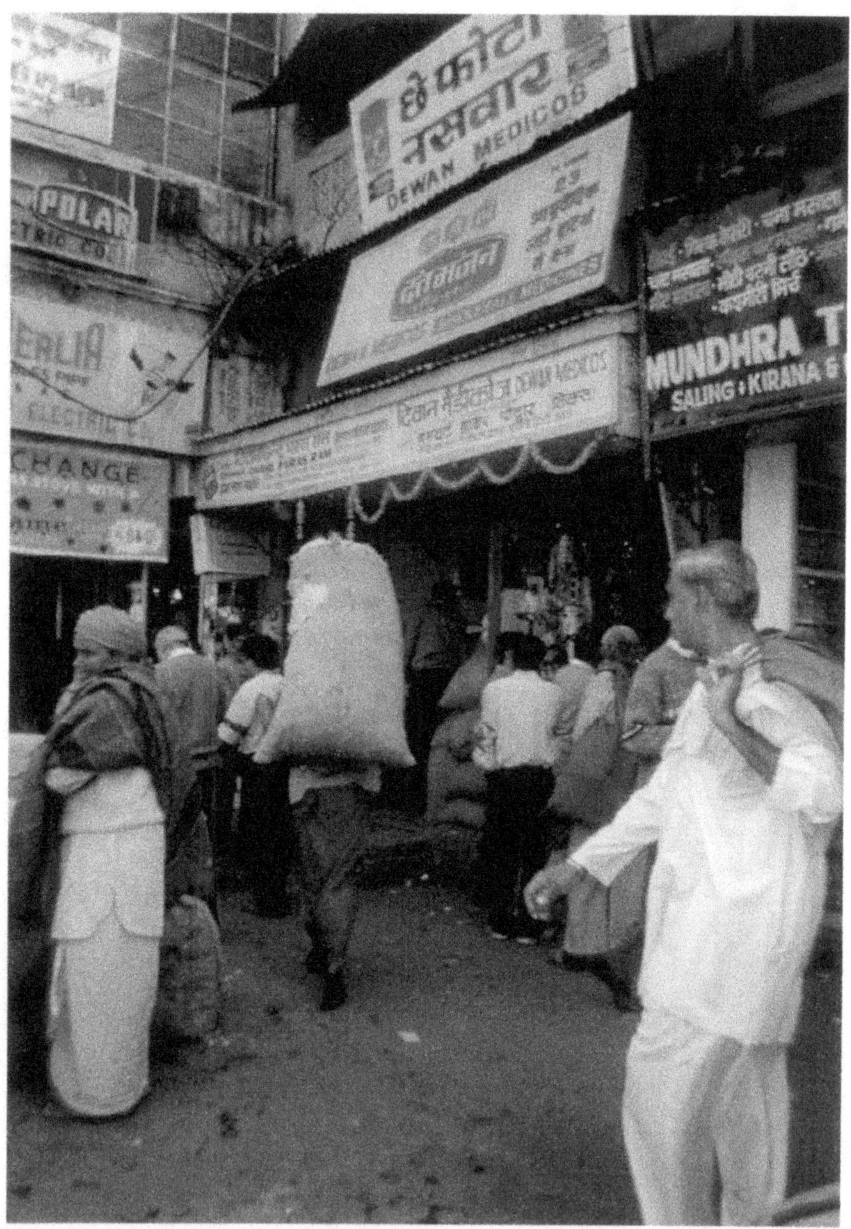

Sacks of wild-harvested medicinal plants from across India and South Asia are carried into the herb market in Chandni Chowk in Old Delhi. From here they make their way to markets throughout India and the world. (*Photo courtesy of G. Bodeker.*)

CHAPTER 6

MEDICINAL PLANT BIODIVERSITY AND LOCAL HEALTHCARE: SUSTAINABLE USE AND LIVELIHOOD DEVELOPMENT[1]

Gerard Bodeker and Gemma Burford

6.1. Background

6.1.1. *Biodiversity and Human Health Linkages*

The environmental impact of landscape changes on health is now gaining attention in both public health and conservation arenas, where it is recognised that environmental disturbance impacts the ecological balance of the hosts of diseases as well as of disease-causing pathogens and parasites. The World Health Organization has recorded over 36 new emerging infectious diseases since 1976, many of which, particularly malaria and dengue, are the direct result of the influence of landscape on the ecology of disease (Taylor *et al.*, 2001).

In the developing world, a large proportion of the rural population depends on biodiversity for livelihood, nutrition and health. Changing forest

---

[1] This chapter builds on work originally published as: Bodeker G, Burford G. Medicinal plant biodiversity and local healthcare: sustainable use and livelihood development. *J Trop Med Plants* (in press).

land to agriculture may, in the short term, slightly enhance the nutritional status of the population, but also leads to a loss of important medicinal plants and can expose people and livestock to diseases resulting from ecosystem imbalance. Furthermore, the role of intact ecosystems in promoting mental, emotional and spiritual health should not be overlooked. Many traditional societies, especially in India (Gadgil & Vartak, 1976) and sub-Saharan Africa (Burford, 2002; Byers *et al.*, 2001; Johnsen, 1996; Lebbie & Guries, 1995) reserve specific areas of forest as sacred groves for healing and other rituals. And in a desert setting, the indigenous people of the Sonora Desert in Arizona maintain a conceptual association between 'the wilderness world' and health (Nabhan, 1997). The new discipline of ecopsychology highlights the importance of early contact with living plants and animals for child development and for mental health in later life (e.g. Kaplan & Kaplan, 1989; Roszak *et al.*, 1995; Shepard, 1982). Hence, the connection between environmental health, on one hand, and immune function as related to mental and spiritual well-being, on the other, has important implications for disease management.

As has been noted by the Harvard Project on Biodiversity and Health, human health, biodiversity, and poverty reduction represent a nexus of inter-related issues that lie at the centre of human development, with biodiversity in turn being dependent upon human health (Epstein *et al.*, 2003). Evidence on the impacts of the December 26th, 2004 tsunamis indicates that those coastal communities with intact mangrove and/or re-afforested coastal strip areas were least affected by tsunami impacts while those where such tree and mangrove barriers had been lost suffered extreme devastation to life, health and property (Commonwealth Forestry Association, 2005). It is a clear implication, then, that conserving forest biodiversity by valuing it and harnessing it as a health resource is consistent with poverty reduction and community health objectives.

6.1.2. *Materia Medica: Supply and Demand*

The surge in global demand for herbal medicines has been followed by a belated growth in international awareness about the dwindling supply of the world's medicinal plants. Over-harvesting for commercial purposes, destructive harvesting practices, habitat loss resulting from forest degra-dation and agricultural encroachment have all been recognised as con-tributing factors. Recent policy interest (WHO, 2002) in the importance of traditional medicine in meeting the health needs of indigenous peoples, rural communities and the poor throughout the developing world has underscored the significance of this topic for the health of the poor and indigenous groups as well as in meeting the pluralistic health requirements of more affluent consumers internationally.

More than a decade ago, a WWF/UNESCO report noted that in Africa, which has the highest rate of urbanisation in the world, the larger the urban settlement, the larger the traditional medicine markets tend to be, thus placing pressure on rural stocks through unsustainable harvesting practices to meet burgeoning demand. The report noted, *'There is significant evidence to show that the supply of plants for traditional medicine is failing to satisfy demand'* (Cunningham, 1993). In South Africa, between 400 and 550 species have been found to be sold for use in traditional medicine, of which an estimated 99% originate from wild sources (Williams, 1996).

Despite recent awareness of the supply-side challenges of the herbal medicine boom, it is now almost two decades since these issues were first given a global profile in the Chiang Mai Declaration of 1988 (Akerele *et al.*, 1991). The Chiang Mai Declaration stated its recognition that medicinal plants are essential in primary health care, both in self-medication and in national health services, and expressed alarm at the consequences of loss of plant diversity. Expressing grave concern that many medicinally important plants were under threat, the Chiang Mai Declaration highlighted 'the urgent need for international cooperation and coordination to establish programs for conservation of medicinal plants to ensure that adequate quantities are available for future generations'.

The Chiang Mai Declaration was followed in the subsequent decade and a half by several other declarations and sets of recommendations calling for the conservation, cultivation and sustainable use of medicinal plants.[2]

---

[2]These include the Arusha Declaration (Mshegeni *et al.*, 1991); the WWF/UNESCO People and Plants Initiative statement on the causes of medicinal plant biodiversity loss and possible remedial strategies (Cunningham, 1993); the 1995 recommendations of the Global Initiative For Traditional Systems (GIFTS) of Health (Bodeker, 1996); the Bangalore Declaration of 1998 (http://ece.iisc.ernet.in/ernet-members/frlht.html); the Neemrana Vision Statement of November 1999 (http://source.bellanet.org/medplant/infodoc.php?op=showdoc&infodoc_id=4); the Nairobi Declaration of 2000 (Burford *et al.*, 2000); the Joint Declaration for the Health of People and Nature resulting from the WWF/ TRAFFIC symposium at the Hannover 2000 Expo, whose signatories include representatives of industry, practitioners' associations, the International Council for Medicinal and Aromatic Plants, WWF, IUCN and TRAFFIC (http://www.traffic.org/news/expo2000b.html); and the 2001 Global Plant Strategy of the CBD (http://www.iucn.org/themes/ssc/news/globalplantstrategy.html).

Consistent themes have been: the need for coordinated conservation action based on both *in situ* and *ex situ* strategies; community and gender perspectives in the development of policies and programs; the lack of information on the medicinal plant trade; the need to establish systems for inventorying and monitoring the status of medicinal plant stocks, involving indigenous taxonomies and para-taxonomists where possible; sustainable harvesting practices; micro-enterprise development by indigenous and rural communities; and the protection of traditional resource/intellectual property rights.

Most recently, WHO, IUCN — The World Conservation Union, the World Wide Fund for Nature (WWF) and TRAFFIC have collaborated to produce a revised set of guidelines on medicinal plant conservation, released in draft form in December 2004 and scheduled for final release in 2006. The guidelines seek to complement and support both international conservation commitments, such as the Convention on Biological Diversity, and global health initiatives, such as the WHO Traditional Medicine Strategy 2002–2005. They apply to a cross-section of stakeholders, including governments, businesses, research institutes, NGOs and communities, and aim to provide broad principles that reflect the varying needs and interests of these diverse parties.

6.2. Issues Relevant to Local, National, Regional and International Communities

6.2.1. *Local*

Throughout the non-industrialised world, hundreds of millions of rural households are estimated to use medicinal plants, both for self-medication and at the recommendation of traditional health practitioners. While reliable data are scarce, it has been estimated that in India approximately two million traditional health practitioners use over 7500 species of medicinal plants (FRLHT, 2002). Community-based methodologies for gathering reliable data on patterns of use of medicinal plants, along with baseline data on their local conservation status, do exist and are pre-requisites for establishing effective strategies for sustainable use.

Unsustainable harvesting practices by herb gatherers, often for commercial purposes, have resulted in the depletion of many medicinal species in otherwise healthy forests. This shift from subsistence to a commercial focus in harvesting is also accompanied by a lengthy marketing chain, which offers very low rates of return to gatherers. Gatherers of the bark of *Prunus africana* in Madagascar, for example, are paid negligible rates compared to the rates received by middlemen in the trade chain from where it is bought by Spanish and French companies for use as a herbal medicine for benign prostatic hypertrophy (Walter & Rokotonirina, 1995). In Mexico, collectors are reported to receive a mere 6% of the consumer price for medicinal plants (Parrotta, 2002). With such low rates of return, gatherers feel a financial pressure to harvest large volumes of plant material. Low prices also discourage cultivation as, with less effort, plants can be gathered for the wild and sold at the same rate.

Traditional knowledge can be a fundamental starting point in conservation strategies. In characterising the medicinal properties of plants, indigenous taxonomies often ascribe identity and spiritual values to plants (Posey, 2000). The apparently polar values of honoring and using, revering and understanding, harvesting and conserving are seen as compatible partners. Andean shamans, for example, characterise plants in their own gardens with a greater degree of discrimination and more diverse information than is found in Western botanical categories. Their gardens at the same time reflect knowledge of ecosystem management and represent symbolically the interrelationships between plants, humanity and the cosmos (Pinzon and Garay, 1990). Such indigenous knowledge and value systems may have a central role in providing the value base necessary for the acceptability and viability of local medicinal plant conservation strategies, and it is important to ensure that they are not superseded by market-oriented systems that value plants solely in economic terms.

6.2.2. *National*

In many countries, the development of effective policies on medicinal plants is hampered because separate aspects, such as utilisation, trade and conservation, are under the remit of different ministries. There is a need to coordinate cultivation and sustainable use programmes, which may be overseen by ministries of forestry, agriculture and/or environment, with strategies to promote human well-being and commercial benefits from medicinal plants, usually the responsibility of ministries of health and industry respectively. The guidelines issued by WHO, IUCN and WWF in 1993 recommend cross-sectoral collaboration at the national level, and it is expected that this issue will be further emphasised in the revised version, due for release in 2006.

The role of ministries of education in medicinal plant conservation efforts has, to date, been largely unrecognised. There is a need for them to work in partnership with local communities to develop curricula for formal education, from pre-primary to postgraduate levels, which affirm the importance of indigenous knowledge and traditional systems of health care; promote cultural and spiritual values of biodiversity; and empower citizens to play an active role in the conservation of their medicinal plant heritage. Similar issues should also be incorporated into recognised national training programmes for traditional health practitioners, where they exist. One national initiative to develop secondary school curricula relevant to medicinal plants and their conservation is already in progress in Vanuatu, with the support of UNESCO's Local and Indigenous Knowledge Systems (LINKS) project (http://www.unesco.org/links), but elsewhere this type of activity tends to be the domain of civil society.[3]

Within the forestry sector, policies have tended to focus on trees and the forest canopy as priorities for conservation, largely overlooking the forest under-storey and ground level non-timber forest products (NTFPs). Some national forestry departments have devised mechanisms for regulating unsustainable removal of NTFPs, based on both their wider commercial value and their local economic value. Clearly there is a need for forestry and environment departments to assign priority to the promotion of medicinal

---

[3] A 2003 regional report compiled by UNEP–WCMC (United Nations Environment Programme, 2003) recommended the establishment of education and training programmes to ensure that traditional knowledge is passed on to new generations. The report cites a case study from the Tanzanian NGO Aang Serian, which has developed a research- and seminar-based model: students interview grandparents and other community elders on topics related to indigenous knowledge and health, then return to the classroom to discuss their findings. Courses based on this model have since been implemented alongside the Tanzanian national curriculum in a rural secondary school in the Maasai village of Eluwai, Monduli District, Tanzania (Burford & Ole-Ngila, in preparation).

plant diversity within programmes such as tree planting and the rehabilitation of forest and boundary areas. Historic mistrust between communities and forestry departments, stemming from the exclusion of local communities from forests, represents a significant barrier to be overcome if partnerships for joint conservation efforts are to be established. This requires a genuine commitment on the part of national governments to strengthening local tenure, respecting relevant traditions and ensuring access rights to resources.

Improved transportation networks near and into areas of tropical forest biodiversity have increased trade, thus creating national supply chains and collection points for what was previously more of a locally-based market system. One report from Nepal noted that 'Hundreds of varieties of herbs in all incarnations — leaves, roots, stems, extracts — continue their journey from remote crags to staging posts in the hills and then to the Tarai. Through a time-tested network of legal and illegal routes, the bundles and sacks are heaved onto trucks, they hop on international flights, board trains and find berths in cargo vessels' (Aryal, 1993).

If local gatherers are to secure a fair price for their work and participate willingly in sustainable harvesting and local cultivation, new models of trade are called for, to shorten marketing chains. These may include cooperatives of gatherers, or producer-owned companies, supplying direct to manufacturers, or linked chains of local bio-enterprises combining cultivation with managed wild harvesting and value-added processing. Such models could offer enhanced levels of returns to local communities, and hence a sounder basis for the sustainable management of medicinal plant resources. This approach to bio-enterprise development is promoted by the UN Conference on Trade and Development (UNCTAD) and is viewed as a novel way of converting the economic potential of biodiversity into conservation initiatives and sustainable development opportunities (UNCTAD, 1998).

Other national factors of significance include inadequate regulatory infrastructure for both conservation and traditional health care itself; absence of legal protection, including intellectual property rights (IPR) protection (Bodeker, Chapter 17 of this volume); and inadequate access to appropriate technology for harvesting and plantation development. Steps to redress this could include identification and protection of threatened species through national legislation and implementation of international trade regulations via CITES, as well as promotion of good-practice regimes within industry that support long term sustainability rather than simply short term production.

6.2.3. *Regional and International*

There is high medicinal plant use across regions, with Asia representing the greatest volume of medicinal plants use, both domestically and for export. India, which reportedly harvests 90% of its medicinal plants from uncultivated sources, has an estimated 9000 manufacturing units. These use almost 1000 of the 7500 known medicinal species in the country. The annual domestic market is valued at almost US$1 billion, and export of raw material and finished herbal products is valued at around US$100 million per year (FRLHT, 2002). Due to habitat loss and over-exploitation, approximately 1000 medicinal species are under threat in India. China, which harvests an estimated 80% of its medicinal plant material from wild sources, exports an estimated 32,600 tons of medicinal raw material each year (Parrotta, 2002). Extensive and historic trade routes exist, with the trade itself characterised by secrecy and generational control over territory, gatherers and access to purchasers.

Increased global demand has brought traders into contact with international regulatory regimes, not least the Convention on International Trade in Endangered Species (CITES). This has led to the recognition that endangered species cannot be exported, and that conservation and cultivation strategies must be established as a matter of urgency in order to at least maintain export levels. In 1994, the Government of India banned export of more than 50 species believed to be threatened in the wild (Government of India, 1997). This was subsequently reduced by about a third following strong representation from the herbal industry, which argued that such restrictions would damage a lucrative area of India's trade with the West.

In response to this situation, new approaches to medicinal plant production have emerged. In Asia, these are large-scale programs of commercial production, while in other regions, activity is more piecemeal and on a project basis. Critical factors influencing regional development are the presence or absence of policy awareness, the volume of international trade in medicinal plants, the political will to forge necessary partnerships between the public and private sectors and civil society, and the presence or absence of dedicated funding to catalyse such action.

Regional and international issues have been identified and responded to by major institutional actors:

- The IUCN Medicinal Plant Study Group has focused on the identification, management and protection of regionally and globally threatened species;
- TRAFFIC and CITES focus on the monitoring and regulation of international trade;
- WWF and the Rainforest Alliance promote education and the regulation of international production-to-consumption chains, e.g. via certification schemes;
- WWF, People and Plants, IDRC, and others concentrate on the development of capacity and best practices.

The Global Environment Facility (GEF) appears to be the leading source of international support for broad-based programmatic development. Of at least eight GEF medicinal plant conservation projects, four are in Africa (Egypt, Ethiopia, Ghana and Zimbabwe), one is in the Eastern Mediterranean region (Jordan), two are in Asia (India and Sri Lanka) and one multi-country project is in the Caribbean. Other organisations and funders long active in supporting model medicinal plant conservation and sustainable use projects include TRAFFIC, IUCN, the International Development Research Centre of Canada (IDRC), the Rainforest Alliance, the Medicinal Plant Specialist Group (MPSG), the Danish International Development Agency (DANIDA) and WWF/UNESCO's People and Plants Program. The model projects of the 1990s are now waiting to be expanded into full regional strategies for comprehensive, ecosystem-based management of medicinal plant biodiversity in the 21st century. The path to this is as yet unmapped, but it is undoubtedly a priority need.

Although the GEF is the major supporter of large projects in the medical plant field, the investment is miniscule in comparison with the scale of demand. The GEF website lists total expenditure for six of eight funded projects at: US$18,211,000 over approximately eight years. At the same time, the value of the global trade in medicinal and aromatic plants — the vast majority of which are wild-sourced — has been estimated by WHO (2002) at over US$60 billion, and may be as high as $80 billion (Mathur, 2003). Clearly, sustainability management cannot rest as the responsibility of international and national donors. The disparities between available resources and size of the trade are too great. Responsibility must come back to industry itself.

6.3. Emerging and Current Trends

There is now broad consensus that cultivation offers the best prospect for conserving many medicinal plants currently harvested from the wild. In addition to maintaining or expanding supply, cultivation is seen as facilitating enhanced species identification and improved quality control, as well as species improvements. A World Bank commentary has observed that *'while commercial cultivation of medicinal plants is taking place on a miniscule scale, this activity is poised for "dramatic growth" in the coming decade'* and favours organic and mixed cropping to ensure 'good agricultural practices' (World Bank, online; undated).

The Chinese Ministry of Agriculture has identified 1000 species of medicinal plants that are important and has begun cultivating species that are in high demand. Over 300,000 hectares are now under cultivation with seabuckthorn (*Hippophae rhamnoides*), employing 10,000 people. The berries alone generate revenues in the vicinity of $40 million annually. *Eucommia ulmoides*, which is used for medicinal tea as well as for a natural rubber used for insulation, is grown in 260 counties of 16 provinces. Around 5000 tons of bark and more than 5000 tons of leaves are produced annually (Lambert *et al.*, 2001).

In Namibia, Devil's Claw (*Harpagophytum procumbens*) has been harvested by poor and marginal communities for the international market for use in a range of conditions including arteriosclerosis, neuralgia, gastrointestinal disorders, diabetes and hepatitis. *H. procumbens* is now under threat on communal lands as gatherers secure low revenues for unsustainable harvesting of secondary storage tubers, which have the highest concentration of active pharmacological agents. Processing does not take place locally, but in importing countries; thus, no revenues are gained through value addition. While cultivation projects do exist in Namibia, South Africa and possibly

Morocco, the quantities produced play a minor role in international trade (Hachfeld & Schippmann, 2000). To redress this situation, the Namibian Non-governmental organisation (NGO) CRIAA SADC assists rural communities to ascertain the quantity of their resource and to establish quotas and sustainable harvesting techniques for the production of high quality products. Direct and economically feasible access to the market is aimed at, in order to generate as much income as possible for the harvesters in the rural and almost exclusively marginalised and poverty-stricken communities. Results indicate that despite conditions of extreme poverty, communities are willing to sustainably harvest their resource (Lombard, 2000).

In South Africa, parts of Asian and the Caribbean, manufactures of herbal medicines and of plant-derived pharmaceuticals have entered into contracts with local communities for large volume production of certain species. Such projects can reduce pressure on wild stocks and create new local enterprises. At the same time, many are based on vertically integrated corporate control of production. Plants are provided along with agricultural inputs and a guaranteed buy-back. However, farmers have little control over what is grown, how it is grown and the price at which the crop can be sold. By contrast, an emerging trend towards cooperative development aims to enable gatherers and small farmers to sell through their cooperative direct to manufacturers and receive not only a fair price for their produce but a dividend on any profits of the cooperative.

In India, the Gram Mooligai Company Ltd. (GMCL) was established in 2000 to ensure more equitable participation of rural medicinal plant suppliers. The majority shareholding of the company is limited to suppliers of medicinal plants who, through collection and/or cultivation, supply direct to GMCL. Rural cultivators and collectors organise into groups, which then become eligible to buy shares. The board of the company is drawn from these groups and a resource pool of professionals is available for technical advice. NGO partners organise the collectors and cultivators into small groups, which undertake the collection or cultivation of medicinal plants according to the demand of the industry. Training is provided in group building, sustainable harvest methods, agro-techniques, cleaning, quality control, accounts and record keeping. The material collected at the village level is then transported to the respective buyers, who are assured of a supply of quality raw drugs. During 2000–2001, GMCL organised cultivation of 400 acres consisting of *Cassia augustifolia*, *Catharanthus rosea*, *Bacopa monneri*, *Mucuna pruriens*, *Phyllanthus amarus* and *Aloe vera*. Collection from non-forest areas supplied about 40 tons of *Eclipta prostrata*, *Boerhavia diffusa*, *Aloe vera* suckers, *Tribulus terrestris*, and *Ocimum sanctum*. GMCL mobilised around 1000 acres in 2002 (http://www.frlht-india.org).

Yet there are risks in reducing the number of players in the supply and marketing chain. Increased government controls at the *in situ* and in-transit levels can impact negatively on local livelihoods, while controls at the storage, manufacturing and trade stages can hurt commercial stakeholders.

In a move away from the demonstration projects of the 1990s towards integrated national conservation, GEF funding in India is helping develop a network of an anticipated 300 *in situ* forest reserves of medicinal plants across different biodiversity zones, linked to decentralised nurseries and a state level seed centre. This will serve as the gene bank for a sustainable national cultivation program (FRLHT, 2002). As a further step towards integrated national policy and practice, the Government of India has established an independent institution known as the 'Medicinal Plants Board' to oversee, coordinate and manage all aspects of medicinal plant biodiversity and its use.

NGOs are playing the lead role in this work, with countless small projects underway constituting an as-yet-undocumented series of models for *ex situ* conservation. Clearly, a strategic international audit of this field is needed in order to establish a frame of reference within which decisions can be made as to the conditions and strategies needed for optimal conservation and production. More than a decade ago, TRAFFIC found that *'The point of view of UK traders appears to be that any conservation considerations (specifically, cultivation as opposed to wild harvesting) are largely an unaffordable luxury'* (Lewington, 1993: 29). Now, there are moves towards certification of sustainably sourced medicinal plant products and eco-labelling to bring consumers in as a market force in support of conservation. If supply is to be guaranteed, industry growth must be stimulated, with incentives being given to companies which can demonstrate that their raw materials are either sustainably harvested or are cultivated commercially in a manner that supports, rather than undermines, the sustainability of the wild resource. A great deal more effort needs to go into evaluation of existing experience, as well as examination of the many assumptions that are currently being made about the relationships between production, resource sustainability, and the consequent impacts on equity and benefits. Such a move will need to be incremental as supply of cultivated material needs to grow exponentially to meet demand, but this would represent a significant step towards accountability on the part of industry.

Important emerging trends and relevant experience include:

- International acknowledgement of the fundamental importance of plants to human well-being, including health, and the threats to their conservation. The recent adoption of the global strategy for plant conservation under the CBD will alter the policy environment for work on medicinal plants, as there is now more emphasis on contribution of traditional management systems and on the need for basic conservation efforts.
- Community-level resolution of conflicts between use and protection of resources, as currently promoted by the IUCN/WWF People and Plants Working Group.
- Adaptation of global threat assessment criteria and methods to support threat assessment and management at the local, national and regional levels (for example, the FRLHT Community Assessment of Medicinal Plants (CAMP) programme, and the IUCN-SSC Red List Programme).

6.4. Research Needs and Gaps

Clearly, such a diverse field calls for a range of interdisciplinary perspectives to be represented in coordinated international and national research agendas. Many of the assumptions that underlie existing policies have not yet been reviewed, nor has the impact of related activities been assessed, as Table 6.1 shows. There is also an urgent need for the results of past research in a variety of disciplines to be collated, systematically organised and — where feasible — delivered to NGOs, government extension workers and local communities in a usable format. This can be illustrated by the example of *Acacia nilotica*, a popular multi-purpose tree species that is widely cultivated for timber, fuel wood, charcoal and paper. A review of ethnobotanical and medical literature reveals that the tree is widely

Table 6.1. Some Common Assumptions and Key Research Questions.

	Research Questions
ASSUMPTION 1: Cultivation supports conservation: long-term sustainability of the resource.	• What evidence-experience exists that supports, or fails to support, this assumption? • What are the important variables and conditions that should influence selection of production-conservation options?
ASSUMPTION 2: *Ex situ* conservation methods as applied to crop species are relevant and adequate to meet the needs for medicinal plants and to address demand.	• What do *ex situ* conservation efforts (e.g. community gardens, botanic garden living collections, seed banks, cryopreservation, tissue culture) contribute to conserving the genetic diversity of medicinal plants required for species viability? • To what extent to do existing *ex situ* models of production impact on the trade in wild-harvested plants? • Which methods are most effective, which least? • What are the advantages and limitations of single species plantation versus inter-cropping and integrated farming? • What conservation systems and organisational strategies would be required to place *ex situ* methods as the lead sources of medicinal plant material?
ASSUMPTION 3: When cultural and economic values are structured along with gender equity into project development, conservation strategies are more likely to succeed and endure.	• Where is the evidence for such an assumption in the case of medicinal plant conservation? What are the lessons from field experience? • How do community-owned and based strategies compare with commercial/industrial models of cultivation and harvesting, in terms of their respective effects on long-term sustainable use? What blends of these approaches exist and to what effect?
ASSUMPTION 4: Knowledge needed for the sustainable management of medicinal plant biodiversity is inadequate, and should be addressed by reviews of best practice and database development of medicinal plant biodiversity and related traditional knowledge.	• To what extent is existing knowledge of the international experience on sustainable use of medicinal plants available and utilised by NGOs and communities? • What are the lessons from the international experience across a range of categories: conservation methods, community participation and ownership, industry partnerships? • Which means of information dissemination have most impact on practice and policy?

used in local communities worldwide for treating a variety of diseases, and exhibits many different pharmacological effects (including antiviral, antibacterial, antifungal, antiparasitic, anti-inflammatory, analgesic, hypoglycaemic, hypotensive and immunomodulatory activities) in *in vitro* studies. Preliminary toxicology studies indicate low toxicity and a possible hepatoprotective effect (Bodeker *et al.*, 2001). Such findings are largely inaccessible to the agroforestry sector, which might benefit from the integration of a human health dimension.

Other priority research needs relate to current gaps in knowledge, which include the following:

- Baseline studies: inventories of national medicinal plant stocks, ethnomedical sources, field surveys, community rapid assessment methods, etc.
- Ecological studies — extent of harvesting, red areas, 'red book' species, volume of harvest, capacity of ecosystem, estimates on viability of the species under current and projected harvest rates.
- Social and cultural research — e.g. gender dimensions of resource use in traditional contexts and within specific programmes, local values and priorities ascribed to species, etc.
- Economic research: studies on enterprise development; trade studies, micro-economics of community-level utilisation and trade with respect to their impact on patterns of use and sustainability.
- Evaluation of conservation measures that may be effective in ensuring the maintenance of genetic diversity, both *in situ* and *ex situ*.
- Identification of viable incentives for sustainable harvesting, together with assessment, monitoring, and regulatory systems for managing sustainable harvesting.
- Agro-technology trials for priority species, including support for tissue culture protocols on medicinal plants.
- Assessment of electronic and other global information resources on medicinal plants, balancing potential benefits against the risk of exposing traditional knowledge to uncontrolled commercial exploitation.

It is not merely plants that are affected by social change, but complex webs of plant-animal-human interactions that may not yet be fully appreciated. Nabhan (1997), citing an unreferenced work by Nancy Turner, reports:

> *'[T]he Salish people of the coastal rain forests of Washington have used banana slugs as a poultice for cuts and wounds because these slugs consume a certain set of plants that have medicinal value. But there are fewer than ten Salish speakers left in this world; the details of which medicinal plants the slugs love are passing out of local knowledge'.*

Thus, research on medicinal plants alone is not sufficient. Attention must be paid not only to indigenous health care systems in their entirety, but also to the transmission of knowledge between generations, and how it is altered by ongoing processes of globalisation.

6.5. Recommendations and Conclusions

There is now a need to move beyond the demonstration projects of the 1990s towards comprehensive conservation of the world's medicinal plant biodiversity — to maintain the resource that has sustained human health for time immemorial; to meet the prospects for new enterprise with viable actions at the local level; and to support the economic hopes of nations for participating in a burgeoning new industry. Future initiatives should link the management and conservation of medicinal plants (and other non-timber forest products) with the commercial development of these resources.

In this spirit of inter-sectoral development, new forestry projects should be designed to have a significant effect on the sustained use of non-timber forest products. A certification system is needed to demonstrate sustainability of harvesting — this is already done with timber, and can be done with medicinal plants. Consumers need to be educated on this issue so that they choose products with the sustainable harvesting label.

Management and conservation must be integrated with programs in other sectors: in health, to foster better use of plant materials; in education, to build awareness of the need for protection and judicious development; and in agriculture, to strengthen farmer extension methods for plant cultivation. Such a strategy would give priority to ensuring affordability in

Table 6.2. Recommendations for Stakeholders, with a View to Boosting the Quality of Plant Resource Management and Increasing Supplies.

Stakeholder(s)	Recommendation(s)
Agricultural support agencies	Strengthen extension efforts to farmers.
Research institutions	Improve basic knowledge about cultivation practices and dissemination of plant species.
Conservation agencies/NGOs	Promote conservation of vulnerable species at grassroots level.
Community organisations	Adopt sustainable collection and management practices on public lands.
Private companies	Develop profitable and ethical enterprises for processing, transport and marketing of medicinal plant products.
Multi-stakeholder groups	Strengthen government institutions to regulate medicinal plant resources and, at the same time, foster their sustainable development and conservation. Develop a sustainable harvesting label and provide relevant consumer education. Collate existing information and ensure its 'repatriation' to local communities in a usable format.

local health care through sustainable medicinal plant production and for contributing to poverty alleviation through micro-enterprise development. Table 6.2 outlines specific recommendations for various stakeholders.

While small scale projects are the crucible for new direction and progress at the community level, the importance cannot be underestimated of developing networks of projects across biodiversity zones, reflecting integrated and well managed local, national and regional integrated strategies. Dedicated research centres for the diverse bio-climatic zones, such as high altitudes, arid zones and the humid tropics, would contribute greatly to the global coordination of efforts. New funding mechanisms and commitments will be needed to support such developments. Nothing less than this is called for if the promise of 'saving the plants that save lives', rather than the threat of their loss — so poignantly outlined in the Chiang Mai Declaration in 1988 — is to become a reality.

References

Akerele O, Heywood V, Synge H (eds.) *Conservation of Medicinal Plants*. Cambridge: Cambridge University Press, 1991.

Aryal M. Diverted wealth: the trade in Himalayan herbs. *HIMAL Kathmandu* 1993;6(1):10.

Bodeker G (ed.) Special issue on traditional health systems and policy. *J Altern Complement Med* 1996;2(3):317–458.

Bodeker G. *Cardozo J Int Comp Law* 2003;11:785–814.

Bodeker G, Burford G, Chamberlain J, Bhat KKS. *Int For Rev* 2001;384: 285–298.

Burford G. *Linking Healthcare and Natural Resource Management: The Ritual of Olpul Among Ilkisongo Maasai in Monduli District, Tanzania*. MSc dissertation, University of Kent, Canterbury, 2002.

Burford G, Bodeker G, Kabatesi D, Gemmill B, Rukangira E. *J Altern Complement Med* 2000;6(5):457–472.

Byers BA, Cunliffe RN, Hudak AT. *Hum Ecol* 2001;29(2):187–218.

Commonwealth Forestry Association, 2005. http://www.cfa-international.org/ CFC2005.html. Accessed 12.04.2006 at 22:00.

Cunningham AB. *African Medicinal Plants: Setting Priorities at the Interface Between Conservation and Primary Health Care. People and Plants Initiative Working Paper 1*. Nairobi: UNESCO, 1993. http://www.peopleandplants.org/whatweproduce/working%20papers.html. Accessed 12.04.2006 at 22:07.

Epstein PR, Chivian E, Frith K. *Environ Health Perspect* 2003;111(10): A506–A507.

FRLHT. *Unpublished Report of the Foundation for Revitalization of Local Health Traditions* Bangalore: FRLHT, 2002.

Gadgil M, Vartak VD. *Econ Bot* 1976;30:152–160.

Government of India. *Report of the National Consultation on Medicinal Plants*. New Delhi: Government of India, 1997.

Hachfeld B, Schippmann U. Conservation data sheet 2: Exploitation, trade and population status of *Harpagophytum procumbens* in southern Africa. *Medicinal Plant Conservation: The Newsletter of the Medicinal Plant Specialist Group of the IUCN Species Survival Commission* 2000;6:4–8. Published on the Internet and accessed 17.10.2005 at 11.23: http://www.iucn.org/themes/ ssc/sgs/mpsg/news_download/mpc6.pdf

Johnsen N. *Folk* 1996;38:53–82.

Kaplan R, Kaplan S. *The Experience of Nature: A Psychological Perspective.* Cambridge: Cambridge University Press, 1989.

Lambert J, Srivastava J, Vietmeyer N. *Medicinal Plants: Rescuing a Global Heritage, 1997. World Bank Technical Paper No. 355.* Washington D.C.: World Bank, 2001.

Lange D. *Europe's Medicinal and Aromatic Plants: Their Use, Trade and Conservation.* Cambridge, England: TRAFFIC International, 1998.

Lange D. *Newsletter of the Medicinal Plant Study Group of the World Conservation Union.* Gland, Switzerland: IUCN, 1996.

Lebbie AR, Guries RP. *Econ Bot* 1995;49(3):297–308.

Lewington AA. *A Review of the Importation of Medicinal Plants and Plant Extracts Into Europe.* Cambridge, England: TRAFFIC, 1993.

Lombard C. The sustainably harvested devil's claw project in Namibia. *Medicinal Plant Conservation: The Newsletter of the Medicinal Plant Specialist Group of the IUCN Species Survival Commission* 2000;6:9. Published on the Internet and accessed 17.10.2005 at 11.23: http://www.iucn.org/themes/ssc/sgs/mpsg/news_download/mpc6.pdf

Mathur A. *Who Owns Traditional Knowledge?* Working Paper No. 96, Indian Council for Research on International Economic Relations, January 2003, pp. 1–33.

Mshegeni KE, Nkunya MHH, Fupi V, Mahunnah RLA, Mshiu EN (eds.) *Proceedings of an International Conference of Experts from Developing Countries on Traditional Medicinal Plants.* Dar es Salaam: Dar es Salaam University Press, 1991.

Nabhan GP. *Cultures of Habitat: On Nature, Culture and Story.* Washington D.C.: Counterpoint, 1997.

Parrotta J, *Conservation and Sustainable Use of Medicinal Plant Resources — An International Perspective.* Paper presented at the World Ayurveda Congress, Kochi, Kerala, 1–4 November 2002.

Pinzon C, Garay G. Por los senderos de la construccion de la verdad y la memoria. In: *Por Las Rutas de Nuestra America.* Bogota, Colombia: Universidad Nacional de Bogota, 1990.

Posey D. *Cultural and Spiritual Values of Biodiversity.* Nairobi: UNEP and Intermediate Technology Publications, 2000.

Roszak T, Gomes ME, Karmer AD (eds.) *Ecopsychology: Restoring the Earth, Healing the Mind.* San Francisco: Sierra Club Books, 1995.

Shepard P. *Nature and Madness.* San Francisco: Sierra Club Books, 1982.

Sinha S. Islamic Organisation for Medical Sciences, Kuwait, in collaboration with the WHO/EMRO and ISESCO (Islamic Educational, Scientific and Cultural

Organisation) — international seminar on *Integration of Traditional Medicine (Complementary/Alternative Medicine) and Modern Medicine* (Cairo, 2002).

Taylor LH, Latham SM, Woolhouse ME. *Philos Trans R Soc Lond* 2001;356: 983–989.

United Nations Conference on Trade and Development. *Partners for Development Summit: The Biotrade Initiative*. Geneva: United Nations Conference on Trade and Development, 1998.

United Nations Environment Programme. *Traditional Lifestyles and Biodiversity Use. Regional Report: Africa. Composite Report on the Status and Trends Regarding the Knowledge, Innovations and Practices of Indigenous and Local Communities Relevant to the Conservation and Sustainable Use of Biodiversity. UNEP/CBD/WG8J/3/INF/3*. Geneva: Convention on Biological Diversity, 2003.

Walter S, Rokotonirina JCR. *L'Exploitation de Prunus Africana a Madagscar*. Antananarivo, Madagsacar: PCDI Zahamena et Direction des Eaux et Forets, 1995.

WHO, IUCN, WWF *Guidelines on the Conservation of Medicinal Plants*. Gland, Switzerland, 1993.

Williams VL, The Witwaterrand muti trade. *Veld Flora* 1996;82:12–14.

World Bank (undated). *Medicinal Plants: Local Heritage with Global Importance* (via World Bank website — Regions and Countries — South Asia). Published on the Internet, accessed 19.05.2005 at 06:34. http:// wbln1018.worldbank.org/sar/sa.nsf/a22044d0c4877a3e852567de0052e0fa/ fae63d87e2bdl4038525687f0057e0d1?OpenDocument

World Health Organization (WHO). *Traditional Medicine Strategy 2002– 2005*, 2002. WHO/EOM/TRM/2002.1. Geneva: WHO. Published on the Internet, accessed 12.04.2006 at 22:12: http://www.who.int/medicines/ publications/traditionalpolicy/en/

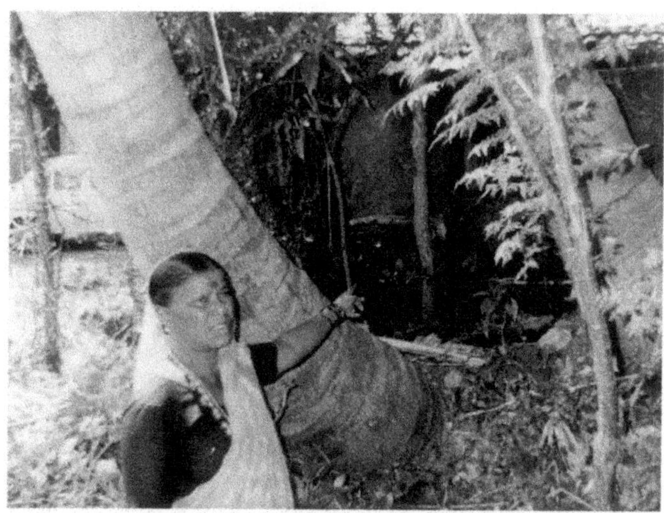

Tucked away in a tangle of tropical plants, a family's herbal home garden in South India has been cultivated for use in primary healthcare and disease prevention. (*Source*: Foundation for Revitalization of Local Health Traditions, Bangalore, India.)

CHAPTER 7

HOME HERBAL GARDENS — A NOVEL HEALTH SECURITY STRATEGY BASED ON LOCAL KNOWLEDGE AND RESOURCES

G. Hariramamurthi, P. Venkatasubramanian, P. M. Unnikrishnan
and D. Shankar

7.1. Introduction

7.1.1. *Home Herbal Gardens and Their Paramount Social Relevance*

Primary Health Care (PHC) is essential health care based on methods and technology made universally accessible to individuals and families in the community through their full participation and at a cost that the community can afford to maintain at every stage of their development in the spirit of self-reliance and self-determination.

Alma Ata Declaration
World Health Organization, Geneva (1978)

In India, the Government's share of health expenditure is 21.7% whereas that of the private sector is 78.3% (World Development Report, 1993). This means that in India, the majority of the citizens pay out of their pockets for health care. Costs of health care are rising due to emerging international trade and Intellectual Property Rights (IPR) regimes. According to the 10th plan document of the Planning Commission of the Government of India (2001), the second highest cause of rural indebtedness arises from health expenditures; the first is due to livelihood needs. As insurance companies do not find health coverage for the rural poor a viable business, the current and future health status of the rural masses is far from secure.

Indians spend about 6% of their GDP on health care, inclusive of both private and public expenditure, which is comparable to most developed nations and more than almost all developing countries. However in absolute terms, it is low. For example, an Indian spends on an average Rs. 250 per person per year, while in England it is Rs. 2500 per person per year, and in Asian countries it is Rs. 1000 per person per year (Health for All, Now!, 2004). Clearly, then people in India can afford to spend relatively less on their health care.

Over 80% of the need for health care is in rural areas, where only 25% of the existing services are located (Lambert, 1998). This is typically so, in the case of village communities in India. The State Government of Karnataka, for example, allocates an annual budget of Rs. 30,000 (660 USD) per PHC Centre for the purchase of medicines (Chandrasehkar, 2000). With population coverage of 30,000 persons per PHC, only Rs. 1 worth of medicines per person per year is available from the Karnataka PHC centres. Due to ineffective Government PHC centres and unaffordable private health care facilities, it has not been possible for the poor, especially in rural areas, to obtain primary health care.

7.1.2. *A Perspective on an Indigenous Approach to Enhancing Health Security*

Common health problems frequently encountered by rural communities, such as cold, cough, fever and diarrhoea, can be readily addressed through traditional solutions. WHO and UNICEF estimate that more than one billion people lack access to safe drinking water (WHO/UNICEF, 2000a) and that the global burden of diseases associated with poor water supply and sanitation equalled two billion cases of diarrhoea and an annual death toll of 2.2 billion (WHO/UNICEF, 2000b). Finding safe, effective local health traditions and ecosystem-based solutions can contribute immensely to the health security of billions of the most vulnerable among the world's population.

In India, Local Health Traditions (LHTs) exist in rural communities. There are hundreds of millions of households and more than a millions of village healers who know about the use of ecosystem resources of plants, animals and minerals for human, veterinary and plant health. It has been documented that in India, 4635 ethnic communities, including one million folk healers, use around 8000 species of medicinal plants (All India Coordinated Research Project, 1990). Many of these health traditions are sound, some are incomplete and a few may be distorted.

Local Health Traditions are embedded in the lifestyle, customs, diet and health practices of thousands of local communities all over India. These traditions prevalent in millions of households are eroding mainly due to economic, cultural and political reasons and not on account of ineffectiveness or inefficiency. This large-scale erosion and loss of local health cultures across thousands of ethnic communities represents a profound cultural loss with implications for civilisation itself (Shankar, 1998).

Indian health traditions are based on epistemologies different from that of the modern western medical science. They have different foundations, world-views, philosophical framework, logic, concepts and categories (Fig. 7.1) and merit conservation as treasury of medical heritage and as a means to preserve cultural diversity. While traditional knowledge can no doubt contribute to and be enriched by modern science, it is important to note that it has existed independently and been enormously productive for centuries, without the aid of the latter.

The concern over side-effects of pharmaceutical drugs coupled with a search for more holistic management of illness, has motivated nearly half of the citizens in most industrialised countries to use some form of traditional medicines as a complementary system of health care. In most countries, this demand has also outstripped the capacity of national health policy (Bodeker, 1998). At the same time, this has led to short-supply of herbal products for the poor at affordable prices (Lambert, 1998).

Traditional health care systems, using ecosystem-specific resources, for human, animal and plant health, are both culturally and economically sustainable, while services through the modern health care systems are becoming increasingly more expensive, particularly for developing nations.

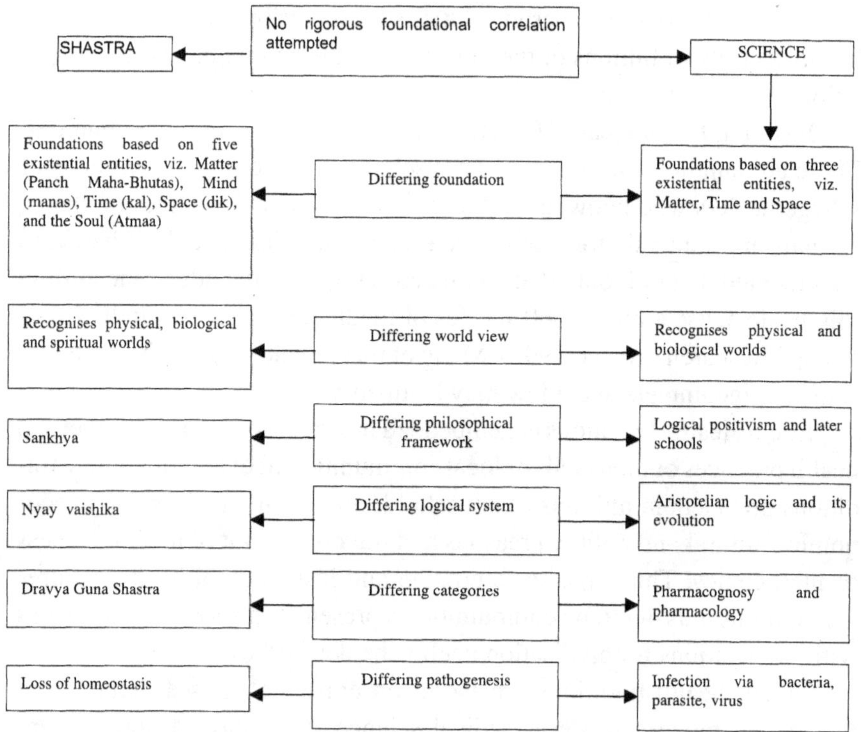

Fig. 7.1. Distinct epistemological foundations of two different knowledge systems both of which have universal applications.

7.1.3. *Health Security Through Home Remedies*

The Foundation for Revitalisation of Local Health Traditions (FRLHT), Bangalore, has pioneered a programme known as the Home Herbal Garden Programme (HHG). *The Home Herbal Garden Programme is designed to promote self-help in PHC among rural populations using medicinal plants.* This programme was initiated in three south Indian states: Karnataka, Kerala and Tamil Nadu. Community-Based Organizations (CBOs), Non-Governmental Organizations (NGOs) and State Forest Departments along with the support of the local communities are the implementers of this ongoing initiative that has been coordinated by FRLHT since 1998.

The objectives of the HHG programme are:

- to increase public awareness about the value of ecosystem-specific plants and local knowledge for solving specific PHC conditions,
- to promote self-help for PHC problems among rural populations using herbal home remedies, and
- to train women village resource persons in the growing and use of ecosystem-specific packages of medicinal plants for common PHC-related complaints, particularly for women's health conditions.

This programme is based on the hypotheses that:

- revitalisation of medicinal-plant-based local health cultures holds the key to enhancing 'health security' of resource-poor rural people,
- use of ecosystem-specific medicinal plants is a fundamentally important poverty alleviation, health and livelihood strategy, and
- biodiversity and cultural diversity go hand in hand and the strengthening of local health cultures will also contribute to the conservation of local biodiversity.

This chapter discusses the defining features of the HHG programme including the methodology adopted and also the impact of the programme on the health security of selected communities.

7.2. Operational Features of the HHG Programme

7.2.1. *Prioritisation of Health Conditions*

This is done through a Participatory Rural Appraisal approach. To begin with, community-based NGOs in a selected district bring together the Women's Self-Help Groups (WSHGs) and other stakeholders to prioritise common health conditions faced by their community. The criteria for prioritisation vary across communities. Some of the commonly used criteria are:

- frequently encountered health conditions
- conditions for which there are well established home remedies
- cost of outside-of-home treatment

- gynaecological problems for which women hesitate to seek outside help
- conditions that cause loss of daily wages
- ease of diagnosis
- conditions for which self-management is possible.

Conditions addressed through the HHG programme include cold, cough, fever, diarrhoea, dysentery, cuts and wounds, irregular menstruation and other menstrual conditions, joint pain, insect bites, indigestion and gastric complaints, mouth ulcer and micturition disorders.

In a few areas, the home remedies are also used to treat common health problems of cattle, with the support of District Milk Unions.

7.2.2. *Selection of Medicinal Plants for the HHG Programme*

Each of the communities and the stakeholders 'decide' on the best set of medicinal plants that are needed for their HHGs. A participatory methodology called Documentation and Rapid Assessment of Local Health Traditions (DALHTS) developed by FRLHT is used for the decision-making. The methodology is used to assess the safety and efficacy of the herbal medicines to be used by the community for their prioritised health conditions (Hafeel *et al.*, 2002). The DALHTS method is inspired by the Conservation Assessment and Management Plan (CAMP) methodology, which is used by IUCN as a rapid assessment tool for threat assessment of plants in the wild. CAMP guidelines designed by IUCN have demonstrated their use in conservation studies undertaken in India, Costa Rica, Panama, Indonesia, Thailand and other countries (Walker & Molur, 1998). Such participatory methodologies have also been used extensively by Government Organisations (GOs) and NGOs involved in watershed development, joint forest management and health education programmes in India, Bangladesh, the Philippines, Indonesia and other countries in Asia, Africa, and South and Central America.

In a DALHTS exercise, the coordinating CBO first brings together the various stakeholders of a community to document local herbal remedies used in treating the prioritised health conditions. The name of the herbs, parts used, preparation of the formulation and dosage levels are recorded for each remedy. Subsequently, a panel comprising community representatives, local healers and traditional and modern doctors assesses the safety

Table 7.1. Assessment of Herbal Remedies Documented by a Community for Specific Conditions Using DALHT Method.

Area Code	No.	Condition	No. of Remedies	Comments on Remedies by Different System of Practice					
				LC	F	A	S	U	Allo
AURO	1	Fever	3	3Y	2Y	3Y	2Y	2Y	1Y
					1DD		1DD	1Y*	1Y*
							1DD		1DD
	2	Gas trouble	3	3Y	3Y	2Y	3Y	2Y	3DD
						1DD		1Y*	
	3	Jaundice	1	1Y	1Y	1Y	1Y	1Y	1Y

LC: Local community, F: Folk, A: Ayurveda, S: Siddha, U: Unani, Allo: Allopathic, Y: Effective remedy, *: Should be used with modification specified by the group, X: Should not be advocated and are not effective, DD: Data deficient/not able to comment.

and efficacy of each of the herbal remedies for the specified condition. 'Traditional physicians' include qualified doctors from the Indian Systems of Medicine (ISM) namely Ayurveda, Siddha and Unani while the 'modern doctors' are qualified physicians from Western biomedicine. Each of the herbal remedies is thus graded for safety and efficacy as shown in Table 7.1.

The bases for selection of a herb for the HHG programme are:

(i) Community feedback on efficacy and safety of a remedy for a specific condition.

(ii) Confirmation of evidence from traditional physicians and experts (local healers).

(iii) Literature evidence from the pharmacopoeias of Indian Systems of Medicine.

(iv) Available evidence from modern pharmacology.

Of the above (i) and (ii) are obtained from DALHTS exercise, and (iii) and (iv) through literature-based research. Item (iv) is generally not available for the plants used by rural communities and is, therefore, not mandatory for the selection of plants for the HHG programme.

The list of plants for the HHG programme is finalized based on the DALHTS exercise. Table 7.2 provides examples of common complaints and medicinal plants selected for HHG households to relieve these conditions.

Each package of HHG contains 15–20 seedlings of medicinal plants suitable for 15–20 health conditions.

Table 7.2. Example of a Medicinal Plant Package for HHG Programme and Its Application.

S No.	PHC Conditions	Medicinal Plants Used	Parts Used	Form of Home Remedy Used
1.	Cold and cough	*Adhatoda zeylanica*	Leaves	Decoction
2.	Cold and cough for children	*Coleus aromaticus*	Leaves	Juice
3.	Fever with cold and cough	*Adhatoda zeylanica*	Leaves	Decoction
4.	Fever with indigestion	*Tinospora cordifolia*	Stem	Decoction
5.	Minor cuts and wounds	*Aloe vera*	Pulp	Fresh pulp applied over the affected parts
6.	Abdominal pain during menstrual cycle	*Aloe vera*	Pulp	Fresh pulp consumed internally
		Asparagus racemosus	Tubers	Hot milk decoction
		Hibiscus rosa-sinensis	Flower	Fresh flower without calyx
7.	Excess bleeding during menstrual cycle	*Aloe vera*	Pulp	Fresh pulp consumed internally
		Asparagus racemosus	Tubers	Hot milk decoction
		Hibiscus rosa-sinensis	Flower	Fresh flower without calyx
8.	White discharge	*Asparagus racemosus*	Tubers	Hot milk decoction
		Hibiscus rosa-sinensis	Flower	Fresh flower without calyx
9.	Diarrhoea	*Punica granatum*	Fruit rind	Decoction
10.	Joint pain	*Vitex negundo*	Whole plant	Medicated oil

7.2.3. *Cost of the Programme*

The average cost of an HHG package containing 15–20 seedlings works out to Rs. 100 (US$2.2). This includes the costs of raising and supplying the plants to the households (Rs. 30), training of the user by the CBO (Rs. 40) and the administrative costs of the CBO/NGO (Rs. 30). On average, the one-time cost of conducting a DALHTS exercise in a community is Rs. 30,000 (approximately $660) which can be recovered over a period of time through the sale of HHG package to the households.

7.2.4. *Raising Seedlings*

The local CBO identifies Women's Self-Help Groups (WSHGs) in the villages who are interested in setting up a medicinal plant nursery enterprise. The CBO then assists the WSHGs in identifying interested users in the villages and in propagation of seedlings in the nurseries. Subsequently, the CBO/NGO trains the women nursery entrepreneurs in establishment and management of medicinal plant nurseries. Each WSHG identifies an enterprising woman in their group who acts as the Village Resource Person (VRP). The VRPs play a pivotal role in the delivery and promotion of the programme to the rural households.

7.2.5. *Distribution and Training*

The VRP selected by the WSHG is trained by the NGO/CBO in aspects of how to grow and use the medicinal plants so that she in turn trains the households. The VRP conducts the village-level training of household women interested in establishing and using HHGs for PHC complaints. She also supports the nursery entrepreneurs in establishment and management of medicinal plant nurseries including monitoring of fencing, waste water course and digging of pits prior to supply and planting, maintenance of medicinal plant seedlings and collection of money in advance and balance amounts from households.

Training of households by the VRP focuses on how to grow, maintain and use the plants in the HHG package. Most of the gardens are designed to fit in the back or front yards of houses to which wastewater from household use is routed (Fig. 7.2).

7.2.6. *Extent of Outreach*

Between 1998–2005, FRLHT has designed and implemented the Home Herbal Garden (HHG) programme across three south Indian states: Kerala, Karnataka and Tamil Nadu (Fig. 7.3). More than 6000 villages and hamlets have been covered under this programme; 150,000 Home Herbal gardens have so far been promoted.

G. Hariramamurthi et al.

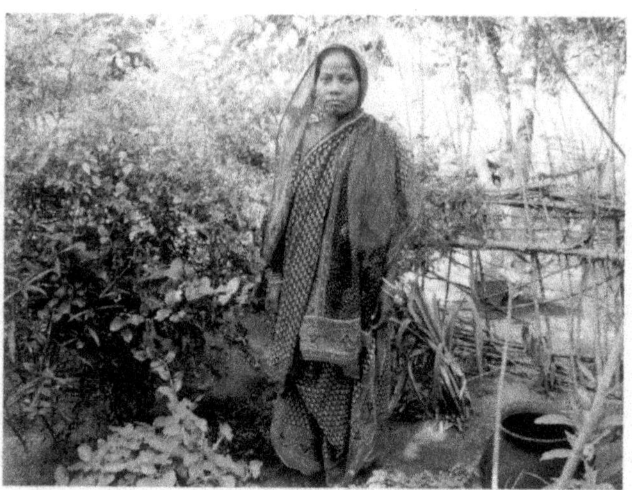

Fig. 7.2. A Home Herbal Garden in the backyard of a village house.

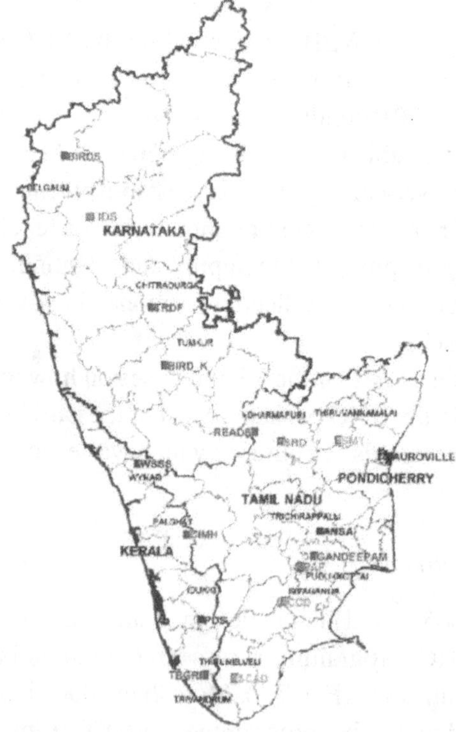

Fig. 7.3. Extent of outreach of HHG programme in South Indian states of Kerala, Karnataka and Tamil Nadu.

Since 2004, HHG programme has been extended to the states of Maharashtra, Andhra Pradesh, Chattisgarh and Orissa. An urban HHG programme has also been initiated in the city of Bangalore at the request of city dwellers.

7.3. Assessment of Impact of the Programme

An impact study was commissioned in 2004 with the help of the Family Health and Development Service Foundation, Madurai. The sample for the study comprised all the households who had adopted the HHG programme for more than seven years, in all the NGO areas selected for the study.

The main objectives of the study were to assess the impact of HHG programme on

- health of women and their families,
- cost-effectiveness of the programme, and
- economic welfare of women and their families due to HHG intervention.

Qualitative and quantitative methods of data collection programme were employed.

Qualitative assessment through interviews of *adopters and non-adopters* of HHG was done via focus group discussions involving all stakeholders in the programme. This was conducted in 21 villages. The women adopters of HHG, community-based organisations (CBOs) to which they belonged, the CBO leaders, the VRPs, and the programme and executive staff of the NGOs and of FRLHT were considered as stakeholders.

Design of the quantitative study was through stratified random sampling where one revenue block was selected from every district covered during the programme. The use of series of strata through a process of multistage sampling was employed to divide the population into relatively homogenous groups and to ensure that each of the groups was represented in the sample. The groups sampled were well represented by different economic and social groupings from 5% of villages in each block. Within each village 5% of HHG adopters and an equal number of non-adopters were sampled.

A total of 871 households were interviewed during the study including those from adopter and non-adopter households from programme villages as well as non-adopters from non-programme villages (Table 7.3).

                    G. Hariramamurthi et al.

Table 7.3. Distribution of Sample Households for Impact Study on Non-adopters.

State	No. of Adopter Households Interviewed in Programme Villages	No. of Non-adopter Households Interviewed in Programme Villages	No. of Non-adopter Households Interviewed in Non-Programme Villages	Total No. of Adopter and Non-adopter Households Interviewed in Programme and Non-Programme Villages
Karnataka	50	61	48	159
Kerala	11	19	24	54
Tamil Nadu	166	166	326	658
Total	227	246	398	871

The findings of the impact study have been summarised below.

7.3.1. *Qualitative Evaluation*

Qualitative evaluation revealed that most of the adopters used home remedies for common complaints such as cold, cough, fever, body pain, stomach ache, dysentery, diarrhoea, headache, constipation, skin diseases and minor gynaecological problems such as white discharge and menstrual problems.

Adopters interviewed across many NGOs confirmed economic benefits in the form of savings from PHC-related expenses by use of home remedies. They also reported that the home remedies were easy to prepare, that the frequency of doctor visits had reduced and that medical expenses have come down after adopting home remedies through HHG.

Saving of health expenses has been projected as a benefit of HHG across all NGOs. People across all NGOs recognised that remedies could be made at home with the help of HHGs.

A few adopters expressed the view that while home remedies do not provide immediate relief for certain symptoms, they were seen as being harmless. Those who sought modern medical treatment cited reasons such as quicker relief and time constraints, for not using home remedies. An NGO staff member stated that modern medical treatment was preferred by the younger generation. A few women non-adopters interviewed reported that their husbands prefer allopathic treatment. A woman adopter said that her children did not like the taste (e.g. bitter) of home remedies. From Focus Group Discussions (FGDs) in the Belgaum District, at the very outset, it became clear that users consisted largely of women and children. According to a researcher who was involved in the coordination of the impact study, women spoken to during some of the FGDs reported that given the high mobility of men, they had a high level of access to 'doctors' and home remedies may only be additional measures. She suggested considering the involvement of men in the future extension strategy.

7.3.2. *Quantitative Study*

Ninety per cent of the adopters felt that home remedies are useful for primary healthcare. The HHG programme had increased awareness among the communities about herbal home remedies and local health traditions. Forty-nine per cent of those interviewed had heard of home remedies before initiating the HHG programme while 93% of both adopters and non-adopters in the programme villages had heard of home remedies after the HHG programme.

The majority of HHG adopters belonged to highly disadvantaged or disadvantaged families. This assessment was based on their land ownership, caste affiliations and ownership of assets including house and cattle. Assessment of disadvantage also factored in access to drinking water and the type of cooking fuel used. The HHG programme was adopted by the poorest of the poor, namely landless (33%), marginal landholding (37%) and small landholding (21%) farmers. Eighty-six per cent of adopters belonged to socially deprived communities, 93% used firewood as cooking fuel, 82% depended on a public tap for drinking water, only 39% had irrigation pump sets for irrigating their agricultural lands, and 72% were affiliated to Women Self-Help Groups.

The HHG programme presented a cost-effective strategy to empower the rural communities in their health practices. The health expenditure incurred by non-adopters was approximately five times more than that of adopters. HHG adopters spent Rs. 92 on an average in three months towards their family's PHC while the non-adopters spent Rs. 478 in that time (Kitchen Herbal Programme, 2004). The cost of an HHG package at Rs. 100 (for the plants) and maintenance cost of Rs. 50–60 per year would still cost a household only Rs. 160 (US$3.5). The benefits from one HHG are shared by not only the family members throughout the year but by friends and neighbours as well. This can therefore be an important means to alleviate poverty due to health expenditure-related indebtedness of the rural poor.

The study found that the HHG programme has mainly benefited women and children in poor communities as a first response to conditions that are recognised as common, e.g. cold, cough and fever. Rural women with gynaecological problems such as leucorrhoea and dysmenorrhoea benefited particularly from the programme since they otherwise were shying away from approaching male doctors at PHC centres.

The VRPs earned at least Rs. 500 (US$11.11) per month through the sale of seedlings and training of households in growing and using the plants, thereby promoting income generation.

A people-to-people process had also set in since it was found that the *non-adopters* of the programme were using the raw drugs from their *adopter* neighbours and were benefiting from it. Belief in home remedies among adopters was 92% and was equally high among the non-adopters (91%) in programme villages.

The study acknowledged the cost-effectiveness of implementation of HHG programme, at Rs. 100 per HHG household. The study recommended that the HHG programme should be integrated into a Public Health Awareness and Education Programme through PHC centres and sub-centres. It has also suggested that a long-term goal needs to be pursued for collective action by both the Government Departments and Non-Governmental Organisations.

7.4. Discussion

Apart from social, health and economic benefits in terms of savings of health expenditure, the Home Herbal Garden Programme based on local health traditions can contribute to health security, without putting additional pressure on the depleting resources from the wild, which are currently extracted in an unsustainable manner by the trade and industry.

The programme can contribute to poverty alleviation by reducing the cost burden and indebtedness due to health expenditure. It can also support local livelihoods, through small-scale nurseries and processing of medicinal plants.

Quite a lot can be done to improve the programme including refining the validation processes and standardisation of form and dosage of HHG medicines. Since regular clinical trials are prohibitive due to costs involved, there is a need for novel culturally and paradigmatically sensitive 'clinical trial' methodologies to be developed to test the HHG solutions and rebuild confidence in traditional medicines.

HHGs can be designed to be multi-faceted to include herbs for veterinary and agricultural care as well as for water purification. Although wide scale promotion of traditional water purification techniques unlike the case of the HHG programme has not yet been undertaken, we believe that it is relevant to mention an extremely significant lab study that FRLHT has carried out to evaluate the effect of storing water in traditional copper vessels. The study revealed that *Escherichia coli*, a bacteria which accounts for over 70% of water borne diseases, is totally eradicated in six to eight hours of storage. The levels of copper leaching into water due to the storage were far below the permissible levels. Copper water had no effect, however, on other organisms such as *Salmonella typhi* and *Bacillus* spp, nor does it contribute to removing chemical residues in water. Further research is ongoing in FRLHT to use copper in combination with selected herbs in order to provide decentralised, safe water purification methods to the resource poor. FRLHT is designing a campaign to reinforce this traditional practice of water storage that was widespread in rural India.

Government, non-government and community-based organisations can participate together in using this sustainable traditional knowledge-based strategy for PHC to benefit a larger number of people in India as well as in other developing countries such as Africa, South America and other Asian countries where the local health traditions are present but fast eroding, due to lack of state support.

In developing countries such as India, where mobilising additional financial resources to provide effective public health care coverage to its citizens has remained a problem that has escaped solution thus far, the Home Herbal Gardens programme provides a sustainable strategy for enhancing health security in primary health care.

Acknowledgements

The Home Herbal Gardens programme was designed and implemented from 1993 to 2001 in collaboration with 18 NGOs and CBOs affiliated to them, in the states of Karnataka, Kerala and Tamil Nadu under a bilateral agreement between Ministry of Environment and Forests, Govt. of India and Danish International Development Agency, Denmark. A similar programme namely Home Herbal Garden programme was implemented from 2001–2004 in the districts of Dakshina Kannada, Kolar, Hassan, Shimoga and Tumkur, Karnataka, in collaboration with the BAIF Institute of Rural Development and District Milk Unions in the above districts with the support of the National Medicinal Plants Board, New Delhi. Presently, a programme for health and livelihood security is under implementation in collaboration with NGOs and CBOs affiliated to them in the tribal areas of peninsular Indian states of Andhra Pradesh, Chattisgarh, Karnataka, Kerala, Orissa, Maharashtra and Tamilnadu, supported by the Department of Science and Technology, Government of India. Folk healers, village resource persons, women in the programme villages of the above states and staff members of all the above organisations have been mainly responsible for the successful implementation of the Home Herbal Garden programme, and are acknowledged for their cooperation. We acknowledge the contribution of Dr. Abdul Hafeel and Ms. Suma Tagadur who developed the DALHTS methodology. Mr. G. Raju, presently the Chief Executive Officer of Gram Mooligai Company Limited, and Mr. Abdul Kareem, FRLHT, have provided enormous support in implementation of the up-scaling of the Home Herbal Garden programme between 1998–2001 and are also acknowledged for their contribution.

References

All India Coordinated Research Project on Ethnobiology. Regional Research Institute, Central Council for Research in Ayurveda and Siddha, Government of India, 1990.

Approach Paper to the 10th Five-Year Plan of the Government of India. New Delhi, India: Planning Commission, 2001.

Bodeker G. Linking healthcare and biodiversity conservation: implications for research and policy on medicinal plants and traditional health systems. In: *Medicinal Plants: A Global Heritage*, Proceedings of the International Conference on Medicinal Plants for Survival, 16–19 February 1998, Bangalore, India.

Chandrasehkar CR. *Presidential Remarks at the Karnataka State People's Health Assembly, Davangere, 26 November 2000*. Bangalore: National Institute of Mental Health and Neuro-Sciences. 24.

Hafeel A, Suma TS, Unnikrishnan PM. In: Shankar D, Unnikrishnan PM (eds.) *Challenging the Indian Medical Heritage*. Ahmedabad: Centre of Environment Education, 2002.

Health for All, Now! *The People's Health Source Book*, 2nd edn. Bangalore, India: People's Health Movement, January 2004.

Kitchen Herbal Programme: Evaluation of Impact. A Report Submitted by the Family Health and Development Service Foundation, Madurai, to FRLHT, 2004.

Lambert JDH. Medicinal plants: their importance to national economies. In: *Medicinal Plants: A Global Heritage*, Proceedings of the International Conference on Medicinal Plants for Survival, 16–19 February 1998, Bangalore, India.

Shankar D. Local health traditions of India. In: *Medicinal Plants: A Global Heritage*, Proceedings of the International Conference on Medicinal Plants for Survival, 16–19 February 1998, Bangalore, India.

Walker S, Molur, S. Training demonstration on conservation assessment and management plan workshop. In: *Medicinal Plants: A Global Heritage*, Proceedings of the International Conference on Medicinal Plants for Survival, 16–19 February 1998, Bangalore, India.

WHO/UNICEF. *Mid-Term Assessment of Progress in the Joint Monitoring Programme: Meeting the MDG Drinking Water and Sanitation Target*. Geneva, 2000a.

WHO/UNICEF. *Global Water Supply and Sanitation Assessment 2000 Report*. Geneva, 2000b.

World Development Report. Washington: World Bank, 1993.

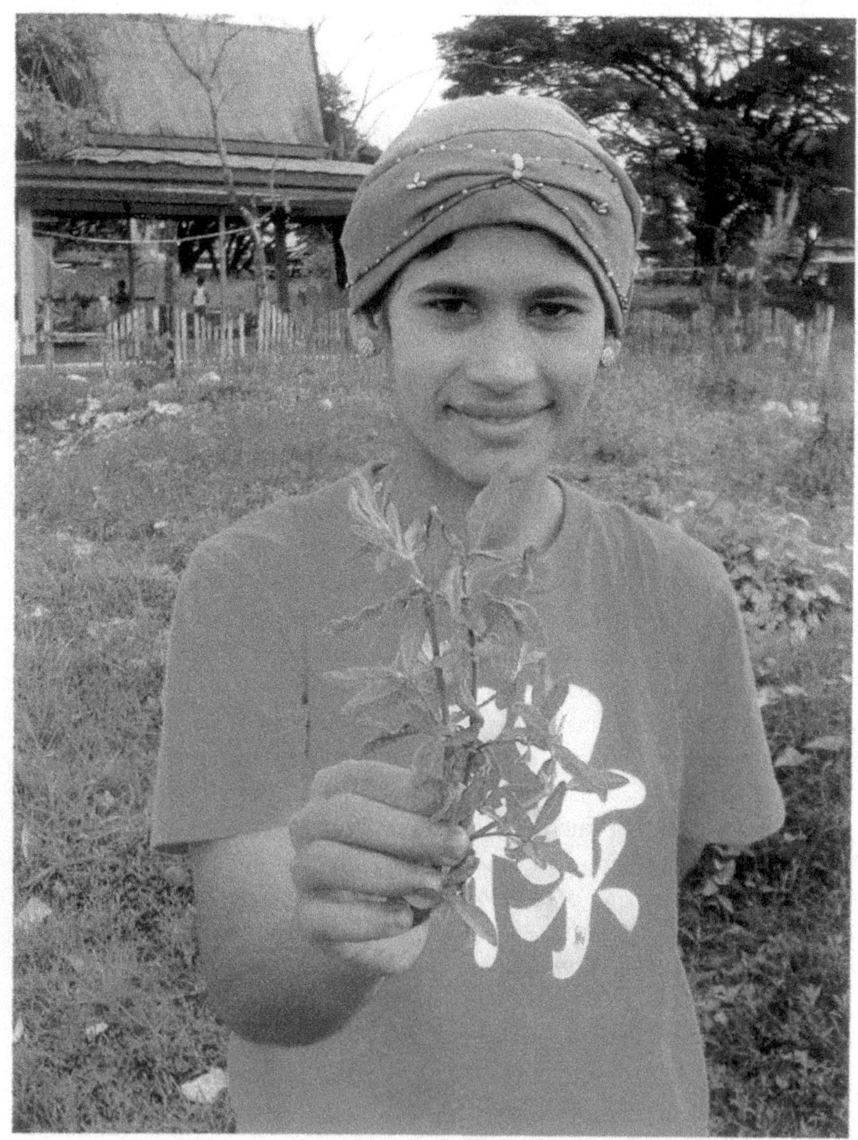

A Burmese Muslim woman in a refugee settlement at the Thai-Burma border with a plant used by her community for urinary tract infections. (*Photo courtesy of C. Neumann.*)

CHAPTER 8

HUMANITARIAN RESPONSES TO TRADITIONAL MEDICINE FOR REFUGEE CARE

Cora Neumann and Gerard Bodeker

8.1. Introduction

Currently, there are over 17 million refugees and 20–25 million internally displaced persons worldwide who have been forced to flee their homes due to civil wars, political oppression, economic inequalities, natural disasters and development projects (UNHCR 2004). These totals include only UNHCR-mandated 'persons of concern', and unofficial estimates total up to 130 million displaced persons worldwide (Castles, 2003). Though emergency health care is necessary upon arrival in host settings, various studies among refugee populations suggest that lack of access to previously available traditional health resources and practitioners may also compound these complex health risks.

According to the WHO, up to 80% of populations in developing countries rely on traditional medicine for their primary health care (WHO, 1995). As the majority of the world's refugees and migrants stem from the developing world, traditional health knowledge and practices play an important role in refugees' understanding of health, and may serve as a resource for improved health service delivery, as well as increased cooperation between aid agencies and refugee populations.

In recent years, international public health and humanitarian aid agencies have made recommendations to increase focus on local resources such as traditional health practitioners and practices, but there is little evidence that these recommendations are being enacted. In this chapter, we will explore traditional health resources possessed by refugee populations, and whether humanitarian and refugee aid agencies may begin to harness and cooperate with these resources in order to provide more effective health care delivery. We will examine the major forces shaping Western aid's approach to traditional health resources, survey case studies from the field, and recommend ways in which these potentially rich traditional health resources may be better developed, leading to improved refugee health, well-being and more sustainable approaches to refugee care.

Humanitarian and refugee aid agencies currently set the global agenda for refugees, and ultimately determine the fate of refugees' health and well-being. In disregarding traditional health systems, these agencies may be overlooking a valuable sustainable resource, as well as contributing unknowingly to a loss of important cultural and health knowledge. Safety remains a central issue in the use and evaluation of medical interventions, especially in high-risk populations such as refugee and migrant populations. At the same time, thoughtful and, where possible, research-based development of traditional health resources may lead to more culturally appropriate and sustainable health care systems, as well as to the preservation of refugee identity and valuable medicinal knowledge.

8.2. The Humanitarian Model

Each year, an estimated 15 million people seek political asylum or become refugees and forced migrants worldwide (Cookson *et al.*, 1998). Major health issues faced by refugees during flight and upon arrival in host settings include acute health care needs relating to communicable disease, respiratory infections, malnutrition, reproductive health and psychosocial trauma; issues of shelter, sanitation and vaccination; legal protection; and as many situations become protracted, issues of resettlement and development emerge.

Over 60% of refugees and forced migrants flee from developing countries into other, often neighbouring low-income countries (UNHCR, 2002). This movement poses substantial health service challenges to host country infrastructures, often times calling for outside intervention in the form of 'humanitarian aid'.

The field of humanitarian aid emerged in the late 19th century in response to major international conflicts, under the First Geneva Convention mandate to alleviate suffering of combatants and non-combatants during war (American Red Cross, 2004). With the emergence of domestic and non-conflict humanitarian crises such as famine and widespread civil conflict, these humanitarian protocols expanded to cover the humane treatment of all persons affected by conflict, but the focus on saving lives and emergency care has continued to shape the humanitarian approach.

The emergency approach is vital during the initial phase of most refugee migrations. The ability to successfully construct, manage and delegate large-scale nutrition, vaccination and sanitation campaigns saves thousands of refugees' and migrants' lives each year. Yet in order to facilitate local cooperation and compliance, as many of these situations move into less acute phases, and as cases of protracted refugee situations become more and more prevalent, issues of culture, identity and traditional practice emerge. Substantial evidence shows that psychosocial and reproductive health interventions are best managed by local leaders and traditional health practitioners within refugee communities, and that neglect of traditional practices can contribute to or exacerbate primary, gender-based and mental health concerns.

Current critiques of this emergency approach scrutinise the 'professionalisation' of the field; the transfer of Western, biomedical standards onto traditional communities; and the subordination or neglect of local (traditional/indigenous) resources. The 'professionalisation' of the humanitarian field is most poignantly described by Castles in his critique of the international humanitarian regime. According to Castles, aid workers are no longer ruled by ethical and human interest in aid, but by their professional roles within the dominant donor structure, which has itself become part of the 'bureaucratic mainstream of national and international governance' (2002). This professionalisation has dehumanised and fragmented the formally morally-driven humanitarian field, projecting Western business-like and impersonal priorities onto much more complex and often long-term situations. The agenda of the developed and donor countries, the dominant power in this relationship, largely defines the structure and priorities of aid programmes, including the strictly Western biomedical approach to refugee health care.

Western biomedical services are often the treatment of choice for acute and rapidly spreading epidemics such as cholera and measles. But, as refugees stem largely from developing countries where traditional medicine use predominates (up to 80% in some regions), neglecting traditional practices can lead to cultural misunderstandings about best practice, as well as delays in vital health-seeking behaviour.

A number of studies among Asian and African refugees highlight the cultural misunderstandings faced when Western doctors attempt to address culturally-specific needs within spiritual and reproductive health care. In a number of studies among Burmese, Cambodian, Lao, Mien, Hmong, ethnic Chinese, Ethiopian and Mozambique refugees, it was found that Western physicians and treatments were not able to address cultural disease constructs or traditional practices, in some cases resulting in false diagnoses and inappropriate or ineffective care (Hiegel, 1990; Buchwald *et al.*, 1992; Gilman *et al.*, 1992; Frye & D'Avanzo, 1994; Schreiber, 1995; Hodes, 1997; Howana, 1998; Ito, 1999; Eyber & Ager, 2002; Mollica *et al.*, 2002; Dhooper, 2003; Bodeker & Kronenberg, 2002). These lapses in understanding and care can and have compromised refugee health. Such oversight of cultural perceptions and practices has also deterred refugees from seeking timely and often vital Western health services for fear of misunderstandings or stigma attached to traditional practices.

One of the main obstacles faced by Western practitioners attempting to understand and integrate traditional practices into refugee care is created by the evidence-based model used in biomedicine. This model requires that all medicines undergo rigorous safety evaluations, which call for extensive funding, clinical testing facilities, Western-trained medical experts, and single, testable active ingredients. Traditional practices and medicines are most commonly made of complex plant compounds, involve spiritual practices and are based in ancient medical texts or indigenous traditions rather than in biomedical scientific principles. Because there are few culturally-sensitive models for evaluating efficacy and safety in biomedicine (see Chapters 4 and 15 of this volume), traditional practices are often dismissed as ineffective or too risky.

The paternalism inherent in this relationship between Western and traditional health systems echoes Castles' critique of the dynamic between the humanitarian 'business-like' emergency model, and a more community-based, development approach, one which involves a 'global framework for dealing with forced migration which is understood and managed locally.' According to Castles, in order to facilitate this, *'we need methods of research that highlight the voice of locals, and we need to involve humanitarian workers into research so research is not just driven by policy'* (Castles, 2003). Alternative evaluation models, ones which involve local voices and traditional evaluation practices, may allow and encourage Western aid workers to usefully assess and incorporate locally-accepted traditional practices.

A number of refugee and humanitarian aid agencies have begun to recognise shortfalls in the strictly emergency and Western-centric approach, recommending the integration of local practices and practitioners in health care delivery (MSF, 1997; Sphere Guidelines, 2004). Though it has been highlighted as a growing priority, the integration of traditional knowledge and local participation in refugee health settings continues to be marginalised. Through our own action research programme at the Thai-Burma border and from research by others in the field, it is clear that traditional health practices continue to prevail and be sought out by refugees irrespective of humanitarian inputs. Accordingly, humanitarian agencies the opportunity is present for aid agencies to encourage this existing health care resource to address gaps in care and to support more sustainable, self-sufficient forms of refugee health services (Hiegel, 1990; Mollica *et al.*, 2002; Bodeker & Kronenberg, 2002).

8.3. Integration of Traditional Health Resources

Traditional (indigenous) medicine, as defined by WHO, is *'the sum total of the knowledge, skills and practices based on the theories, beliefs and experiences indigenous to different cultures, whether explicable or not, used in the maintenance of health, as well as in the prevention, diagnosis, improvement or treatment of physical and mental illnesses'* (2000).

Many studies on psychosocial and primary health practices among refugees validate the effects of integrating traditional practices into refugee care. One of the first examples of such integration efforts was seen in the 1980s, when Dr. J. P. Heigel of the International Committee for the Red Cross (ICRC) helped Cambodian refugees in Thailand set up Traditional Medicine Centres. Western clinicians and traditional practitioners cooperated to build a dual treatment system with effective, mutual referral procedures. Refugees were allowed to pass freely between the traditional and Western health care facilities as well as elicit simultaneous care from both sources. Through this process it was believed that refugees were able to bridge the gap between pre- and post-migration cultures, resulting in improved health and wellness (Hiegel, 1990).

Another leading example is seen in Cambodia, where the Harvard Center for Refugee Trauma has shown that refugee trauma can be reduced by re-introducing traditional healing systems to dislocated communities, and in framing refugee health care within a culturally familiar context (Mollica *et al.*, 2002). The study found that traditional therapies are effective in improving refugee health, and made the recommendation to policy-makers 'to create programmes that support work, indigenous religious practices, and culture-based altruistic behaviour among refugees' (p. 158).

Our work on the Thai-Burma border, detailed in the next section, includes training of refugee community health workers and clinic staff in herbal medicine; research on refugee patients' use of and belief in traditional medicine and spiritual practices; and initial work on the development of networks of herbalists in the Thai-Burma border region. During follow-up research and involvement, we found that our initial training programmes have contributed to stimulating several grassroots initiatives and to the development of herbal clinics and training programmes along the border region.

These examples of integrating and supporting traditional health resources within refugee interventions demonstrate new strategies for care, and highlight the need for increased international awareness regarding existing health resources within refugee populations. The challenges to this perspective are considerable, as Hiegel has noted: *'many doctors and nurses condemned (our integrative health programme without trial. Had it not been for the support, the caution and authority of the ICRC, the inception and development of this experiment would never have been possible'* (1990: 254). At the same time, these cases highlight the potential for mitigating the effects of dehumanising and culturally inappropriate 'humanitarian' practices through the reinforcement of traditional health care networks and knowledge.

8.4. Thai-Burma Case Study

8.4.1. *Background*

Burmese refugees and forced migrants have been entering Thailand since 1984. In 2003 there were an estimated 150,000 refugees in 11 refugee camps spread north and south along the Thai-Burma border (Hynes, 2003), and an estimated two million forced migrants are currently living through-out Thailand as 'illegal immigrants' (Caouette & Pack, 2002; Broadmoor, 2001).[1] The majority of refugees fleeing into Thailand stem from northern Burma, and are predominately of Karen, Karenni, Mon and Shan ethnicities.

Burmese refugees arriving in Thailand suffer from a range of health conditions, including one of the most highly drug-resistant strains of cerebral malaria in the world (Nosten *et al.*, 1991). Other conditions include high rates of respiratory infections including tuberculosis, malnutrition, and psychosocial disturbances resulting from violence and displacement. HIV is also an increasing health concern among this population. These health conditions often arise from lack of access to adequate clinical health care, but our research at the Thai-Burma border suggests that they may also be exacerbated by lack of access to previously available traditional health networks and providers.

8.4.2. *Training Programme and Research*

Begun in early 2001, the programme on traditional medicine in Mae Sot, Thailand, included the training of clinic staff in herbal medicine; research

---

[1] It should be noted, however, that the Memorandum of Agreement signed between Thailand and Burma in June 2003 has resulted in new policies under which the Thai government is now reported to be deporting 400 Burmese refugees and migrants every month, as well as 'exporting' an additional 10,000 migrant workers every month (Zia-Zarifi, 2004).

on Mae Tao Clinic outpatients' use of and belief in traditional medicine; and initial work on the development of networks of herbalists along the Thai-Burma border region. This work has also generated a medicinal plant and traditional medicine database for community and health worker use. In order to protect the intellectual property rights of customary knowledge holders, the actual plants and methods of preparation reported by respondents have not been identified in this article (see Bodeker, 2003).

The Mae Tao Clinic, located in Mae Sot, Thailand, was founded by Dr. Cynthia Maung in 1989 to serve Burma's refugee and forced migrant population. Dr. Maung, known locally as 'Dr. Cynthia', is a Burmese physician who fled Burma in 1988. Mae Tao is a free clinic supported with international aid and serving a patient base that has been growing by almost 40% per year.

In 2001, the clinic treated over 30,000 cases to a total beneficiary population estimated to be between 150,000 – 200,000. Conditions treated fell into seven major categories: acute respiratory conditions (49%), followed by malaria (19%), anaemia, skin disease, diarrhoea, gastric and urinary conditions. Malaria resulted in the highest fatality rate. The clinic provides outpatient health services, including pharmacy and laboratory services. Inpatient services include obstetrics and long-term care for chronically ill and terminal patients. Many of the clinic's 60 volunteer health workers and students also live at the clinic compound and are on 24-hour call.

8.4.2.1. Training Programme

Our work in the Thai-Burma border region began in response to the apparent presence of traditional medicine use among refugees and the corresponding lack of awareness and information about this by mainstream refugee health workers. At the request of key refugee medical personnel in the border region, our involvement began with designing a training programme to orient Back Pack Healthworkers (BPHW) to herbal medicine use by their patient populations. BPHWs are young health workers who carry medical supplies in backpacks to remote villages along the border and within Burma.

The inaugural five-day training session, organised jointly by the BPHW programme, the Burma Medical Association and the Global Initiative For Traditional Systems (GIFTS) of Health, Oxford, UK, with support from the Burma Refugee Care Project (now Planet Care www.planetcare.org), was held in August 2001 and involved traditional Burmese medicine practitioners and Back Pack Healthworkers. While serving Burma's displaced peoples, BPHWs can be cut off from their base for weeks or months due to weather, conflict, political difficulties, etc., and find themselves unable to provide further medical support. It was reasoned that with some basic knowledge of local medicinal plants, ultimately guided by handbooks on the identification of species and their preparation as medicines, a local approach to managing common ailments could be evolved.

Traditional health practitioners (THPs) were contacted and brought into Mae Sot from outlying villages to train BPHWs in safe and effective traditional health practices, including how to identify and prepare locally available medicinal plants.

Workshop participants included an experienced modern medical doctor with a family background in herbal medicine; a woman herbalist; a trained midwife; a coordinator from the Health Department of a local women's organisation; five experienced herbalists; two Buddhist monks, both highly experienced and educated in both the theory and practice of herbal medicine; and a meeting facilitator trained in international public health and traditional medicine policy and research.

Topics covered included: food poisoning and vomiting; diarrhoea and dysentery; HIV/AIDS; tuberculosis; malaria; wounds and skin disease. These were addressed from both a modern medical perspective and from the viewpoint of the contribution that traditional medicine could make either as adjuvant therapy or to manage conditions in the absence of available pharmaceutical drugs. General issues addressed included diagnostic issues, differentiation between plants, safety of herbal drugs, ethics — including intellectual property rights pertaining to traditional medical knowledge, plant rarity and conservation, and the theoretical framework of Burmese traditional medicine which has its origins in the Ayurvedic health care system of India (MacDonald, 1879). There was also a field trip to the rural monastery of the two monks, where detailed discussions were held on rare and important medicinal species conserved in the monastery's medicinal plant garden.

Through this training, clinic staff learned practical skills in traditional medicine for use in refugee and fieldwork settings, as well as valuable traditional health knowledge to complement their Western training. As a result, BPHWs have become new members of the networks of those offering traditional health care to their communities.

8.4.2.2. Research Programme

Through involvement in this training programme, further questions arose on the extent to which Burmese refugee patients and community members were themselves engaging in traditional health practices. In December 2002, we designed and developed community surveys on Mae Tao patients' use, knowledge and perceived need for traditional health resources within the refugee setting. The survey consisted of 59 semi-structured interviews conducted in Mae Tao's outpatient and inpatient departments. Respondents were 71% female and 29% male, the majority of the respondents were Karen, followed by Burman, Mon, and other such as Pa-O, Shan and Indian.

After analysing the results, it was found that a total of 145 responses were given about traditional Burmese remedies used to treat the clinic's most common conditions. The majority of these remedies were rated by respondents as effective. Of the 59 respondents we interviewed, 37 believed traditional medicine was to some degree effective for their current condition, but due to issues of displacement or severity they had to come to the clinic at that time. Except for the cases of severity (13 out of 59), these displacement issues indicate that traditional Burmese medicine is often a treatment of choice, but due to displacement, the insecure status of refugees, and the danger in returning home to access traditional practitioners, many turn to Western medical care (Bodeker & Kronenberg, 2002).

Safety remains a central issue in the use and evaluation of medical interventions, especially in high-risk populations such as refugee and migrant populations. At the same time, thoughtful and, where possible, research-based development of traditional health resources may lead to more culturally appropriate and sustainable health care systems, as well as to the preservation of refugee identity and valuable medicinal knowledge.

In response to questions on spiritual and psychosocial health, refugees' identified spirit entities, witches and spiritual healers as possessing the ability to influence health and illness. In this study, 74% of respondents questioned about spirits (17) believed that traditional Burmese spirits, or Nats, if not adequately respected, were able to cause mental, gastrointestinal and febrile illnesses. As Nat worship (respect) is integral to refugees' beliefs, people reported risking their lives to cross border conflict zones to make Nat donations in their home villages. Belief in ghost- and witch-induced illnesses was also a distinct reality for some of the refugees interviewed, illnesses which can only be neutralised through the power of spiritual healers and Buddhist monks. However, in the refugee setting, many people are separated from their original villages which would normally offer access to a spiritual healer.

In the case of Burmese refugees who cross back from Thailand into Burma to 'pay respect to their Nats', i.e. perform ceremonies to protect themselves from witches and ghosts, there is apparently no structure implemented to incorporate their beliefs into a therapeutic framework. There is clearly a need for sensitive ethnographic investigation of refugee mental health beliefs and traditional methods of dealing with these, in order to tailor interventions which, in addressing the conceptual framework and therapeutic expectations of refugees, are more likely to be culturally relevant and hence effective.

Fifty-three of the 59 respondents indicated that if they knew of or were able to access a traditional health practitioner (THP) within the immediate border area, they would be eager to seek treatment from them. The recent development of grassroots initiatives that have emerged along the border seem to indicate that traditional practitioners and refugees are working to meet these needs, and highlights the value traditional medicine continues to play in refugees' and THPs lives, and in their ability to meet their own health care needs, even where Western medical services are available.

8.4.3. *Evolution of Community-Based Traditional Health Networks and Services*

Following the initial training sessions, the Mae Sot Herbal Forum was established with funding from BRCP to build a network of herbalists, establish a database of significant medicinal plants and from this to prepare booklets in local languages for use by BPHWs and local village communities in the preparation of simple plant-based medicines.

This work also led to the planning of an Association of Herbalists among the Karen, Mon and Karenni refugee populations; and to the creation of two traditional medicine clinics at refugee camps along the border. The

Mae Tao Clinic is seeking the establishment of the training programme for clinic workers as well as for BPHWs as a regular and integrated part of the training curriculum for health workers in the area.

Using data from the workshops and from Burmese traditional medical texts, a herbal database was begun in mid-2002 by students working with GIFTS of Health. This work was done using the database and IT facilities at the Queen Sirikit Botanical Garden (QSBG) in Chiang Mai, Thailand. A CD-ROM of important medicinal species was developed with data on plants, formulae for their preparation as medicines and images of the plants and their habitats. This has been further developed in 2004 – 2005 in partnership with QSBG as the source of instruction booklets for communities and health workers. The database currently includes approximately 200 species of medicinal plants commonly available throughout northwest Thailand and the border region, including information on preparation, safety and use. With respect to considerations of indigenous intellectual property rights (Bodeker, 2003), the database has been prepared in partnership with refugee community representatives with full consideration given to prior informed consent on use of the material, protection of indigenous knowledge through non-disclosure of the contents of the database, and ensuring that the content and format of the database is checked with community leaders and representatives at each stage of development.

Follow-up discussions in late 2002 with the leading herbalist in the area revealed new herbal programme activities resulting from the original Mae Sot herbal meetings. A senior herbalist reported setting up a new herbal clinic in a remote jungle setting at the Thai-Burma border. Here he had trained four herbalists and had plans to integrate their work with that of the modern medical clinic in the area. He also reported that another herbalist, who attended the Mae Sot herbalists' meetings, had established a herbal clinic in another remote refugee camp, with 15 volunteer staff all of whom are herbalists with some degree of prior experience. A training course was being planned to enable these health workers to further develop and share skills and knowledge. The project, open to all community members, was initially being funded by small donations of 10–15 Thai baht (US$0.05) from people who had been successfully treated by the herbalists in the past. From this they built a group clinic. In another area, herbalists were developing a herbal garden for demonstration and training purposes. Subsequently at least two aid agencies provided support and advice on developing the herbal programme in conjunction with the existing mobile health clinic service.

In a meeting with the BPHW team in November 2003 and from a subsequent report prepared in December 2003 by the staff at a traditional medicine clinic in one of the refugee camps, it was learned that a new herbalist programme had begun within another border camp and an earlier one had been expanded. The new programme included a herbal clinic with about 16 staff, most of whom are herbalists. The clinic is staffed on a roster basis and sees 10–15 people each day. It has a medicinal plant exchange with the monks who had participated in the early training programme, particularly with the abbot and senior traditional physician. Herbalists and Western health workers have agreed on referring patients to the herbalist clinic when either: (1) patients prefer herbal medicine, or (2) patients are untreatable with modern medicine, such as those suffering with diabetic conditions or liver pathology arising from hepatitis or cirrhosis of the liver. A one-year training programme was established by senior herbalists in one camp for five trainees. Curriculum included theoretical foundations of Burmese traditional medicine in the first term of four months; traditional pulse and other diagnostic procedures in the second term, lasting two months; and medical plant identification, herbal medicine preparation, and herbal medicine treatment strategies in the third term, which lasted six months and concluded in early 2004. Interest by trainees was reported as high and their services are viewed by the refugee health workers in the camps as offering a low cost, safe and effective treatment option in a setting where access to medical care is difficult. The programme was funded via a combination of grant money from the Burma Humanitarian Mission, the NGO Free Friendly Asia (FFA), and patient contributions. In December 2004, it was reported that an additional new clinic had been established in a remote jungle setting staffed by four herbalists who had been trained through the herbalist training programme.

These developments are expressions of refugee interest, receptivity and perceived need for traditional health services within the refugee context. These services are locally available and offer affordable medicines and treatments to a severely underserved population. They highlight the existence of indigenous networks in refugee communities that are largely overlooked by aid agencies and workers, yet which serve as powerful sources of continuity and identity among people who have few external links back to their original culture and social identity.

8.5. Discussion

The Mae Sot example reported on in this chapter shows how community-based and initiated development can lead to improved service delivery as well as sustainable health programmes. The unexpected grassroots response from herbalists who, through the herbalist training programme, have come to take their role as partners in community health care in a more focused and organised manner, has demonstrated the value of supporting existing resources through integration and knowledge exchange. The resultant emergence of networks of herbalists sharing knowledge, planning new remote-area clinics, and planting new herbal gardens in villages where basic medical supplies are unavailable is a grassroots response that embodies elements of sustainability, cultural appropriateness and community-based and managed development.

Despite recent recommendations to incorporate local resources into humanitarian interventions, humanitarian agencies' interest in traditional medicine use among refugees is mainly reserved for psychosocial health interventions and reproductive health programmes, as these post-emergency phases are more flexible in their consideration of culturally-appropriate practices. Though the reproductive and psychosocial aspects of traditional health care are indeed vital areas of care, the primary health care aspect has been rarely examined within the humanitarian context. This is due in part to the fact that Western medicine has widely adopted evidence-based medicine in its approach, and in doing so excludes traditional and non-Western medicine due to the costly and lengthy process of safety and efficacy standardisation. Though this policy makes sense in the Western context, where standardisation and legalisation are required for all clinical care, it may prove detrimental in environments where traditional medicine is the common or most accessible form of health care, as in some acute and most protracted refugee settings.

An important insight gained through the Thai-Burma research, and one that is shared in the Cambodian examples cited earlier (Mollica and Hiegel), relates to refugee beliefs that many traditional medicines are effective and longer lasting. Though safety studies and clinical evaluation are needed for treatments for such serious conditions as malaria, acute respiratory conditions and HIV-related illness, this wider range of treatments may include trusted remedies for more common conditions, such as certain skin diseases and gastric conditions. These treatments may be more culturally familiar, accessible, affordable and potentially effective for certain illnesses, in particular those which are culturally based. In the broader context of refugee care, where conventional treatments may be less accessible or culturally unfamiliar, commonly used traditional therapies can address unmet needs in primary care.

Another important outcome of the research has been the perspective gained that refugees' deeply held spiritual beliefs clearly affect their notions of disease which in turn impacts on therapeutic outcomes. These beliefs appear to have cultural and identity dimensions that need to be understood in the context of creating effective mental health programmes and in managing conditions that are unresponsive to conventional treatment.

Refugees themselves may provide clues for sustainable health care delivery, as seen in our Mae Sot example. By harnessing this knowledge and moving beyond a crisis mode towards models of self-sufficient local health services, refugee aid agencies could help facilitate new global strategies for sustainable refugee health care, contributing at the same time to cultural continuity and refugee identity.

8.6. Towards More Integrated and Community-Based Refugee Health Care

The international health focus on 'humanitarian aid', relating to acute refugee situations, has resulted in the rapid emergence and professionalisation of numerous humanitarian aid organisations and programmes.[2] At the

---

[2]The largest players in humanitarian aid (service-delivery) include UNHCR, Office for the Coordination of Humanitarian Affairs, USAID, WFP/FAO, Medecins Sans Frontieres, International Rescue Committee, International Committee of the Red Cross, CARE International, Concern, Catholic Relief Services, and various other NGO and religiously-affiliated charity organisations worldwide.

Eighth Conference of the International Association for the Study of Forced Migration, held in Chiang Mai, Thailand, in January 2003, participants and coordinators argued that 'for reasons of self-preservation', UNHCR and international aid agencies have a vested interest in the relief model over initiatives for a community based development approach which could lead to sustainability (Nadig, 2003: 370).

This professionalisation of humanitarian aid hinders the ability of both refugees and aid workers to develop and explore traditional forms of health care. Donor-recipient roles formalise the aid process, neglecting valuable community resources and leading to longer term effects on health, well-being and identity.

According to Colson, refugees within camp and self-settle settings often succumb to depression and apathy, affecting their abilities to thrive. To counter-balance these detrimental outcomes, Colson suggests support-ing existing refugee resources: '... the loss of role structures means that (refugees) cannot know who they are or who anyone else is until new roles are constructed and people assigned to them'. If possible, traumatised indi-viduals prefer to make minimal short-term changes so that they may rapidly return to their own identities, becoming 'themselves' again. This return of identity is crucial in the health and well-being of refugees (Colson, 2003: 8). Traditional health networks provide refugees the ability to preserve and resume their pre-migration roles.

Therefore, engaging local practitioners in the aid process benefits these practitioners as well as their communities, as indigenous health care practi-tioners are often in the best position to serve as a bridge in planning strate-gies for incorporating traditional health and psycho-spiritual dimensions into health care programmes for refugees.

These topics of culturally appropriate care and refugee identity have further implications for strategies in international aid. At present, humani-tarian responses to refugee health do little to support cultural and traditional health resources of most refugee populations. As a source of self-care, indigenous networks, such as those in traditional health, indicate what civil society can do in the context of influencing globalisation, potentially reduc-ing dependence on foreign aid and the 'professionalisation' which threatens to undermine the practices and efficacy of health interventions within the field of humanitarian aid.

References

American Red Cross. *The Geneva Conventions, the International Committee of the Red Cross and the Rights of Prisoners of War*. Accessed 10 November 2004: http://www.redcross.org/museum/gc.html.

Bodeker G. Traditional medical knowledge, intellectual property rights and benefit sharing. *Cardozo J Int Law* 2003;11:785–811.

Bodeker G, Kronenberg F. A public health agenda for complementary, alternative and traditional (indigenous) medicine. *Am J Public Health* 2002; 92(10):1582–1591.

Broadmoor T. Labor pains: the Thai government's latest resolution to control the growing migrant worker population lacks resolve. *Irrawaddy* 2001;9(7):7.

Buchwald D, Panwala S, Hooton TM. Use of traditional health practices by Southeast Asian refugees in a primary care clinic. *West J Med* 1992; 156(5):507–511.

Burmese Border Consortium. *Program Report: July–December 2001*. Bangkok: Author, 2002.

Caouette TM, Pack ME. Pushing past the definitions: migration from Burma to Thailand. Report prepared for Refugees International and Open Society Institute, 2002.

Castles S. *The New Global Politics and the Emerging Forced Migration Regime*. Paper for Refugee Studies Seminar Series, Oxford, 2002. http://www.jcwi.org.uk/resources/globalisation_refugees.PDF (05/20/03).

Castles S. *Presentation on Forced Migration Trends*. Conference of the International Association for the Study of Forced Migration (IASFM), January 2003, Chiang Mai, Thailand.

Colson E. Forced migration and the anthropological response. *J Refugee Stud* 2003;16(1):1–18.

Cookson S, Waldman R, Gushulak B, Macpherson D, Burkle F Jr, Paquet C, Kliewer E, Walker P. Immigrant and refugee health. *Emerg Infect Dis* 1998;4(3):427–428.

Dhooper SS. Health care needs of foreign-born Asian Americans: an overview. *Health Soc Work* February 2003;28(1):63–73.

Eisenbruch M. The survival of Cambodian culture through the traditional healer: a responsibility in international mental health. Paper for World Congress, World Federation for Mental Health, 18–23 August 1991, Mexico.

Eyber C, Ager A. Conselho: psychological healing in displaced communities in Angola. *Lancet* 2002;360(9336):871.

Frye BA, D'Avanzo C. Themes in managing culturally defined illness in the Cambodian refugee family. *J Commun Health Nurs* 1994;11(2):89–98.

Gilman SC, Justice J, Saepharn K, Charles G. Use of traditional and modern health services by Laotian refugees. *West J Med* September 1992;157(3):310–315.

Hiegel JP. Do traditional healers have a role in refugee camps? *Refugee Participation Network*, Vol. 8, Oxford Refugee Studies Program, 1990.

Hiegel JP. *The ICRC and Traditional Khmer Medicine.* International Review of the Red Cross, No. 224, pp. 251–262, Geneva, 1981.

Hodes R. Cross-cultural medicine and diverse health beliefs. Ethiopians abroad. *West J Med* 1997;166(1):29–36.

Howana A. Trauma and healing in Mozambique. *Accord: An International Review of Peace Initiatives*, 1998.

Hynes P. *Research Guide on Burma.* Forced Migration On-Line, 2003: http://www.forcedmigration.org/guides/fmo019/ (02/15/04).

Ito KL. Health culture and the clinical encounter: Vietnamese refugees' responses to preventive drug treatment of inactive tuberculosis. *Med Anthropol Quart* 1999;13(3):338–364.

Macdonald KN. *The Practice of Medicine Among the Burmese*, 1979 reprint. Edinburgh: Machlachlan and Stewart, 1879.

Medicins Sans Frontieres. *Refugee Health: An Approach to Emergency Situations.* London and Oxford: Macmillin Education Ltd., 1997.

Mollica RF, Cui X, Mcinnes K, Massagli MP. Science-based policy for psychosocial interventions in refugee camps: a Cambodian example. *J Nerv Mental Disord* 2002;190(3):158–166.

Nadig A. Forced migration and global processes. Report of the Eighth Conference of the International Association for the Study of Forced Migration, Chiang Mai, Thailand, 5–9 January 2003. *J Refugee Stud* 2003; 16(4):361–375.

Nosten F, Ter Kuile F, Chongsuphajaisiddhi T, Luxemburger C, Webster HK, Edstein M, Phaipun L, Thew KL, White NJ. Mefloquine-resistant falciparum malaria on the Thai-Burmese border. *Lancet* 1991;337(8750):1140–1143.

Schreiber S. Migration, traumatic bereavement and transcultural aspects of psychological healing: loss and grief of a refugee woman from Begameder county in Ethiopia. *Br J Med Psychol* 1995;68(Pt 2):135–142.

Sphere Project. *Evaluating Food and Relief Programmes on the Burma/ Thailand Border*, 2000. Sphere Case Studies. Accessed June 2002: www. sphereproject.org/practices/cs_burma.htm.

Sphere Project. *Humanitarian Charter and Minimum Standards in Disaster Response.* Geneva, Switzerland: Sphere Project.

UNHCR. *Basic Information About UNHCR*. Refugees by Numbers (2004 Edition), accessed at www.unhcr.org on 15 November 2004.

United Nations. *Situation of Human Rights in Myanmar*. Report of the Special Rapporteur of the Commission on Human Rights presented at the 58th session of the UN General Assembly, UN Document A/58/219, 5 August 2003.

United Nations Development Program. *Human Development Indicators 2003: Myanmar*. Human Development Report 2003, UNDP website, 3 April 2003: www.undp.org/hdr2003/indicator/cty_f_MMR.html.

WHO. *Traditional Practitioners as Primary Health Care Workers*. Division of Strengthening of Health Services and the Traditional Health Program, 1995, p. 10.

WHO. *Traditional Medicine Strategy 2002–2005*. World Health Organization, Geneva. http://www.who.int/medicines/organization/trm/orgtrmmain.shtml).

World Bank. *Myanmar at a Glance*. World Bank website, accessed 10 April 2004: http://www.worldbank.org/data/countrydata/aag/mmr_aag.pdf.

Zia-Zarifi S. Thailand: harsh policy towards Burmese refugees. *The Nation*, 2004: http://www.hrw.org/english/docs/2004/01/27/thaila7075.htm (02/16/04).

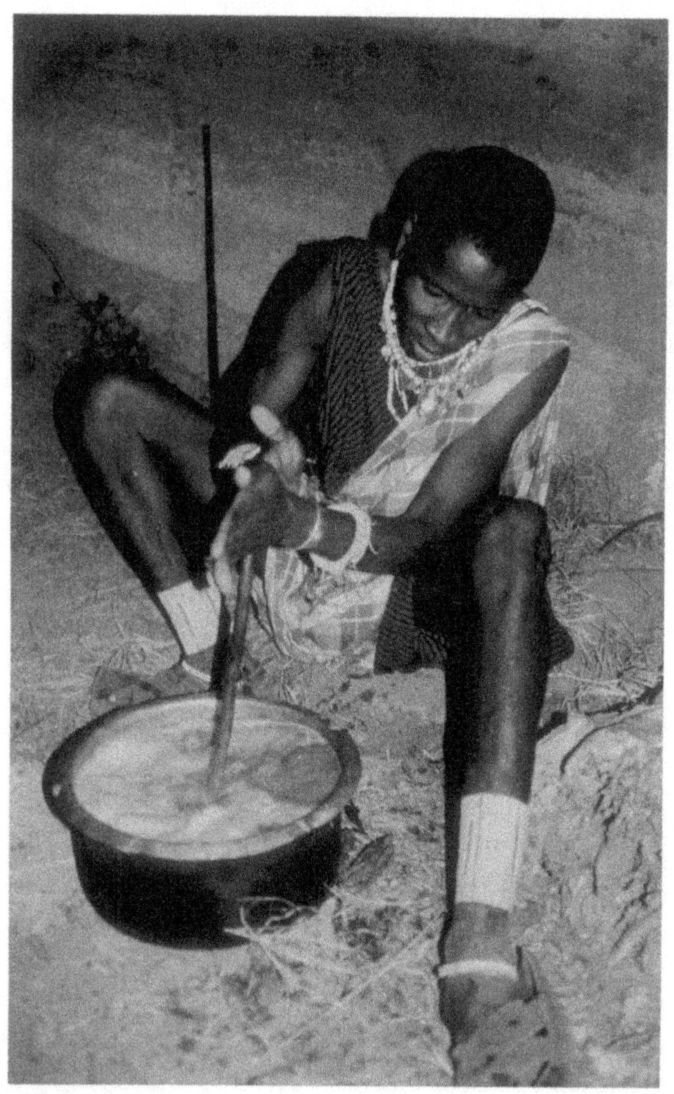

A Maasai youth stirring a medicinal broth used in traditional coming of age ceremonies. (*Photo courtesy of B. Webzell.*)

PUBLIC-PRIVATE PARTNERSHIPS FOR THE DEVELOPMENT OF TRADITIONAL HEALTH CARE: CASE STUDIES FROM EAST AFRICA

Patrick M. Mbindyo

9.1. Background

The increase in global health expenditure from an average of 3% of GDP in 1950 to 8% (US$3 trillion) in 1999 (WHO, 2000) has been driven by rising income, changing demographic and epidemiological trends, and costly new pharmaceuticals and technology. Public funding has not kept pace with the growth in spending. Much of the increase has been financed from private sources (out-of-pocket payments and private insurance), while the share funded publicly (by tax revenue and national insurance) declined by 6% between 1977 and 1997 (Taylor & Blair, 2002).

For many countries, the process of solving this problem has led to the restructuring of health systems and finding the best form of public–private mix in service provision. The traditional provider of health infrastructure and services in developing countries has been the public sector. Of late, it has been extremely constrained in its ability to maintain and improve, as well as expand, current facilities due to inadequacies on the part of the public sector owing to lack of resources and management capabilities (Nishtar, 2004). This has resulted in various problems such as increased costs (direct and indirect) of doing business, poor access to essential services and lower standards of living.

Developing countries carry the burden of some of the world's most fatal diseases and conditions on the one hand, and face shortage or lack of essential goods and services on the other. Governments, international health organisations and non-governmental organisations, once the central actors in addressing the burden, are looking to the private sector for help (Taylor & Blair 2002). At the same time, private for-profit organisations have come to realise the importance of public health goals, and to take a broader view of social responsibility for their immediate and long-term objectives as part of the corporate mandate. Multi-sector partnerships involving various actors, both in the public and private sector domains, can help to deliver broad health interventions that reduce disease burdens.

A major component of private health care provision is the service offered by traditional medical practitioners. It is recognised that the traditional medical sector constitutes an important part of private health services in many African countries (Kasilo *et al.*, 2005; UNAIDS, 2002; Leonard, 2001), considering that nearly 80% of the population in developing countries relies on these systems for their daily primary health care needs (WHO, 2002). Traditional medical practitioners offer care, support and prevention alternatives that are readily available, accessible and affordable. They take into account the feelings of patients, their ability/inability to pay for the health services and their socio-cultural and economic realities (UNAIDS, 2002; Mbindyo, 2001). This is in addition to having specialised knowledge for treating physical, cultural and psychological ailments (Scheinman, 2002; Mbiti, 1969).

9.1.1. *The Nature of Traditional Medicine in Africa*

Traditional health practitioners occupy a critical role in African societies, and make a valuable contribution to health care (Bodeker *et al.*, 2000; KWG, 2002), especially in areas where Western medicine is not an option (Molvaer, 1981). For example, in Madagascar, 32% of people first sought the care of a traditional healer (Hanson & Berman, 1994). Traditional healers often have greater credibility than do village health workers, especially with respect to social and spiritual matters. Further, as the services provided are client-centred and personalised, this makes traditional healers important communication agents for health and social issues (UNAIDS, 2002).

The case studies used in this chapter illustrate, however, that the real scope of African traditional health care is much broader than straightforward healer-patient relationships. It incorporates traditional methods of preventing disease, such as using plants to repel or kill mosquitoes (as in the ICIPE-Biop example, Section 9.3.2), or the use of charms and amulets; and promoting beneficial cultural practices that reduce the burden of disease (as in the WOFAK example, Section 9.3.1). It also encompasses a substantial lay sector — health care provision by non-specialist 'families and friends' — that often constitutes the first line of response to illness, especially in rural societies. Research carried out among Tanzanian Maasai has shown that almost all adults, and many children, have at least a basic knowledge of plant-based remedies for common ailments such as fever and cough (Burford *et al.*, 2001). The same findings have been noted among the Luo of Kenya (Geissler & Meinert, 2000). The support of community members through prayer, 'healing songs', storytelling, counselling and assistance with practical issues such as food provision and childcare, among others, adds a vital psychosocial dimension to health care. Furthermore, there is often a conceptual association between health and the natural environment, as when specific forest sites are used for healing rituals (Burford *et al.*, 2001; Burford, 2002).

In contrast to the 'symptom/drug' approach of Western biomedicine, African traditional health care places illness and wellness firmly within their social contexts. Research and development activities, however, often focus on two aspects: the isolation of specific medicinal plants and their 'active ingredients', and/or the involvement of individual practitioners — usually herbalists or traditional birth attendants — in partnerships with biomedical personnel. An over-emphasis on these two approaches may lead to the marginalisation of other traditional mechanisms for improving well-being, such as the preventative and psychosocial interventions noted above. This, in turn, could alter the nature of traditional health care so that it more closely resembles the biomedical system, with traditional herbal preparations marketed as 'herbal drugs' and practitioners re-branded as paramedical staff — to the possible detriment of consumer satisfaction. To prevent this, there is a fundamental need for interdisciplinary research, involving medical anthropologists as equal partners with clinicians and laboratory scientists.

9.1.2. *The Health Situation in Kenya*

Kenya recognises that good health is a prerequisite for the socio-economic development of the country. As such, the vision for the health sector is to create an enabling environment for the provision of sustainable quality care that is acceptable, affordable and accessible to all Kenyans (CBS, 2003). In order to promote and improve the health status of all Kenyans by making all health services more effective, accessible and affordable (Kimalu, 2002), the country's health policy revolves around two critical issues, namely:

- how to deliver a basic package of quality health services to a growing work force and their dependants; and
- how to finance and manage these services in a way that guarantees their availability, accessibility and affordability to those most in need of them.

To achieve this, the Kenyan Government since independence has initiated or encouraged and supported public-private partnerships in the health sector. This was mostly carried out with the not-for-profit sector (especially mission hospitals) to provide health care to rural area residents in their jurisdiction through subsidies. Further, the Government also utilised the motto of *harambee*[1] to bring together Kenyans of different persuasions to construct and maintain hospitals, especially in the rural areas (GOK, 1983) while the government became responsible for providing medical personnel, supplies and equipment. As a result of this, private sector and NGO contributions in the provision of health services amounted to 42% of the recurrent and development expenditure of the health sector in 1988 (GOK, 1988), with similar levels in most years (Hanson & Berman, 1994).

---

[1] *Harambee* denotes collective effort, cooperative enterprises and all forms of community self-reliance (Mbithi & Rasmusson, 1977: 14).

As a result, Kenya made substantial gains in the health status of its population. By the late 1980s, health and fertility indicators were better than those of most other countries at similar levels of development, as reflected in longer life expectancy and lower infant mortality rates (Tostensen & Scott, 1987). Socioeconomic factors coupled with the rapid expansion of government-financed health and family planning programs during this period played a major role in these advances.

By the early 1990s, however, pressure on the economy caused the government to pursue tight fiscal policies (outlined in the structural adjustment programme adopted during this period). This led to a slowdown in government expenditure (Owino, 1997) in various sectors, including the health sector. A major component of the programme was the removal of government subsidies and the introduction of user fees in public health facilities, among other sectors. The reduction was contrary to intended government spending in the health sector (GOK, 2000: 18) as revealed by the 1997 and 2003 Public Expenditure Reviews (PERs) (GOK, 2004: 64). For example, health care spending as a percentage of the GDP stood at 4.5% in 2004. The PERs also revealed that the available resources are poorly distributed, exemplified by high spending on curative rather than preventative health care, unpredictable funding and often a mismatch between allocations and actual cash releases (GOK, 2004: 64).

Various changes have been proposed to improve health care in the country. These include increasing health care spending to over 10% of the GDP to have the desired effect, implementing a National Social Health Insurance Fund (NHSIF, which is a contentious issue and thus may not be implemented in the near future), considering giving subsidies and tax concessions to investors in the health care system (GOK, 1988), revitalising health care delivery systems in rural and marginalised areas of Kenya, and improving terms of service for medical staff in public hospitals (Gichira, 2004). These form an important backdrop to the development of partnerships for traditional medicine growth.

9.1.3. *Traditional Medicine in Kenya*

Traditional medicine in Kenya encompasses a diverse range of practices, including herbalism and spiritualism. The term 'traditional healers' covers a range of individuals who call themselves diviners, priests, faith healers or bone-setters, among others (Sindiga, 1995a; Hanson & Berman 1994). This is a reflection of the variety of cultures and belief systems in the country, and the equally varied experiences, training and educational backgrounds (UNAIDS, 2000). This diversity is further enhanced by traditional healers adapting to the dramatic social changes that have affected much of the region since colonisation, such as urbanisation, globalisation, population migration and displacement, and civil conflicts (Good, 1987; Sindiga, 1995a).

The Kenya Government has stated its intention to adopt appropriate traditional diagnostic, rehabilitative and therapeutic control technologies (GOK, 1989). As little has been achieved since this proclamation, the World Health Organization (WHO) published a Traditional Medicine Strategy for the period the period 2002–2005 to provide standards by which traditional medicine would be developed (WHO, 2002).

The University of Nairobi will soon offer an undergraduate course in traditional medicine. This is due to the growing interest in traditional medicine, accompanied by interest in funding such studies, and also to reverse the current trend of having studies on traditional medicine being carried out only at graduate level (masters and doctoral). The course is proposed to focus on pharmacognosy (Ithula, 2004b).

Raw botanical materials fetched US$8 billion while natural product extracted pharmaceuticals alone contributed an estimated US$120 billion (or 40% of global pharmaceutical sales) in 1997 (KWG, 2002). Considering that Africa is home to 25% of the world's biodiversity, it is clear that the continent can derive huge benefits from the commercialisation of traditional medicine.

Despite this, the traditional medicine sector has not received much attention. While there is a proposed traditional medicine bill in development in Kenya, there has been some opposition to it by traditional healers due to lack of involvement in formulating it (Ithula, 2004b). This relates to the perception that the Ministry of Health (mainly comprising of physicians, pharmacists, and nurses) makes decisions on their behalf which may lead to the medicalisation of their practice (Bodeker *et al.*, Chapter 1 of this volume). This could potentially result in further marginalisation and a perception that traditional healers are doctors for the poor rather than providers of much needed health care. As such, many biomedical practitioners in the country will not be willing to collaborate with traditional healers.

9.1.4. *Public-Private Partnerships*

Definition:

While various definitions of public-private partnerships exist, for our purposes, PPPs are defined here to refer to the situation where the public sector (federal, tribal, state, and/or local officials and agencies) joins with the private sector (employers, philanthropies, media, civic groups, families, individuals and service providers) in pursuit of a common goal (NCCIC, no date). This includes partnerships between communities, individuals and either private sector organisations or non-governmental organisations, so long as these serve a public need (such as poverty alleviation, development of low cost medicinal products, etc.) and the benefits derived from the relationship accrue to both partners.

Most public-private partnerships aim to promote improvements in financing and provision of services from both the public and private sectors but not to increase the role of one over the other (Wang, 1999). Others have increasingly targeted the improvement of existing services provided by both sectors with an emphasis directed on professional, technical, financial assistance, system efficiency, effectiveness, quality, equity and accountability. As such, three types of partnerships are identified (Walt, 2001):

- *Partnerships for service delivery* initiated to improve services and/or provide alternative sources of health care.
- *Product development partnerships* initiated by the public sector in response to market failure.
- *Systems/issues partnerships* such as the Roll Back Malaria initiative, which involves coordination of different groups.

These variations point to the variety of PPP arrangements in terms of size, form and scope at a global, regional or country level (Nishtar, 2004). Although each public-private partnership is unique in its membership and structure, all share the following characteristics (NCCIC, no date):

- They bring together representatives from the public sector who derive their authority from federal, state, or local governmental entities; and representatives from the private sector (e.g. business, philanthropy, parents, individuals, community organisations) around shared goals.

- Each partner contributes time, money, expertise or other resources to the partnership.
- Partners work together toward common goals or objectives.
- Decision-making and management responsibilities are shared among the partners.

Evolution of Partnerships:

Walt (2001) states that the types of partnerships being pursued have changed over time. For example, in the 1970s there was a stand-off between the public and private sectors which resulted in a separation of their activities. The political climate of the time ruled out any possibilities of partnership and instead there was a feeling of hostility, antagonism and conflict between the two. In the 1980s, the private sector began to expand and gain influence. Public sector institutions began holding discussions with commercial enterprises, though often in secret. Most recently, the 1990s have ushered in an era in which the private sector has grown dramatically. This has encouraged governments and international organisations to work much more closely with industry and civil society in an effort to achieve health goals.

9.2. Public-Private Partnerships for the Development of Traditional Health Care

9.2.1. *Introduction*

A health system is a framework of ideas that have been generated in response to causes of illness and the treatment of these illnesses, as well as cultural aspects underlying a society's response to health needs which form relationships, roles and institutions (Nigenda *et al.*, 2001). Health systems differ from one country to another as they address different health goals that have arisen due to the country's development history.

Health systems have three fundamental objectives, which are to improve the health of the population they serve; respond to people's expectations; and provide financial protection against the costs of ill-health (WHO, 2000). Because these objectives are not always met, public dissatisfaction with the way health services are run or financed is widespread

(WHO, 2000), resulting in patients seeking health care from alternative sources (Sindiga, 1995a). It is for these reasons that the key issues concerning policies to improve the performance of health care systems include health status, raising clinical effectiveness, improving safety or reducing medical errors, raising responsiveness of the system, improving efficiency or containing costs, and equity need to be addressed (Orr, 2002).

In Kenya, there exist two subsectors — Western (biomedicine or allopathic) and African traditional healing systems. Within each subsector, there are a variety of service providers both in the public and private domains. Though these have existed side by side for quite a long period of time, there is little contact between them in spite of various efforts by the government to integrate them (Sindiga, 1995a; Bodeker, 2004). This situation needs to be amended: as the WHO (2000: 9) notes, changes in the way currently available interventions are organised and delivered can reverse the spread of an epidemic and dramatically reduce the cost of saving a life. This can be exemplified by the response to HIV/AIDS epidemic by traditional healers and AIDS patients (Bodeker, 2004; Scheinman, 2002).

As such, though the formal health sector has been reluctant in joining with the traditional medical sector, there exist a number of reports which indicate genuine interest and enthusiasm of traditional healers to collaborate with their biomedical counterparts (Sindiga, 1992; UNAIDS, 2002). These reports indicate that when there is a mutual willingness on the part of traditional healers and conventional health practitioners to collaborate, and when there is a genuine interest in the beliefs and values of traditional healers, as well as a respect for their practices, a bridge can be built between the two complementary health systems (Sindiga, 1992 and 1995a; UNAIDS, 2002). This can be attributed to the realisation that partnerships with traditional healers avail a mechanism to provide effective HIV/AIDS prevention messages and have wider reach than conventional as these healers reside close to their patients. The next section attempts to describe reasons for this.

9.2.2. *Drivers of Public-Private Partnerships*

Public-private collaboration in health care delivery is not new (Hursh-César, 1994). The non-profit mission sector, for example, has existed for many years in developing countries, and has a sound relationship with government. According to Johnson & Collins (1998), there are various reasons for the emergence and growth of PPPs in health care. The first is as a result of the complexity of the health and social problems coupled with increasing pressure on resources. This requires collaboration among organisations from many sectors and at many different levels. For this reason, some 91 international partnership arrangements have been initiated in the health sector to find cures for problems such as malaria, HIV/AIDS and tuberculosis, among others (Nishtar, 2004).

Additionally, despite the worldwide effort to increase access to primary health care for people everywhere, coverage in some developing countries still does not exceed 30% to 40% of the population (Taylor & Blair, 2002). Traditional medicine can supplement government health services by ensuring access to services in areas or for groups that a government is unable to cover adequately, work in partnership with the government and with large employers to provide services in under-utilised facilities and thus ease pressure on public health resources. The private sector can also help by partnering with the traditional medicine sector and government to manufacture and distribute needed medicines, supplies, and equipment.

Finally, partnerships are not only a mechanism for enhancing cooperation and collaboration among the public, NGO, and private business sectors; they are also a way to involve people from the community in the public health issues that affect them.

9.2.3. *Why Pursue Public-Private Partnerships in Traditional Medicine?*

A major reason for the pursuit of PPPs is improved and increased access to alternative sources of financing to fund infrastructure development, improve service delivery as well as managerial capabilities, and increase access to services and facilities. This is based on the idea that the private sector can supplement or complement the services provided by the public sector, especially when there is a need for more options and services that are not provided by governments (Wang, 1999). This is especially true of traditional medicine, which offers a number of advantages for service delivery on public health/government terms. Hursh-César (1994) states that this can be achieved through the following:

Financing

Current levels of health expenditure in many poor countries are far below those needed to provide the bare minimum of services to their populations (WHO, 2004). This is attributed to shrinking budgetary resources, increasing demand for health services, rising health care costs and inequalities in the distribution of the available finances. Further, in a survey of public financing mechanisms for TCAM, it was found that these were present in only 58 of 212 surveyed countries (Burford *et al.*, Chapter 2 of this volume), where a very high proportion of TCAM expenditure is still covered by out-of-pocket payment or private health insurance. In light of this, increasing spending on health to overcome deficiencies of inputs and strengthen management systems (WHO, 2004) may be difficult. In addition, the poor economic performance has resulted in the loss of employment for many people who are further deterred from seeking health care from public health facilities as these facilities have instituted cost recovery measures (user fees). These persons have instead resorted to traditional healers. As such, encouraging the use of alternative delivery systems and health service providers from outside government may help to address deficiencies associated with low levels of financing.

Improving and Increasing Service Delivery

The traditional medicine sub-sector has been offering services in both rural and urban areas where formal health services have been absent (Sindiga, 1995a). This is due to the spatial inequity of public and private health facilities (GOK, 2002: 64, 68; Sindiga, 1995a), poor service delivery (Owino, 1997; Sindiga, 1995b; GOK, 2001a), poor ratio of doctors to patients, and poor access to health care facilities with the exception of Nairobi and Mombasa (GOK, 2002). If provided with additional training, traditional health practitioners can make a significant contribution to organised health care interventions that focus on disease prevention. For example, Green (1995) found that the traditional medical practitioners trained in sexually transmitted diseases had a greater effect on the reduction of STDs than formal health services due to their cultural acceptability.

Drugs

Research has revealed that a major reason for seeking treatment from health facilities is drugs (Owino, 1997). For example, 58% of the rural poor and 56% of the urban do not seek public health care because of the unavailability of drugs (GOK, 2001b: 15). In comparison, traditional healers have almost never lacked medicines to heal their patients. While there may be questions on the preparation, packaging, storage and efficacy of these drugs, it is appreciated that patients seeking treatment from traditional healers do get affordable medicines readily (WHO, 2002: 13).

9.3. Examples of Public-Private Partnerships in Traditional Medicine in Kenya

The reasons for setting up the public-private partnerships described here-after were different (UNAIDS, 2002). In Nairobi, Women Fighting AIDs in Kenya (WOFAK) was set up to address the issue of gender imbalance, as well as the rejection and marginalisation of women infected with HIV, which motivated healers to set up a programme to help infected and affected women cope with their situation with an economically feasible treatment option. The ICIPE-Biop partnership in Kilifi District (Coast province in Kenya) was established to help farmers and communities to improve their economic situation by marketing products derived from the neem tree.

9.3.1. *Women Fighting AIDS in Kenya (WOFAK)*

WOFAK was initiated as an AIDS support organisation by ten infected and affected women in 1993 to bring poor women living with HIV/AIDS together to share experiences and provide mutual support, as well as helping them to access the limited services available (UNAIDS, 2002). WOFAK is registered as an NGO with its head office located in Nairobi's city centre, an outreach office at Homa Bay (Nyanza Province in Kenya) and a drop-in centre at Kayole (a peri-urban residential area located to the east of Nairobi, about 30 km from the city centre). Activities undertaken by the organisation include counselling and psychosocial support for infected and affected children and adults; traditional medicine for the relief of opportunistic infections at its drop-in centre; HIV/AIDS education and awareness to different groups, including youth throughout Kenya; reproductive health services; home-based care; advocacy for the rights of women with HIV/AIDS; training in counselling, education and home-based care for WOFAK members and traditional healers; training in income-generating projects (UNAIDS, 2002).

Following the First International Meeting on Traditional Medicine and AIDS held in Senegal in 1999 and with funds from the Ford Foundation, WOFAK embarked on a new adventure to support the discussion and use of traditional therapies for HIV-associated opportunistic infections. WOFAK's mission with regard to herbal medicine is: *to sustain and promote various forms of traditional medicine and to develop ties with beneficial cultural practices throughout the country.* In relation to this, WOFAK established a working agreement and collaboration with the Kenyan Forestry Research Institute (KEFRI) to grow, process and conduct safety assessment and analyses of some medicinal herbs. Up to date, useful herbal therapies have been identified for herpes zoster, diarrhoea, malaria, skin rash, cough, fever and joint pains (UNAIDS, 2002).

A core outcome of the partnership between WOFAK and KEFRI (UNAIDS, 2002) is the identification of herbal therapies for herpes zoster, diarrhoea, malaria, skin rash, cough, fever and joint pains. This partnership is reinforced by a KEFRI herbalist who serves in the WOFAK drop-in centre twice a week. Additionally, WOFAK facilitates the identification of traditional medicines through training seminars and workshops. During these sessions, members bring samples of plants that they have been using and discuss with biomedical experts the various uses of medicinal plants. They are in turn taught how to properly collect and store them. WOFAK documents the names of the plants and their uses, and helps the KEFRI herbalist to collect and process them. The organisation also provides technical assistance to projects of value to traditional medicine.

This is supported by the development of a databank on Kenyan traditional healers and their areas of expertise by WOFAK as well as training them in HIV/AIDS counselling and education skills (UNAIDS, 2002). In these training sessions, participants were taught their role in AIDS control, traditional medicine in the management of opportunitistic infections, access to treatment for HIV/AIDS, and counselling, among other topics. WOFAK also provides AIDS education (for religious groups, youth groups and other NGOs) and education against harmful traditional practices (such as widow inheritance, early marriage and female genital mutilation).

WOFAK also enables collaboration between biomedical doctors and traditional healers at its drop–in centre at Kayole. In a single structure, WOFAK provides two clinic rooms-one for traditional medicine and another for biomedicine; the main purpose being to encourage cross-referral. The clinic has one community nurse, one traditional healer, one-part-time doctor and two herbal nurses. The nurse or doctor refers to the herbalist and *vice versa*, depending on the condition, the medicine available, or the patients preference. Despite the useful features of this service especially to the poor living in areas with high HIV prevalence, official recognition that will enable collaboration with biomedical practitioners at the national level is yet to occur.

WOFAK recognises that most of its members are poor and has initiated several income generating activities (fruit and vegetable vending, shopkeeping) to help these members acquire some income. The organisation has contracted two herbalists to supply herbal medicine for WOFAK patients. WOFAK members pay a monthly fee which entitles them to free treatment, but non-members pay a small fee.

Other collaborating partners include African Medical Research and Education Foundation (AMREF), traditional healers, Kenya AIDS Society (KAS), Kenya AIDS NGO Consortium (KANCO), Kenya Medical Research Institute (KEMRI), Ministry of Health (MoH), National AIDS Control Council (NACC), Society for Women with AIDS in Kenya (SWAK) as well as individual members of society (UNAIDS, 2002).

9.3.2. *ICIPE-Biop Company Ltd.*

Biop Company Limited was incorporated in Kenya in the late 1990s to commercialise the International Centre of Insect Physiology and Ecology's (ICIPE) research on tropical plants to produce eco-friendly natural products for the agricultural, beauty care and health care markets. Biop's core objective to produce safe and affordable natural products capable of improving human, animal, plant and environmental health by replacing the harmful synthetic products available in the market. The long-term plan of Biop is to create awareness among rural communities on the need to nurture plants that have medicinal value and turn them into cash crops. One such plant is the neem tree that grows abundantly in Lamu and Kilifi (towns long the Kenyan Coast). The plant is reputed to have many human, veterinary and agricultural applications. Some of these include healing fungal infections, treating hypertension and urinary disorders among humans, manage infestations in pets, and controlling agricultural pests (Ithula, 2004a and b).

In order to directly benefit members of the community from which the product originates, Biop Company buys neem tree seeds from cooperatives and women's groups in Lamu, Kilifi and surrounding areas. To increase their earnings, these groups have been encouraged to carry out value adding activities (basic processing of the neem) before selling the product to Biop. Several schools that are carrying out neem tree planting in the area have been turned into small collection points for neem seeds. The effect has been increased incomes for the community, which has in turn resulted in an increase in the number of school going children who would otherwise be engaged in income generating activities. In ecological terms, the region — which is semi-arid — has benefited from the increase in vegetative cover (Ithula, 2004a and b). As a result, many communities in these areas have concentrated their efforts in planting the neem tree.

In keeping with its core objective, Biop initially developed soaps and other skin products made from neem tree extracts, the company also develops herbal tea products made from neem tree leaves. Following clearance by the Kenya Bureau of Standards, the company will also market herbal fertilisers and pesticides in the local and international markets.

Collaborators in this project include ICIPE-Biop, Ministry of Education, Science and Technology (in a proposed development of a Techno-Park), local primary schools and the community (Ithula, 2004a and b).

9.4. Other Relevant East African Case Studies

9.4.1. *The Tanga AIDS Working Group (TAWG), Tanzania*

The Tanga AIDS Working Group (TAWG) was started in 1990 by a German doctor, Dr Elmar Ulrich, who was working at the Government hospital in

Pangani, a coastal town 60 km away from Tanga in Southern Tanzania. He observed that patients delayed reporting to the hospital for treatment and was curious about the reasons behind the delays. He discovered that patients first visited traditional healers, which prompted him to approach the healers. During a workshop, a traditional healer, Waziri Mrisho, an 84-year-old healer, offered to treat a hospitalised AIDS patient with his plant medicines. Although Mrisho explained that his medicines had successfully been used for centuries to treat the symptoms this patient displayed, the hospital staff did not expect to see the patient gain weight and improve after taking Waziri's medicines. The patient surprisingly improved, was discharged from the hospital, and is reportedly alive to date.

From that beginning sprung TAWG (Scheinman, 2002), which was later registered as an NGO in Tanzania in 1994 (UNAIDS, 2002; King, 2000). Through collaborating physicians, TAWG acquired space within the compound of Bombo Hospital, Tanga and has subsidiary offices at Muheza and Pangani (UNAIDS, 2002). Its objectives include providing treatment for people living with HIV/AIDS, minimising the spread of HIV infection in Tanga, and collaborating with traditional healers.

A major outcome of the partnership between traditional healers and biomedical experts through TAWG is increased collaboration between these practitioners (UNAIDS, 2002). Initially, TAWG held a series of sensitisation meetings between Local Government, District Public Health Committees, village health committees, communities and traditional healers to discus how to treat various ailments, when to refer a patient to hospitals, public health issues, and how to cooperate with biomedical personnel (Scheinman, 2002; King, 2000). As a result, traditional healers agreed to have their remedies scientifically examined by scientists at the Lushoto Herbarium located in Lushoto region in Tanzania. The medicines so developed, in the proper form and dosage, have been found to be safe and effective especially if initiated in the early stages of HIV/AIDS (UNAIDS, 2002). For example, the TAWG medicines have been found to increase appetite, help patients gain weight, stop diarrhoea, resolve skin rashes and fungal infections, and treat herpes zoster, among other conditions (Scheinman, 2002).

TAWG also runs seminars for traditional medical practitioners and has an effective education and HIV/AIDS prevention programme (UNAIDS, 2002). For example, since 1994, over 160 traditional healers have been trained in HIV/AIDS and health information (King, 2000). The trained healers have been able to distribute condoms (which they get free from TAWG) and help to identify other traditional healers with useful herbal therapies for HIV/AIDS, besides educating family and community members on HIV/AIDS. Further, health personnel at each health facility in the Tanga region were trained to support the programme, which as only possible due to the close working relationship between TAWG and the Tanzanian Government (King, 2000).

TAWG has also been providing care and treatment for HIV/AIDS patients and their families through its home care service. Activities carried out include monitoring general health, administering traditional medical remedies, and counselling patients and their relatives. Additionally, TAWG provides social support to people living with HIV/AIDS. By 2002, the organisation had approximately 800 HIV/AIDS registered patients (UNAIDS, 2002).

Through its objective of minimising the spread of HIV infection, TAWG established a Community Health Information and Care Centre (CHICC) located in the central business area of Tanga town. The CHICC is staffed by nurses who have additional training as counsellors and community educators. Activities carried out at the centre include HIV testing and counselling; spreading critical information on HIV/AIDS through youth-centred drama and daily video sessions, among other information, education and communication activities; and treatment of sexually transmitted diseases.

At national level, useful developments include the establishment of a Department of Traditional Medicine in the Ministry of Health, which has organised traditional healers at all levels of the district health team. Further, the Institute of Traditional Medicine in Dar es Salaam has established guidelines for collaboration between traditional healers and biomedical practitioners and is now working on a legal framework. In addition, a research network is being established between the National Institute of Medical Research and traditional healer organisations.

Collaborating partners include Ministry of Health (MoH), Bombo Hospital, African Orphans Aid Appeal (AOAA), Afriwag (NGO that helps orphans), Tanga Regional Culture Office Tanga Regional AIDS Coordination Office, and CHAWATIATA (local traditional healer association).

9.4.2. *Traditional and Modern Health Practitioners Together Against AIDS (THETA), Uganda*

THETA was founded to respond to the challenge of providing the health care and prevention challenges caused by HIV/AIDS in 1992 (UNAIDS, 2002). THETA's main goal is to improve and expand access to HIV/AIDS prevention, education and care for disadvantaged populations (such as women and children) through mobilisation and the training of traditional healers in Uganda. THETA's Programmes (currently operational in ten districts in Uganda) include training traditional healers in community mobilisation, prevention education and counselling; AIDS care training for healers; Training of Trainers (TOT) for healers; biomedical health practitioner training to collaborate with traditional healers; information management; herbal processing and packaging; herbal gardening; and clinical and social research on traditional medicine and AIDS.

With the support of the National AIDS Control Programme and the Uganda AIDS Commission, together with The AIDS Support Organisation (TASO) and *Médecins Sans Frontières* (MSF), THETA started two pilot projects in Kampala in 1992 to carry out clinical research on traditional medicine and its effect on AIDS. The outcome of the first project, which aimed at evaluating traditional herbal treatments for some specific AIDS symptoms, demonstrated that herpes zoster and chronic diarrhoea could be successfully alleviated by local herbal preparations. Research work carried out on the effectiveness of THETA's traditional medicines in treating herpes zoster, chronic diarrhoea and weight loss confirmed these findings (Bodeker *et al.*, 2000). In order for these local preparations to be used more widely, THETA piloted a herbal processing and packaging demonstration lab and initiated the growing of useful herbs at a herbal garden near its Kampala offices. This has been further enhanced by THETA's collaboration with the Department of Pharmacology (Makerere University) in the standardisation and packaging of selected herbal treatments.

The second project, which tested the effect of empowering traditional healers as STI/AIDS educators and counsellors through training, showed that traditional healers can be enthusiastic and effective community educators and counsellors for STI/AIDS through their ability to deliver preventive messages in unique ways, such as the use of personal testimonies, stories, song, dance, drama and proverbs. By 2001, nearly 1000 healers had participated in three-day AIDS awareness workshops and approximately

300 traditional healers had gone through an intensive four-year training and certification programme in STI/AIDS counselling and education (UNAIDS, 2002). Post-training initiatives carried out by the traditional healers include training other healers (over 200 have been trained), conducting community AIDS education, condom distribution, carrying out home visits, and individual AIDS counselling and care, especially in disadvantaged and remote areas without access to HIV/AIDS educational activities. Additionally, over 100 biomedical health practitioners have been trained to collaborate with traditional healers.

THETA also established a Resource Centre for Traditional Medicine and AIDS, which facilitates the exchange of information and networking, advocacy and promotions, publications of promotional and educational material and provides library services, both locally and globally.

In recognition of its efforts, THETA was chosen in 2000 as the Regional Secretariat of a Task Force aimed at developing collaboration between the traditional and modern health sectors for HIV/AIDS prevention, care and research for nine countries in Eastern and Southern Africa. A follow on meeting in May 2003 focused on developing minimum standards of practice in TM/HIV/AIDS research and programme implementation. Draft standards were developed in areas such as prevention and care, evaluation of herbal medicine, indigenous knowledge including conservation and propagation, intellectual property rights; and spiritual healing (THETA Uganda, 2003).

Collaborating partners include the National AIDS Control Programme, Uganda AIDS Commission, The AIDS Support Organisation (TASO), Ministry of Health (MoH), National Drug Authority and *Médecins Sans Frontières* (MSF).

9.5. Developing Public-Private Partnerships in Traditional Medicine

9.5.1. *Possible Areas for Development of Partnerships*

Policy

An important area of partnership critical to the development of traditional medicine is policy development. Policymakers' awareness of the importance of traditional medicine can be done if informed through practice, for example by seeing actual ongoing healthy collaboration between biomedical doctors and traditional healers. Collaboration between the two health systems is low in Kenya (Mbindyo, 2001), as in many other countries of East Africa (UNAIDS, 2002). WOFAK, for example, tries to encourage cross-referral through its drop-in centre comprising of a two-roomed clinic where traditional and biomedical practitioners work together.

Participation in national conventions to develop traditional medical policies is also critical. The Kenya Working Group, for example, has drafted a National Strategy and Action Plan for Medicinal and Aromatic Plant Species which is currently under review.

Information, Education and Communication

In a project to test the effect of empowering traditional healers as STI/AIDS educators and counsellors through training, WOFAK found traditional healers to be enthusiastic and effective community educators and counsellors for STI/AIDS through their ability to deliver preventive messages in unique ways, such as the use of personal testimonies, stories, song, dance, drama and proverbs (UNAIDS, 2002). Green (1995) also found this in South Africa, as did THETA in Uganda (UNAIDS, 2002). This needs to be encouraged.

The other area of partnership is training the healers in additional skills such as the identification of traditional medicine and training on how to use them and public health skills to help reduce communicable diseases as well as provide first line treatment where necessary.

Research to Develop Medicines

Various institutions in East Africa have been carrying out research on traditional medicinal plants — such as the Kenya Medical Research Institute (KEMRI) and Kenya Forestry Research Institute (KEFRI) in Kenya, and the Lushoto Herbarium and the Institute of Traditional Medicine in Tanzania, among many others. High collaboration between these players needs to be encouraged to avoid duplication of efforts and spread the research resources to cover more areas.

WOFAK has additionally developed a data bank on Kenyan healers and their areas of expertise, which includes name and full contact address of the healer, a short biography (age, level of education, length of training, etc.), area of operation, area of specialisation and list of herbal remedies used (roots, leaves, herbs, how they are prepared, their dosage and what they treat) (UNAIDS). This is critical in enabling access to the healers besides storing indigenous knowledge. This should be emulated and enhanced.

Infrastructure Utilisation and Development to Increase
Service Delivery

Applying the approach used by TAWG in Tanzania, THETA in Uganda and WOFAK in Kenya, collaboration between legitimate traditional healers and the Government can and should be pursued. This would be helpful in areas where there is poor access to biomedical facilities.

Poverty Reduction

All of the partnerships examined above have a component of income generation for the traditional healer (THETA or WOFAK) and in the case of the ICIPE-Biop project, the whole community. Such an activity coupled with conservation awareness would enable the collection and conservation of traditional medicinal plants having potential income. Those plants having a low potential can be conserved for posterity, as part of larger efforts.

In Kenya, the Forestry Bill 2004 (currently in Parliament for debate) had proposed that each municipal or country council in the country sets aside some 10% of the land available to the authority to create herbariums or arboretums to conserve unique plants in the area. This creates a unique opportunity for communities in such areas to partner with the local authorities to develop projects that can earn income for both parties.

Financing

Public-private partnerships in other sectors of the economy have been found to be useful in meeting the financing gap. The PPPs described in the case studies presented earlier in this chapter were an initiative of individuals or communities that saw a need to address issues which the Government had been constrained to deal with due to various reasons.

With the exception of the ICIPE-Biop example, the PPPs described have not focussed on profit except for the purpose of generating funds to sustain the services provided. Even with the case of the ICIPE-Biop case study, it should be noted that the company was created to market the products developed by the ICIPE researchers for the benefit of the population as well as create a source of supplemental funding. Further, as in the case of WOFAK, a poverty alleviation goal has been pursued as it has been realised that poverty further worsened the health status of its clients (many of whom have HIV/AIDS) as well as placing undue burdens on the rest of family members.

9.5.2. *Benefits of Public-Private Partnerships for Traditional Medical Sector Development*

The most important reason for PPPs in traditional medicine is to improve the capacity of traditional medicine's service delivery to an acceptable standard as outlined in WHO's Traditional Medicine strategy. Such standards can help to instil discipline in the traditional medical sector by rooting out unlicensed practitioners (Mbindyo, 2003) especially if the users of the service know the standards. The pursuit of such partnerships as described in this chapter has led to a better understanding of the role of traditional healers, their cultural practices, development of a number of herbal-based medicinal products and alleviating poverty.

A major reason for pursuing these partnerships is to attract new resources and use them efficiently by focussing attention on neglected health problems such as malaria and tuberculosis, among other diseases; as well as addressing the issues of ethics and corporate responsibility at the international level (Nishtar, 2004). Applying the same thinking to traditional medicine, this would help to focus on the incredible resources available in traditional medicine which are yet to be researched and developed for public use.

In the case of the Biop Company, involving for-profit companies in PPPs has major ramifications relating to intellectual property, benefit sharing and access to knowledge. As a partner or stakeholder in public-private partnerships, the role of the Government might be to provide a measure of public control over the activities of the corporate sector with respect to traditional resource rights. In the case of NGOs and international organisations carrying out research that may lead to inventions that can raise money (e.g. ICIPE), benefit sharing and access to knowledge as well as the products derived from the partnership is critical. This is examined in detail in Chapter 17 of this volume.

As such, involving traditional healers in the national health system, either through integration or collaboration, would increase their incomes as well as their ability to produce better quality drugs while increasing coverage and accessibility to health care (Ithula, 2004a and b). This would help to fill service gaps, raise the profile of traditional medicine and increase access to services for underserved groups. Public-private partnerships can open up substantial opportunities to provide health in a comprehensive manner, enabling joint planning and rational delivery of services (Johnson & Collins, 1998).

9.5.3. *Challenges of Developing and Sustaining Public-Private Partnerships*

Safety

Although traditional health systems are locally accessible and culturally relevant, they must first be rendered safe (Shia, *et al.*, Chapter 4 of this volume). The WHO Traditional Medicines Strategy (2002–2005) outlines four strategies that any country that wishes to enhance traditional medicine should follow — Rational Use; Access; Safety, Efficacy and Quality; and Policy. Within this, poor documentation, a lack of standardisation, and the absence of regulatory mechanisms for traditional health care practice in many countries are impediments to be overcome if traditional medicine is to be more systematically included as a key player in national health systems.

Intellectual Property Rights

Mutual misunderstanding between modern and traditional practitioners due to modern practitioners not accepting traditional healers, among other reasons, has led to poor collaboration between them. Healers' fear that treatment secrets will be stolen, especially in relation to research and intellectual property (Bodeker *et al.*, 2000; UNAIDS, 2002; Sindiga, 1995a) is another point of contention. This may be due to poor past history in ventures involving both, where the traditional healer did not receive any benefits from the research carried out.

Problems in the Perception of Traditional Medical Practice

Traditional medical practice continues to be perceived poorly. This is attributed to weak organisation of healers and sensationalist media reporting (Bodeker *et al.*, 2000). Public-private partnerships may result in loss of identity for some partners, which for traditional healers is a major reason for not agreeing to work with biomedical practitioners (Last & Chavunduka, 1986; Mbindyo, 2003). One partner may feel stifled by another partner's direction of policies, staffing and reporting requirements, and/or close management of activities, and thus be led to believe that the other controls the partnership (Johnson & Collins, 1998). This does not always have to be the case, as shown by the case studies in this chapter (UNAIDS, 2002).

Lack of Political Will

Despite many governments and international agencies calling for 'recognition' of traditional medicine, lack of serious commitment and action on this issue has been seen as a key impediment to identifying effective indigenous approaches and to building strong partnerships for an integrated strategy to the delivery of health services (Sindiga, 1995a; Mbindyo, 2001). As a result, many medicinal plants used daily in Africa that may have potential effectiveness against many diseases remain unknown or uninvestigated, while most Africans with HIV/AIDS, for example, cannot afford modern drugs with proven effectiveness. This may have a serious effect on government credibility to support the development of the traditional medical sector.

9.6. Implications for Policy

From the preceding discussions, it can be seen that PPPs are an important resource and avenue to address the gap between traditional and hospital medicine by providing available, culturally relevant and low-cost treatment (UNAIDS, 2002).

It is important that countries wishing to pursue PPPs with the traditional medical sector develop a legal framework for traditional medicine. Participation by all parties in the development of the legal framework is critical to the acceptance of the policies developed and will ensure adherence.

In the examples of WOFAK and THETA, it is clear that traditional healers can play an important role as information, education and communication (IEC) agents. This is attributed to their knowledge of the traditional and cultural backgrounds of their clients as well as an intimate knowledge of and integration into the communities they serve (Mbiti, 1969; UNAIDS, 2002). This is further exemplified by TAWG, who found that traditional healers tended to form long-term innovative and participatory support groups, which have proven successful in prevention, care and support to HIV-infected and affected people (UNAIDS, 2002). As such, their role as IEC agents cannot be gainsaid.

From the examples given above, traditional healers and biomedical practitioners can collaborate successfully for the benefit of the patient. A combination of the strengths of the two systems by TAWG, for example, has proven to be culturally and economically relevant while enabling it to provide a comprehensive response to AIDS (UNAIDS, 2002). The same can be done for other diseases such as malaria and diarrhoea. In spite of this, it is clear that this is only be possible in situations where the healers are respected as partners in the healing process.

The ICIPE case is of particular interest as it identifies traditional systems of health care as having an important role to play in the prevention of disease, not only in curing. This has been supported by research carried out by ICIPE's Botanicals for Malaria Control programme. The programme takes an integrated approach to malaria prevention, incorporating larvicides, ovicides, mosquitocides, repellents and botanicals for bednet impregnation.

The PPPs created in this way need to be based on local structures that facilitate people's access to health care services. For example, the traditional medicine component given by WOFAK is a valuable addition to the care, support and income generation services of the organisation, which has lead to its clients' empowerment and their ability to care for themselves (UNAIDS, 2002).

It is crucial that healers be encouraged to participate in biomedical research, first as resource persons providing information for the process and as end users of the products developed. This will enable them to provide 'certified drugs' to their clients. Yet, experience has shown that when the healers have given their information, they rarely get to know the results of the research undertaken. Better frameworks to guide research activities should be developed. Additional areas of collaboration include training on skills in the packaging and processing of herbs and methods of increasing the production of medicinal plants for example through the development of traditional medicinal plant nurseries, arboreta or herbaria.

As such, developing a National Resource Centre on traditional medicine which has the ability to organise information exchange through seminars, workshops, publications, networking and appropriate information, educational and communication materials is critical. Such resources do exist, but they are not as yet linked together to form a united front to push the traditional medicine agenda forward. Further, linking this to international efforts in promoting traditional medicine would be invaluable to raising the profile of the sector.

In this process, political goodwill backed by adequate funding would send a clear message of the Government's intentions and pave the way for improving the status of traditional medicine in Kenya and the region.

9.7. Conclusion

The widespread use of traditional medicine in addition to effective collaboration between traditional and biomedical practitioners shows that the practice can help to increase access to medical care, especially in marginalised and disadvantaged areas. The many problems currently besieging formal public health care in Africa only serve to increase the profile of traditional medicine, especially in cases such as AIDS, malaria, diarrhoea and others. Yet, it is recognised that much work needs to be done on the how and why of traditional medicine in terms of diagnostic procedures, treatment processes and drugs.

It is appreciated that this process to improve the profile of traditional medicine will require much broader partnerships than are currently present amongst traditional healers; and between them and the various public-sector organisations interested in these issues. Traditional healers themselves need to be empowered to drive, if not fully participate in, this process. This presents a complex problem that requires a large-scale mobilisation of resources, capacities and skills inherent in national governments, international organisations and civil society organisations to enhance the traditional medicine sector, and thus impact a huge section of the population in Kenya and Africa as a whole.

It is imperative that the public-private partnerships approach be based on an evaluation of basic needs and the opportunity cost of payment strategies, including non-utilisation (Bodeker *et al.*, 2000). Such an approach should be integrated into a more 'political' approach that is interested in the process of impoverishment, and addresses the macro-economic and social causes of poverty and inequity as these are obstacles to quality and accessible health care.

References

Adetokunbo L. *Public-Private Partnerships: Illustrative Examples*. Extracts from a paper presented at a workshop on Public-Private Partnerships in Public Health, Massachusetts, USA, 7–8 April 2000.

Bodeker G. Traditional medicine. In: Cook GC, Zumla AI (eds.) *Manson's Tropical Diseases*, 21st edn. Philadelphia: W.B. Saunders, 2004.

Bodeker G. Lessons on integration from the developing world's experience. *Br Med J* 2000;322:164–167.

Bodeker G, Kabatesi D, King R, Homsy J. A regional task force on traditional medicine and AIDS. *Lancet* 2000;355:1284.

Burford G. *Linking Healthcare and Natural Resource Management: The Ritual of Olpul Among Ilkisongo Maasai in Monduli District, Tanzania*. MSc dissertation, University of Kent, 2002.

Burford G, Rafiki MY, Ole Ngila L. The forest retreat of orpul: a holistic system of health care practised by the Maasai tribe of East Africa. *J Altern Complement Med* 2000;7(5):547–551.

Central Bureau of Statistics. *Kenya Demographic and Health Survey 2003: Preliminary Report*. Nairobi: Government Printer, 2003. Source: www.cbs.go.ke (accessed 18 May 2004).

The Gallmann Memorial Foundation. *Research-Magic Plants (Lelechwa by Africa Botanica)*. Source: http://www.gallmannkenya.org/magicplants.php (accessed 15 December 2004).

Geissler W, Meinert L. *Proceedings of Workshop on People and Medicines in East Africa*, Mbale, Uganda. Denmark: Danish Bilharziasis Laboratory, 2000.

Gerrard MB. Public-private partnerships. *Finance and Development*, Vol. 38, No. 3, September 2001. Source: http://www.imf.org/external/pubs/ft/fandd/2001/09/gerrard.htm (accessed 15 December 2004).

Gichira E. Urgent reforms required to boost public health sector. Health Survey 2004, *The East African Standard*, Wednesday 29 September 2004, Nairobi.

Githae J. Ethnomedical practice in Kenya: the case of Karati Rural Service Centre. In: Sindiga I, Nyaigotti-Chacha C, Kanunah MP (eds.) *Traditional Medicine in Africa*. Nairobi: East African Educational Publishers, 1995, pp. 55–63.

Good CM. *Ethnomedical Systems in Africa*. London: Guilford Press, 1987.

Government of Kenya (GOK). *Public Expenditure Review: Towards Enhancing Efficiency in Public Expenditure Management*. Nairobi: Government Printer, 2004.

Government of Kenya (GOK). *The Economic Recovery Strategy for Wealth and Employment Creation*. Nairobi: Government Printer, 2003.

Government of Kenya (GOK). *Development Plan, 2002–2008*. Nairobi: Government Printer, 2001a.

Government of Kenya (GOK). *Economic Survey, 2001*. Nairobi: Ministry of Finance and Planning 2001b.

Government of Kenya (GOK). *Economic Survey, 2000*. Nairobi: Central Bureau of Statistics, 2000.

Government of Kenya (GOK). *The National Health Sector Strategic Plan*, Health Sector Reform Secretariat. Nairobi: Government Printer, 1999.

Government of Kenya (GOK). *Development Plan, 1989–1993*. Nairobi: Government Printer, 1998.

Government of Kenya (GOK). *The Pharmacy and Poisons Act, Chapter 244 of the Laws of Kenya (Revised Edition)*. Nairobi: Government Printer, 1989.

Government of Kenya (GOK). *Development Plan, 1984–1988*. Nairobi: Government Printer, 1983.

Green EC. *The Participation of African Traditional Healers in AIDS/STD Prevention Programmes*. ADSLINK (a publication of the Global Health Council), No. 36, November/December 1995.

Hanson K, Berman P. *Assessing the Private Sector: Using Non-Government Resources to Strengthen Public Health Goals*. Data for Decision-making Project, Harvard School of Public Health, 1994.

HM Treasury. *Public Private Partnerships: The Government's Approach*, 2000. Source: http://www.hm-treasury.gov.uk/mediastore/otherfiles/PPP2000.pdf (accessed 30 September 2004).

Hursh-César G, Berman P, Hanson K, Rannan-Eliya R, Rittman J, Purdy K. *Summary of Country Studies: Private Providers' Contributions to Public Health in Four African Countries*. Conference — Private and Non-government

Providers, Partners for Public Health in Africa, 28 November–1 December 1994, Nairobi, Kenya.

IFPMA. *Building Healthier Societies Through Partnership*, 2004. Source: http://www.ifpma.org/site_docs/Health/Health_Initiatives_Brochure_May04.pdf (accessed 30 September 2004).

Ithula M. Healing and empowerment: the wonders of the neem tree. Health Survey 2004, *The East African Standard*, Wednesday September 29, Nairobi.

Ithula M. Herbalists Oppose Proposed Bill on Alternative Treatment. Health Survey 2004. *The East African Standard*, Wednesday September 29, Nairobi.

Johnson S, Collins D. Forming partnerships to improve public health. *The Manager*, Vol. 7, No. 4, Management Sciences for Health (MSH). http://erc.msh.org/mainpage.cfm?file=2.2.1b.htm&language=english&module=planning (accessed 30 September 2004).

Kasilo OMJ *et al*. Regional overview: African region. In: Bodeker G, Ong C-K, Grundy C, Burford G, Maehira Y (eds.) *WHO Global Atlas of Traditional, Complementary and Alternative Medicine. Text Volume*. Kobe, Japan: WHO Centre for Health Development, 2005.

Kenya Working Group on Medicinal and Aromatic Plant Species (KWG). *National Strategy and Action Plan for Medicinal and Aromatic Plant Species — 2003–2008*. Kenya Working Group in Medicinal and Aromatic Plant Species, Serindia Agencies, Nairobi, 2002.

Kimalu PK. *Debt Relief and Health Care in Kenya*. Discussion Paper No. 2002/65, Kenya Institute of Public Policy Research and Analysis, Nairobi, 2002.

King R. *Collaboration with Traditional Healers in HIV/AIDS Prevention and Care in Sub-Saharan Africa: A Literature Review*. Joint United Nations Programme on HIV/AIDS (UNAIDS), Geneva, 2000.

Korte R, Heidrichter FM, Gorgen H. *Financing Health Services in Sub-Saharan Africa: Options for Decision Makers During Adjustment*, 1992. Source: http://www.gtz.de/decentralization-health/download/Financing-HS-in-Africa.pdf (accessed 3 November 2004).

Last M, Chavunduka GL (eds.). *The Professionalisation of African Medicine*. Manchester: Manchester University Press, 1986.

Leonard KL. *'Active Patients' in Rural African Health Care Implications for Research and Policy*, 2004. Source: http://www.arec.umd.edu/kleonard/papers/active04.pdf (accessed 2 November 2004).

Leonard KL. *African Healers: Are They as Good at Economics as They are at Medicine?*, 2001. Source: http://www.arec.umd.edu/kleonard/papers/trhl_pd_pr.pdf (accessed 2 November 2004).

Mbindyo PM. *Regulating Traditional Medicine in Kenya: Issues and Options.* Paper prepared for the Second National Congress on Quality Improvements in Health Care, Medical Research and Traditional Medicine, 24–28 November 2003, Nairobi.

Mbindyo PM. *How Does Social Capital Work as Informal Insurance Within Traditional Medicine?* Unpublished MSc. Dissertation, London School of Economics and Political Sciences, 2001.

Mbiti JS. *African Religions and Philosophy*, 2nd edn. Nairobi: Heinemann International, 1969.

Mbithi PM, Rasmusson R. *Self Reliance in Kenya: The Case of Harambee.* Uppsala: The Scandinavian Institute of African Studies, 1977.

McKinsey (2002): *Developing Successful Global Alliances.* Report prepared for the Bill and Melinda Gates Foundation, 2002. http://www.gatesfoundation. org/nr/downloads/globalhealth/GlobalHealthAlliances.pdf (accessed 3 November 2004).

Molvaer RK. *Kibwezi Survey: Report on an Investigation into Health-Related Beliefs and Practices in a Kamba District of Kenya.* Nairobi: African Medical and Research Foundation, 1981.

Muela SH, Mushi AK, Ribera JM. The paradox of the cost and affordability of traditional and government health services in Tanzania. *Health Policy Plan* 2000;15(3):296–302.

Murray A, Duran X. *Factors Shaping Successful Pro-Poor ICT Public Private Partnerships: Inception Phase of a Study in Commonwealth Developing Countries.* Commonwealth Policy Studies Unit, 2002 (http://www.cpsu.org.uk/ downloads/ReportDFID.pdf).

Nigenda G, Mora-Flores G, Aldama-Lopez S, Orozco-Nunez. La Practica de la Medicina Traditional en America Latina y Tolerancia. *Salud Publica Mex* 2001;43:41–51.

Nishtar S. Public-private 'partnerships' in health — a global call to action. *Health Res Policy Syst* 2004;2:5. Source: http://www.health-policy-systems.com/content/2/1/5 (accessed 28 September 2004).

Orr Z. *Improving the Performance of Health Care Systems: From Measures to Action (A Review of Experiences in Four OECD Countries).* Labour Market and Social Policy — Occasional Papers No. 57, Unclassified DEELSA/ELSA/WD (2002), Organisation de Coopération et de Développement Economiques, 2002.

Owino W. *Delivery and Financing of Health Care Services in Kenya: Critical Issues and Research Gaps.* IPAR Discussion Paper Series, DP No. 002/1997, Nairobi, 1997.

PriceWaterhouseCoopers. *Public Private Partnerships: A Clearer View*, 2001. Source: http://www.pwcglobal.com/uk/eng/about/svcs/pfp/pwc_ppp-study.pdf (accessed 30 September 2004).

Private Finance Initiative and Public Private Partnerships: What Future for Public Services? Source: http://www.centre.public.org.uk/publications/briefings/pfi-and-ppp/ (accessed 30 July 2004).

Public-Private Partnership in Health (PPPH): Increasing Private Health Sector Participation in All Aspects of the National Health Programme. http://www.health.go.ug/part_health.htm (accessed 30 July 2004).

Public-Private Partnerships to Promote Essential Health Care http://www.naco.nic.in/nacp/public.html#b1 (accessed 30 July 2004).

Public-Private Partnerships in Public Health, Held on 7–8 April 2000. Co-hosted by the Harvard School of Public Health and the Global Health Council. Source: http://www.hsph.harvard.edu/partnerships/ (accessed 30 July 2004).

Reich MR. Commentary: public-private partnerships for public health. *Nature Med* 2000;6(6):617–620.

Ruster J, Yamamoto C, Rogo K. *Franchising in Health: Emerging Models, Experiences, and Challenges in Primary Care*, 2003. Source: http://rru.worldbank.org/Viewpoint/index.asp (accessed 30 September 2004).

Scheinman D. *Traditional Medicine in Tanga Today: The Ancient and Modern Worlds Meet*. IK Notes No. 51, The World Bank, Washington, 2002.

Schneider P, Diop FP, Bucyana S. *Development and Implementation of Prepayment Schemes in Rwanda*. Technical Report No. 45, Partnerships for Health Reform (PHR) Project, Bethesda, MD, 2000.

Sindiga I. Traditional medicine in Africa: an introduction. In: Sindiga I, Nyaigotti-Chacha C, Kanunah MP (eds.) *Traditional Medicine in Africa*. Nairobi: East Africa Educational Publisher Ltd., 1995a, pp. 1–15.

Sindiga I. African ethnomedicine and other medical systems. In: Sindiga I, Nyaigotti-Chacha C, Kanunah MP (eds.) *Traditional Medicine in Africa*. Nairobi: East Africa Educational Publisher Ltd., 1995b, pp. 16–29.

Sindiga I. *Ethnomedicine and Healthcare in Kenya*. Report to the International Development Research Council, Moi University, Nairobi, 1992.

Taylor R, Blair S. *Public Hospitals: Options for Reform Through Public-Private Partnerships*, 2002. Source: http://rru.worldbank.org/Documents/PublicPolicyJournal/241Taylo-010802.pdf (accessed 12 October 2004).

THETA Uganda. *THETA: Traditional and Modern Health Practitioners Together Against AIDS and Other Diseases*, 2003. Source: http://www. thetauganda.org/ (accessed 5 August 2005).

Tostensen A, Scott JG. *Kenya: Country Study and Norwegian Aid Review. The CHR*. Bergen: Michelsen Institute, 1987.

UNAIDS. *Ancient Remedies, New Disease: Involving Traditional Healers in Increasing Access to AIDS Care and Prevention in East Africa.* Joint United Nations Programme on HIV/AIDS (UNAIDS), Geneva, 2002.

Walt G. Using private money for public health: the growing trend towards partnership. In: *Public-Private 'Partnerships': Addressing Public Health Needs or Corporate Agendas?* Seminar report, HAI Europe, 2001. Source: http://www.haiweb.org/campaign/PPI/seminar200011.html (accessed 12 October 2004).

Wang Y. *Public-Private Partnerships in Health and Education: Conceptual Issues and Options.* Paper prepared for 'Manila Social Policy Forum: The New Social Agenda for the East, Southeast and Central Asia', Joint ADB-World Bank Conference, 9–12 November 1999.

Webb R, Pulle B. *Public Private Partnerships: An Introduction.* Research Paper no. 1 2002–03, Economics, Commerce and Industrial Relations Group, 2002. Source: http://www.aph.gov.au/library/pubs/rp/2002-03/03RP01.htm (accessed 30 September 2004).

What are Public Private Partnerships? Source: http://news.bbc.co.uk/1/hi/uk/1518523.stm (accessed 30 July 2004).

World Health Organization. *The World Health Report 2004 — Changing History.* WHO, Geneva, 2004.

World Health Organization. *WHO Traditional Medicine Strategy* 2002–2005 (draft copy). World Health Organisation, Geneva, 2002. Source: http://www.who.int/medicines/library/trm/trm_strat_eng.pdf (accessed 15 October 2004).

World Health Organization. *The World Health Report 2000 — Health Systems: Improving Performance.* WHO, Geneva, 2000.

PUBLIC HEALTH ISSUES: PRIORITY DISEASES AND HEALTH CONDITIONS

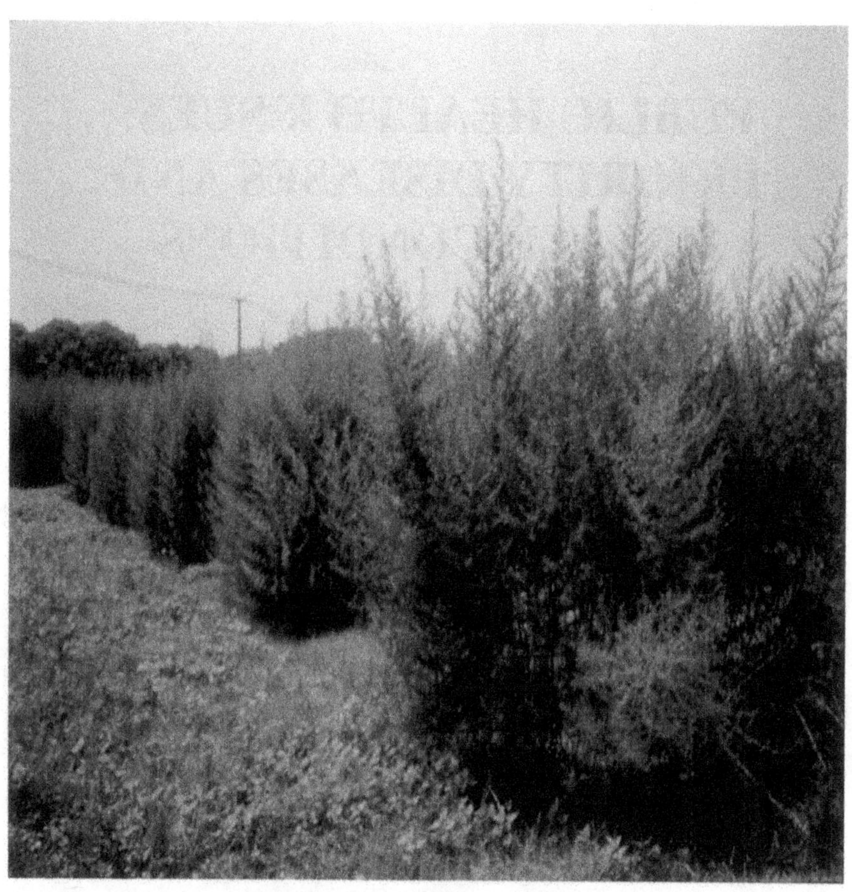

Artemisia annua, the traditional Chinese febrifuge, now the source of the most effective class of anti-malarial drugs. (*Photo courtesy of G. Bodeker.*)

CHAPTER 10

MALARIA

Merlin L. Willcox and Gerard Bodeker

10.1. Introduction: The Importance of Malaria

Although the commonly quoted incidence of malaria infection is around 300 million cases per year, it is estimated that well over two billion febrile episodes resembling malaria occur annually, and a substantial proportion of these are parasitaemic (Breman, 2001); 90% of these cases are in Africa (Breman, 2001). In spite of malaria control programmes and the efforts of 'Roll Back Malaria', the estimated burden of disease due to malaria increased from 39.27 million Disability-Adjusted Life Years (DALYs) in 1999 to 42.28 DALYs in 2001 (WHO, 1999 and 2002). Estimated global malaria mortality increased slightly from 1.110 million in 1998 to 1.124 million in 2001 (WHO, 1999 and 2002). In certain parts of Africa, malaria mortality has increased two- to three-fold since the late 1980s, in tandem with the spread of chloroquine resistance (Trape, 2001). Malaria mortality rates have substantially decreased in most of the world since 1900; but in sub-Saharan Africa, although mortality halved between 1900 and 1970, it has increased again from 107 per 10^5 in 1970 to 165 per 10^5 in 1997 (WHO, 1999). Malaria mortality in under-fives almost doubled in eastern and southern Africa over the period 1990–1998 compared with 1982–1989 (WHO, 2003a). Today, *Plasmodium falciparum* causes more deaths than any other infectious agent in young African children; in Eastern and Southern Africa, it is now responsible for almost 40% of these deaths (WHO, 2003a). Other species of malaria (*P. vivax, P. malariae* and *P. ovale*) hardly ever cause any deaths.

Malaria is not just a disease of poor countries; it is a disease of the poorest people in poor countries, which often strikes at the hardest times (WHO, 2003b); 58% of malaria deaths occur in the poorest 20% of the population (Barat *et al.*, 2004). In India, 60% of cases of falciparum malaria, and 50% of malaria deaths are estimated to occur in 7% of the population, who are tribal people living in remote forested areas (Singh *et al.*, 1998). In Brazil, 99% of malaria cases are transmitted in the Amazon region, where the population consists mainly of tribal people and poor immigrants from other areas (Krettli *et al.*, 2001). Furthermore, malaria often strikes in the season when conditions for the poor are the most difficult. In the highlands of Madagascar, the malaria season occurs just before the rice harvest, when poor farmers have no money left from the previous harvest, and food supplies are at their lowest. In India, hunger leads some tribal people to catch larvivorous fish from pools with high mosquito densities, thus exposing themselves to mosquitoes while killing their natural predators (Singh *et al.*, 1998). For patients from remote areas seeking modern health care facilities, transport is difficult at the best of times; but in the rainy season, when malaria strikes, it can become almost impossible (Reilly *et al.*, 2002).

In these conditions, it is not surprising that under 20% of febrile episodes and deaths due to malaria come to the attention of any formal health system (Breman, 2001). Many of these patients use traditional medicines. At present, an average of 42% of febrile African children under five are treated with an anti-malarial drug, and 80% of these with chloroquine, which has become largely ineffective (WHO, 2003a). Even when anti-malarial drugs are used, the dosage is incorrect in most cases (McCombie, 2002). One of the targets of Roll Back Malaria is that *'60% of those suffering with malaria should have access to and be able to use correct, affordable, and appropriate treatment within 24 hours of the onset of symptoms'* (WHO, 2003b). Even if this very ambitious target is attained, 40% of the population will remain without timely access to effective modern medicines.

Of the currently available anti-malarials, only three cost US$1 per treatment or less (White, 2003), which is the threshold for affordability set by WHO. All of these, chloroquine, amodiaquine and sulphadoxine-pyrimethamine, are fast becoming useless because of drug resistance. The other two, artemisinin and 'lapdap', are not yet widely available. Furthermore, the scientific malaria community is now arguing for the use of artemisinin combinations as first line treatment for malaria, to counteract growing drug resistance (White, 2003). These will cost at least US$1–2 per course.

It has been estimated that an effective global malaria treatment and prevention strategy, including the use of drug combinations where necessary, will cost an extra US$2.5 billion per year (Sachs & Malaney, 2002), whereas international spending on malaria control in 2002 was US$120 million (WHO, 2003b). Provision of artemisinin-based combinations to only the African countries that currently need them would cost an extra US$100–200 million per year (MSF, 2003). Although a Global Fund has been set up to redress these financial deficiencies, in 2002 it only awarded US$14 million to malaria control programmes (Teklehaimanot & Snow, 2002). Its projected malaria spending is US$250 million over the next two years. The total health sector budget for the World Bank, to cover all health programmes in the world, is US$2.4 billion a year, and this is not set to increase (Pannenborg, 2002). It seems that there is a lack of political will to fund the proposed malaria control programmes.

The publication of the genomes of *P. falciparum* and of *An. gambiae* have been hailed as a breakthrough for public health (Morel *et al.*, 2002). Yet the costs of reverse engineering a new drug, vaccine or insecticide from these genomes will be considerable. The cost of the final products is also likely to be considerable, placing them out of the reach of those who most need them. The requirements for registration of traditional herbal medicines are much less extensive than for registration of new chemical entities as drugs, and so new treatments could be developed much more cheaply and quickly. Guidelines have been produced on the requirements for registration of traditional herbal remedies (WHO, 1993 and 1998). Yet traditional medicine, which is one of the only measures available to the poor, is receiving very little attention from the 'big players' in the malaria world. Although further research on herbal anti-malarials was rec-ommended by the International Conference on Malaria in Dakar, Senegal (NIH, 1997; WHO, 1997), there seems to have been very little progress on this front.

History has proven traditional medicine to be the surest source of effective anti-malarials. *Cinchona* and *Artemisia annua* have provided the basis for two of the three main classes of anti-malarials, and there is evidence that many other plants contain useful anti-malarial agents. Herbal remedies have several potential advantages, perhaps most importantly, that they are readily available and affordable. Patients, even in the remotest areas, could be empowered to cultivate, prepare and administer effective herbal anti-malarials, thus freeing them from dependency on unreliable supplies of modern medicine from the outside world.

Traditional medicine is not without its own limitations. Firstly, there is little clinical data on safety and efficacy. Secondly, the concentration of active ingredients in a given plant species varies considerably, depending on a number of factors. Thirdly, there is no consensus, even among traditional healers, on which plants, preparations and dosages are the most effective.

However these limitations are all remediable, through research. Such research is likely to be less costly than sequencing genomes, although it would create more jobs for field workers in malaria-endemic countries than for laboratory scientists in the North. The Research Initiative on Traditional Antimalarial Methods (RITAM) was formed in 1999 by the Global Initiative For Traditional Systems (GIFTS) of Health at Oxford University, with the aims of promoting and facilitating such research (Bodeker & Willcox, 2000). It now has over 200 members from 30 countries, many of whom have helped to produce systematic reviews and guidelines (Willcox *et al.*, 2004b).

10.2. TCAM and Malaria: Current State of Knowledge

10.2.1. *Treatment*

A systematic review of the literature has revealed that over 1200 plant species are used worldwide for the treatment of malaria or fever. Of these, 11 species are used on all three tropical continents, 47 are used in two continents, and 106 are used in more than one country, within the same continent (Willcox & Bodeker, 2004a).

Few of these plant species have been evaluated clinically for their safety and efficacy. A systematic literature review found only ten controlled clinical trials, 34 cohort studies (17 on falciparum malaria), and 18 case studies. Many of these studies enrolled small numbers of patients, and had methodological problems.

None of these studies reported serious side effects. However, minor side-effects can be important. For example, almost half of the patients taking the herbal remedy 'AM' experienced one or more side-effects (Willcox, 1999). In about 8% of cases, these were unpleasant enough to cause patients to stop taking the treatment. Some herbal anti-malarials have a bitter taste, which can make them difficult to administer to children. Doses often need to be taken more frequently, and the volume to ingest is often larger than with conventional drugs.

Of the 17 cohort studies on falciparum malaria, six reported 100% parasite clearance on days 4–7, and a further three reported parasite clearance rates above 90%. However, follow-up data beyond day 7 is only available for two of these nine studies, and only five of them included more than 40 patients (Willcox & Bodeker, 2004b). One problem with cohort studies is that the population chosen may be semi-immune to malaria, and may clear parasites and symptoms even without effective treatment. Therefore high parasite clearance rates are not necessarily indicative of efficacy. In highly endemic areas (as in much of sub-saharan Africa), children are considered to have a good immune response to malaria above the age of five. In areas with high transmission of malaria, achieving complete parasite clearance for any length of time may not be realistic. In these circumstances, WHO recommends that Adequate Clinical Response (ACR) is a more useful measure of treatment efficacy. ACR is defined as absence of parasitaemia on day 14, or absence of fever (regardless of parasitaemia), without previously meeting the criteria for an 'early treatment failure'. Some remedies produce low rates of parasite clearance, but higher rates of ACR.

Of the controlled trials for falciparum malaria, the most promising is that of *Cryptolepis sanguinolenta*, in which parasite clearance took only one day longer than with chloroquine, and in which fever clearance was 12 hours faster (Boye, 1989). However, the number of patients was small, and a larger trial is needed to confirm these results. Also of interest is the trial of *Artemisia annua* infusions compared to quinine (Mueller *et al.*, 2004). The parasite clearance was good at day 7. However, a significant proportion of patients experienced a recrudescence, so that by day 28 only 37% of patients treated with *Artemisia annua* were still free of parasites (compared to 86% in the quinine group). Unfortunately rates of ACR were not reported in this trial.

10.2.2. *Prevention*

Traditional medicine can be used to prevent malaria in a number of ways. First, a herbal medicine may be administered prophylactically on a regular basis. Second, plants with anti-malarial properties may be incorporated in the diet. Third, some plants are used as insect repellents, and fourth, others are used as insecticides.

Fewer studies report use of medicinal plants for the prevention than for treatment of malaria (Willcox & Bodeker, 2004a). However, the dichotomy between curative and preventive medicine is a biomedical concept, which is not ubiquitous among populations at risk of malaria. The Luo of Kenya believe that illness is always present in the body and must be controlled continuously (Geissler *et al.*, 2001). They do not view this as prevention. Food may also function as a prophylactic. The Mende of Sierra Leone increase their consumption of hot peppers in food during the cold season, and these are believed to combat fevers (Bledsoe & Goubaud, 1985). Etkin & Ross (1991) found that many food plants ingested during the malaria season in Nigeria had anti-malarial properties, although they were not consciously being used as prophylactics.

Herbal insect repellents are used in some areas. In one survey in Sudan, about 70% of women used smoke to repel mosquitoes, and about 75% used vegetable oils applied on the skin (A/Rahman *et al.*, 1995). Smoke is the most widely used means of repelling mosquitoes in the tropics, be it from special plants, or from cow dung. There have been few studies to measure whether the use of smoke actually prevents malaria. Snow *et al.* (1987) showed that 'churai' (*Daniellia oliveri*) smoke used as a repellent in the Gambia did not significantly reduce the incidence of malaria in children. However, a study in Sri Lanka found that the use of traditional fumigants did protect against malaria (van der Hoek *et al.*, 1998). The difference in the results of the two studies may be related to erratic use of churai in the Gambia. It is also very likely that the massive entomological inoculation rate (EIR) in the Gambia requires more effective means of personal protection from infected bites than offered by the churai. In Sri Lanka the lower EIR and less anthropophilic vector mosquito, *An. culicifaces*, may mean that burning local plant repellents are a viable means of malaria prevention. In Sri Lanka, Holy Basil (*Ocimum sanctum*), 'tulsi' (Sanskrit name) is commonly burned, as are the seed husks from oil extraction from neem (*Azadirachta indica*) and the butter nut tree (*Madhuca longifolia*) (Silva, 1991). These seeds contain insecticidal and repellent agents.

Traditional use of plants as insecticides is rare, but several plants have interesting insecticidal properties which could be used in vector control programmes. Larvicidal activity is the most widely investigated property of mosquitocidal plants. The third or fourth instar larvae are used. According to Napralert citations from 1941 to 2001, 120 medicinal plants representing 102 genera in 52 families have been tested against *Anopheles*, *Culex* and *Aedes* mosquitoes; 87% of the 162 plant extracts screened for mosquitocidal activities were reported to be active as larvicides (Gbolade, 2004).

10.3. Traditional, Complementary and/or Alternative Medicine (TCAM) in Malaria Control Programmes

10.3.1. *Cinchona: A Historical Perspective*

Cinchona bark, the source of quinine, was the first and longest-lasting anti-malarial to be used on a large scale in 'public health' programmes. As early as 1649, Cardinal de Lugo recommended that 'Jesuit's bark' be distributed to the poor and to missions throughout Europe (Honigsbaum & Willcox, 2004). Its use continued well into the 20th century, when the British disseminated its use in India, and the League of Nations conducted large trials of crude bark extracts (Pampana, 1934). Plantations of *Cinchona* still exist in many tropical countries, and could be used as a source of bark for local malaria control programmes.

10.3.2. *Ayush-64 in India*

Widespread resurgence of malaria in India during 1970s prompted the Central Council for Research in Ayurveda and Siddha (CCRAS) to develop an Ayurvedic remedy for malaria. In 1980 scientists of CCRAS selected four plants used in the treatment of fever including malaria, and prepared a formulation named 'Ayush-64'. CCRAS further developed the drug in collaboration with 20 laboratories in India, and patented Ayush-64 as a new anti-malarial herbal compound. So, it is not really an Ayurvedic treatment for malaria. Rather, it is a phytomedicine produced by scientists based on ethnobotanical leads. The drug was subsequently licensed for production and clinical trials. CCRAS has been producing Ayush-64 in their pilot plant for clinical trials and limited distribution. Twenty-two pharmaceutical companies had purchased the know-how from CCRAS, and at least seven of these are currently manufacturing Ayush-64. The drug is marketed throughout India by the private sector, and dispensed by the central and state governments in the treatment of malaria (Sharma, 2004).

Ayush-64 is marketed in a manner similar to modern medicine and therefore suffers from the disadvantage of distribution at the periphery. The drug is also not cheap compared to chloroquine, as the treatment cost of an adult with both the treatments is Rs.10–15 (=US$0.25–0.30) per case. Ayush-64 has relatively weak anti-malarial activity. All the controlled trials have been conducted in patients with *P. vivax* malaria. The parasite clearance rate is 50%–95% with 17% recrudescence; Ayush-64 has not been tested for its action on the hypnozoites. Ayush-64 was used on a large scale in malaria epidemics in 1994 and 1996 in Rajasthan and Assam, for 3600 and over 2200 fever cases, respectively. It was reported to be effective although there was no formal follow-up of the patients (Bhatia, 1997).

10.3.3. *Traditional Medicine Development in Mali*

Mali is one of the few African countries that has a national policy promoting traditional medicine, and whose National Formulary includes 'improved traditional medicines' (Ministère de la Santé, 1998). One of these is 'Malarial', a formula comprising three different anti-malarial herbs, based on a traditional recipe: leaves of *Cassia occidentalis* L. (Caesalpinaceae), leaves of *Lippia chevalieri* Mold. (Verbenaceae), flowerheads of *Spilanthes oleracea* L. (Asteraceae).

This underwent a series of randomised controlled clinical trials before being marketed. The trials showed that Malarial led to clinical improvement in most cases, although not parasite clearance, and was less effective than chloroquine (Diallo *et al.*, 2004). However, the studies were conducted before the emergence of significant chloroquine resistance in Mali.

The Department of Traditional Medicine, which is part of the Malian Ministry of Health, is continuing research to develop more effective herbal anti-malarials, based on traditional knowledge. The aim is to produce more effective standardised traditional anti-malarials, and also to disseminate knowledge to villagers about plants they can cultivate and prepare themselves, if they have no access to health care.

10.3.4. *Artemisia annua: The New Cinchona?*

Artemisia annua L (Asteraceae) is a herbaceous plant used in China for the treatment of fevers for at least 2000 years. Recent research in China led to the isolation of the most potent active ingredient, artemisinin. This is one of the most potent anti-malarials ever discovered, and its derivatives have been developed into modern pharmaceuticals, which are now used for the treatment of malaria, where they are available. *A. annua* is now widely cultivated, principally for the extraction of artemisinin.

However, interest is growing in the use of the herbal preparation of *A. annua*, which would be easier to grow and prepare locally in areas with no access to modern medicine. ANAMED (Action for Nature and MEDicine) is an NGO promoting the use of traditional medicines (www.anamed.org). It distributes seeds of a recently developed artemisinin-rich genotype of *Artemisia annua* (Delabays, 1997; De Magalhães, 1996) for cultivation and preparation as a herbal anti-malarial. Over 240 partner organisations in developing countries are participating in this programme, and their feedback has helped the organisation to refine its recommendations.

Mueller *et al.* (2000) showed that local cultivation and preparation of *A. annua* are feasible in Africa, and that the traditional preparation is effective for the treatment of malaria in semi-immune patients. If effectiveness in non-immune patients is demonstrated, local cultivation and preparation of *A. annua* could be considered as part of a malaria control strategy, especially in remote areas with poor access to health facilities, and poor availability of effective anti-malarial drugs. Such remote areas (such as the Brazilian Amazon, and remote rural areas of Africa) are particularly problematic for malaria control programmes, and are often neglected. Herbal medicines may not be as perfect as the exact dosages administered in industrially produced formulations, but may be better than no treatment, or treatment with fake artesunate tablets, which are widespread in southeast Asia. If there are no effective local treatments for malaria, early treatment with a herbal preparation of *A. annua* may in some circumstances prove to be life-saving.

One of the principal concerns regarding the use of herbal *Artemisia annua* for malaria is that the ingestion of low doses of artemisinin may accelerate the development of resistance to this drug. There is little evidence to support or refute this claim, and further research is needed. It could be argued that some degree of resistance to artemisinin has already evolved in China. Chinese strains of *P. falciparum* are much less sensitive to artemisinin than African strains. This could be explained by the long-standing local use of *Artemisia annua*, or of artemisinin itself over the last 30 years (Wernsdorfer, 1999). The parasites would find it easier to develop resistance to a single agent than to a battery of anti-malarial compounds such as those contained in whole plant extracts.

Indeed, the traditional preparation of the herb is more effective than would be expected from its low artemisinin content, because other compounds in the plant enhance the efficacy of artemisinin. Furthermore, studies in China have shown that the recrudescence rate can be reduced by combining *Artemisia annua* with the roots of two other plants, *Astragalus membranaceus* (Leguminosae) and *Codonopsis pilosa* (Campanulaceae) (Chang & But, 1986).

On balance, the potential benefits of local *A. annua* cultivation and preparation in poor areas with no other anti-malarial treatments may outweigh the risks of such a programme; therefore some NGOs are already promoting this. However, others argue that it is premature to promote the use of Herba *Artemisia annua* until there is better data on its safety and efficacy. Furthermore, research is needed on the optimal preparation, dose, and length of treatment, and on the best variety to cultivate (Willcox *et al.*, 2004a).

10.3.5. *Traditional Healers and Malaria Control*

In most African countries, traditional healers are the most numerous *de facto* providers of primary health care. Although patients often self-medicate with local plants for uncomplicated malaria, traditional healers are usually the first port of call for severe malaria. It has been assumed that traditional practices are universally harmful in severe malaria. However recent research in Mali has demonstrated that collaboration between modern health services and traditional healers can dramatically improve prompt attendance at modern health facilities, and reduce mortality.

Most national malaria control programmes (and public health programmes) overlook or even denigrate traditional healers. Yet constructive collaboration can yield real benefits for all concerned.

10.4. The Way Forward: Goals and Hurdles

10.4.1. *How Much Research is Needed?*

There is constant debate as to the level of evidence required before a herbal remedy can be recommended or used officially. It has been proposed that good results from a cohort study can justify use at a local level, whereas a randomised trial would be needed to justify recommendation of a herbal remedy on a larger scale (Willcox & Olanrewaju, 2004). Of course this will vary according to national regulations and legislation.

10.4.2. *Clinical Cure or Parasite Clearance?*

There is also debate as to whether the therapeutic goal should be parasite eradication or clinical cure. In patients with no or low immunity, parasite clearance is undoubtedly necessary, but in patients in endemic areas, with well-developed immunity, clinical cure is sufficient. Even if parasite clearance is achieved, re-infection will soon occur. The majority of the population in endemic areas harbour parasites with no clinical symptoms.

10.4.3. *Public Health Niches for TCAM in Malaria Control*

There are clear niches for traditional medicine in malaria control programmes. Firstly, traditional medicines are often the only option in remote rural areas, with no modern health facilities. In these areas, malaria management could be improved by evaluating local remedies, to find the safest and most effective preparation and dosage. Secondly, traditional medicines may prove more cost-effective than modern medicines (especially as more expensive medicines are now being used because of chloroquine resistance) for the management of presumed uncomplicated malaria in older children and adults, in endemic areas. These patients have well developed immunity, and therefore total parasite clearance is not necessary. Treating these patients with effective traditional remedies would free up resources for other important aspects of malaria control, such as providing free treatment for severe malaria. Thirdly, collaboration with traditional healers can help to reduce fatality rates from severe malaria. As up to 75% of patients with malaria opt to use traditional medicine, malaria control programmes ignore it at their peril.

References

A/Rahman SH, Mohamedani AA, Mirgani EM, Ibrahim AM. Gender aspects and women's participation in the control and management of malaria in Central Sudan. *Soc Sci Med* 1995;42(10):1433–1446.

Barat LM, Palmer N, Basu S, Worrall E, Hanson K, Mills A. Do malaria control interventions reach the poor? A view through the equity lens. *Am J Trop Med Hyg* 2004;71(Suppl 2):174–178.

Bhatia D. Role of Ayush-64 in malaria epidemic. *J Res Ayurveda Siddha* 1997;XVIII(1–2):71–76.

Bledsoe CH, Goubaud MF. The re-interpretation of Western pharmaceuticals among the Mende of Sierra Leone. *Soc Sci Med* 1985;21(3):275–282.

Bodeker G, Willcox ML. Conference report: the first international meeting of the research initiative on traditional antimalarial methods (RITAM). *J Altern Complement Med* 2000;6(2):195–207.

Boye GL. Studies on the antimalarial action of *Cryptolepis sanguinolenta* extract. In: *Proceedings of International Symposium on East-West Medicine*. Seoul, Korea, 1989, pp. 242–251.

Breman JG. The ears of the hippopotamus: manifestations, determinants, and estimates of the malaria burden. *Am J Trop Med Hyg* 2001;64(Suppl 1,2): 1–11.

CCRAS. *Ayush-64: A New Antimalarial Herbal Compound*. Delhi: CCRAS, 1987.

Chang HM, But PPH. *Pharmacology and Applications of Chinese Materia Medica*, Vol. 1. Singapore: World Scientific Publishing, 1986.

Delabays N. *Biologie de la Reproduction Chez l' Artemisia annua L. et Génétique de la Production en Artémisinine*. Thèse de Doctorat, Faculté des Sciences, Université de Lausanne, 1997.

De Magalhães PM. *Seleção, Melhoramento e Nutrição de Artemisia annua L. Para Cultivo em Região Inter Tropical*. PhD thesis, UNICAMP-IB., Campinas-SP, Brazil, 1996.

Diallo D *et al.* 'Malarial-5': development of a traditional herbal antimalarial in Mali. In: Willcox ML, Bodeker G, Rasoanaivo P (eds.) *Traditional Medicinal Plants and Malaria*. Boca Raton: CRC Press, 2004, 117–130.

Etkin NL, Ross PJ. Recasting malaria, medicine and meals: a perspective on disease adaptation. In: Romanucci-Ross L, Moerman DE, Tancredi LR (eds.) *The Anthropology of Medicine*, 2nd edn. New York: Bergin & Garvey, 1991.

Gbolade A. An overview of plants used for malaria vector control. In: Willcox ML, Bodeker G, Rasoanaivo P (eds.) *Traditional Medicinal Plants and Malaria*. Boca Raton: CRC Press, 2004, 375–388.

Geissler PW, Meinert L, Prince R *et al.* Self-treatment by Kenyan and Ugandan schoolchildren and the need for school-based education. *Health Policy Plan* 2001;16(4):362–371.

Honigsbaum M, Willcox ML. Cinchona. In: Willcox ML, Bodeker G, Rasoanaivo P (eds.) *Traditional Medicinal Plants and Malaria*. Boca Raton: CRC Press, 2004, pp. 21–42.

Krettli AU, Andrade-Neto VF, Brandão MGL, Ferrari WMS. The search for new antimalarial drugs from plants to treat fever and malaria or plants randomly selected: a review. *Mem Inst Oswaldo Cruz* 2001;96(8):1033–1042.

McCombie SC. Self-treatment for malaria: the evidence and methodological issues. *Health Policy Plan* 2002;17(4):333–344.

Ministère de la Santé, des Personnes Agées et de la Solidarité. *Formulaire Thérapeutique National*. Bamako: Editions Donnaya, 1998.

Morel CM, Touré YT, Dobrokhotov B, Oduola AMJ. The mosquito genome — a breakthrough for public health. *Science* 2002;298:79.

MSF. *Act Now to Get Malaria Treatment That Works to Africa*. Geneva: MSF Access to Essential Medicines Campaign, 2003.

Mueller MS, Karhagomba IB, Hirt HM, Wernakor E, Li SM, Heide L. The potential of *Artemisia annua* L. as a locally produced remedy for malaria in the tropics: agricultural, chemical and clinical aspects. *J Ethnopharmacol* 2000;73: 487–493.

Mueller MS, Runyambo N, Wagner I, Borrmann S, Dietz K, Heide L. Randomized controlled trial of a traditional preparation of *Artemisia annua* L. (Annual Wormwood) in the treatment of malaria. *Trans R Soc Trop Med Hyg* 2004;98(5):318–321.

Pampana EJ. Clinical tests carries out under the auspices of the Malaria Commission. *League of Nations Q Bull Health Org* 1934;III:328–343.

Pannenborg O. *Round Table Discussion on Combination Therapy, 3rd MIM Pan-African Malaria Conference*. Arusha, Tanzania, 17–22 November 2002.

Reilly B, Abeyasinghe R, Pakianathar MV. Barriers to prompt and effective treatment of malaria in northern Sri Lanka. *Trop Med Int Health* 2002;7(9): 744–749.

RBM. *Reducing Malaria's Impact on Child Health, Development and Survival* (WHO/CDS/RBM/2002.38), 2002.

Sachs J, Malaney P. The economic and social burden of malaria. *Nature* 2002;415:680–685.

Sharma VP. Ayush-64. In: Willcox ML, Bodeker G, Rasoanaivo P (eds.) *Traditional Medicinal Plants and Malaria*. Boca Raton: CRC Press, 2004.

Silva KT. Ayurveda, malaria and the indigenous herbal tradition in Sri Lanka. *Soc Sci Med* 1991;33(2):153–160.

Singh N, Singh MP, Saxena A, Sharma VP, Kalra NL. Knowledge, attitude, beliefs and practices (KABP) study related to malaria and intervention strategies in ethnic tribals of Mandla (Madhya Pradesh). *Curr Sci* 1998;75(12):1386–1390.

Snow RW, Bradley AK, Hayes R, Byass P, Greenwood BM. Does woodsmoke protect against malaria? *Ann Trop Med Parasitol* 1987;81(4):449–451.

Teklehaimanot A, Snow RW. Will the Global Fund help roll back malaria in Africa? *Lancet* 2002;360:888–889.

Trape JF. The Public Health impact of chloroquine resistance in Africa. *Am J Trop Med Hyg* 2001;64(Suppl 1,2):12–17.

Van der Hoek W, Konradsen F, Dijkstra DS, Amerasinghe PH, Amerasinghe FP. Risk factors for malaria: a microepidemiological study in a village in Sri Lanka. *Trans R Soc Trop Med Hyg* 1998;92(3):265–269.

Wernsdorfer WH. The place of Riamet® in dealing with drug-resistant falciparum malaria. In: *Novartis Satellite Symposium, 9th June 1999: Controlling Malaria in Non-immune Travellers: Riamet (Artemether and Lumefantrine) as Standby Emergency Treatment*. Basel: Novartis Pharma AG, 1999.

White NJ. Malaria. In: Cook GC, Zumla A. (eds.) *Manson's Tropical Diseases*. London: Elsevier Science, 2003.

WHO. *Research Guidelines for Evaluating the Safety and Efficacy of Herbal Medicines*. Manila: WHO Regional Office for the Western Pacific, 1993.

WHO. *Guidelines for the Appropriate Use of Herbal Medicines*. Western Pacific Series No. 23, WHO Regional Publications. Manila: WHO Regional Office for the Western Pacific, 1998.

WHO. *The World Health Report 1999*. Geneva: WHO, 1999.

WHO. *The World Health Report 2002*. Geneva: WHO, 2002.

WHO. *The Africa Malaria Report 2003*. Geneva: WHO/UNICEF, 2003a. WHO/CDS/MAL/2003.1093 (http://mosquito.who.int).

WHO. *Assessment and Monitoring of Antimalarial Drug Efficacy for the Treatment of Uncomplicated Falciparum Malaria*. WHO/HTM/RBM/2003.50. Geneva: World Health Organization, 2003b.

Willcox ML. A clinical trial of 'AM', a Ugandan herbal remedy for malaria. *J Public Health Med* 1999;21(3):318–324.

Willcox ML, Bodeker G. Frequency of use of traditional herbal medicines for the treatment and prevention of malaria. In: Willcox ML, Bodeker G, Rasoanaivo P (eds.) *Traditional Medicinal Plants and Malaria*. Boca Raton: CRC Press, 2004a.

Willcox ML, Bodeker G. Traditional herbal medicines for malaria. *Br Med J* 2004b;329: 1156–1159.

Willcox ML, Bodeker G, Bourdy G *et al. Artemisia annua*. In: Willcox ML, Bodeker G, Rasoanaivo P (eds.) *Traditional Medicinal Plants and Malaria*. Boca Raton: CRC Press, 2004a.

Willcox ML, Bodeker G, Rasoanaivo P. *Traditional Medicinal Plants and Malaria*. Boca Raton: CRC Press, 2004b.

Willcox ML, Olanrewaju I. Guidelines for clinical trials on herbal antimalarials. In: Willcox ML, Bodeker G, Rasoanaivo P (eds.) *Traditional Medicinal Plants and Malaria*. Boca Raton: CRC Press, 2004.

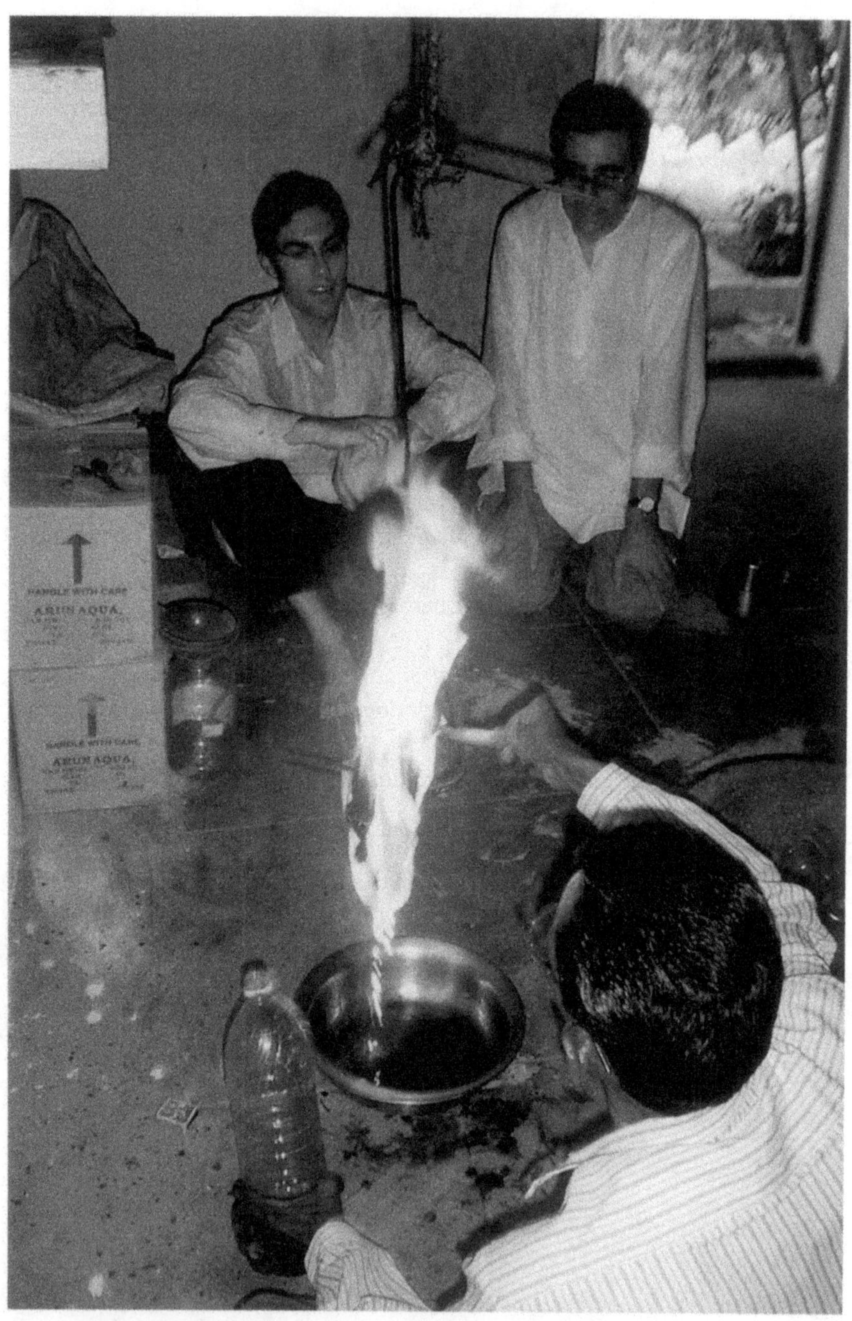

Herbal oil being prepared in a Siddha medicine clinic in Tamil Nadu, India for HIV-related skin conditions. (*Photo courtesy of G. Bodeker and Z. M. Oo.*)

CHAPTER 11

HIV/AIDS: TRADITIONAL SYSTEMS OF HEALTH CARE IN THE MANAGEMENT OF A GLOBAL EPIDEMIC[1]

Gerard Bodeker, Gemma Burford, Mark Dvorak-Little
and George Carter

11.1. Introduction

As the AIDS crisis leads an increasing number of countries to question their priorities in health expenditures, there is an emerging awareness that traditional health care systems can play an important role. The high cost and unavailability of anti-HIV drugs to people living with HIV/AIDS (PLWHA) in the developing world leads many to turn to traditional medicine to manage HIV-related illness. In addition to their high cost, antiretroviral drugs (ARVs) require the support of expensive medical infrastructure not available in many developing countries, and rarely available in rural areas of any developing country. ARVs can also produce significant side-effects, while sometimes being ineffective (NACO, 2002: 29). Adverse effects can

---

[1] This chapter builds on work originally published as: Bodeker G, Dvorak-Little M, Carter G, Burford G. HIV/AIDS: Traditional systems of health care in the management of a global epidemic. *J Altern Complement Med* 2006;12:6.

255

include heart attack, adult diabetes, death of the bone without infection and other serious conditions (Barnett & Whiteside, 2002: 342).

Given the challenges of developing a cost-effective treatment and prevention programme, UNAIDS and WHO have recommended that developing countries harness the potential contribution of local resources and knowledge — specifically, traditional medicine (TRM)[2] and its practitioners. Given that TRM is low cost, widely available (particularly in rural areas) and culturally familiar, WHO has long considered TRM an 'appropriate technology' for developing countries.

UNAIDS (2002) has observed that the TRM establishment is able to offer affordable and effective treatments — especially for opportunistic infections (OIs) and sexually transmitted diseases (STDs) — and has noted the facility with which Traditional Health Practitioners (THPs) serve as effective agents in the dissemination of prevention and education messages.

In this chapter we will consider the potential for partnerships between traditional and modern health care approaches in combating HIV/AIDS and address some of the accompanying socio-cultural, public health and biomedical research issues of significance.

11.1.1. *Widespread Use of TCAM by PLWHA*

In the United States, exceptionally high levels of use of TCAM are reported among PLWHA (Sparber & Wootton, 2000). Studies in Australia have found that more than half of those using ARVs are also using TCAM, and that reported benefits include reduced pain, weight gain and symptomatic relief from a range of HIV-related conditions. More than three-quarters of Australian PLWHA surveyed consider that complementary therapies can improve general well-being, while 41% of respondents stated that TCAM therapies were 'a central part of their HIV treatment' (La Trobe University, 1998).

In South Africa and India, the countries with the highest numbers of people with HIV, the World Health Organization estimates that at least two-thirds or more of the population of these countries rely on traditional medicine for their every day health care needs (Kasilo *et al.*, 2005;

---

[2]The abbreviation 'TRM' is used throughout much of the WHO literature and is followed in this chapter.

Lavekar & Sharma, 2005). By extrapolation, there is likely to be high use of traditional medicine for HIV-related illness among PLWHA.

11.1.2. *TCAM Practitioners in HIV Public Health Education*

Studies consistently show that there are far higher numbers of traditional health practitioners in developing countries than there are modern medical doctors or allied health professionals. Experience has shown that a significant majority are motivated to learn more about HIV, how to recognise it and how best to advise their patients. Traditional health practitioners are often excellent community educators — making important contributions to ongoing HIV/AIDS prevention programmes, increasing condom use, and helping to eliminate risky behaviours. Their high level of community acceptance and respect makes them ideal for such a role. The chapter reports on training efforts in Africa that have resulted in significant outreach with HIV prevention messages through training programmes for THPs. In Asia, such partnerships have yet to begin on any significant level, but offer the same promise of on-the-ground community education for HIV prevention, management and reduction of stigma, that has begun in Africa.

11.1.3. *Herbal Medicines for Managing HIV-Related Illness*

In vitro studies on the antiretroviral and immunostimulant/immuno-modulatory properties of medicinal plant extracts have shown promising initial results, as have preliminary open-label clinical trials of traditional medicines in both Africa and Asia. In India, the findings of nationally-funded research to evaluate the potential of the Siddha medical system in offering a low-cost alternative to HAART have been described by some as 'encouraging', but fiercely contested by others, within a broader political debate about the meaning of such terms as 'evidence' and 'efficacy' in traditional medicine research (Section 11.3). The challenge that remains is to develop methodologically sound clinical trials, which remain faithful to the principles of the respective traditional health care systems while still maintaining 'gold standard' scientific rigour. The issue of research methodology is addressed in more depth by Chaudhury *et al.* in Chapter 15.

The early and effective treatment of opportunistic infections is another vital aspect of care for AIDS patients, as it is ultimately these infections — usually minor conditions when contracted by non-immunocompromised individuals — that lead to morbidity and early death, rather than the retrovirus itself. In practice, PLWHA tend to view their illness symptomatically, and to continue their customary methods of treatment (often herbal) for conditions such as STIs, tuberculosis, weight loss, skin problems, diarrhoeal disease, etc., regardless of whether or not HIV has been diagnosed. As the medicinal compounds in plants have evolved as defences against bacterial, fungal and viral attack, it is self-evident that traditional systems of health care incorporate a vast array of antimicrobial compounds, many of which are already used very effectively in managing HIV-related illness. The combination approach often used in herbal medicine (see also Chapters 10, 12, 13 and 15 of this volume) can help to reduce the problem of microbial resistance to antibiotics, and the emergence of lethal 'superbugs'. While it is beyond the scope of this chapter to review this topic in detail, we will briefly refer to specific infections often associated with AIDS, namely *Candida albicans* and *Mycobacterium tuberculosis*.

In spite of the potential of these various approaches, there are valid concerns about unsafe practices, and a growth in claims of traditional cures for AIDS — the majority of which remain unsupported by clinical evidence. Partnerships between the modern and traditional health sectors are a cornerstone for building a comprehensive strategy to manage the AIDS crisis.

11.1.4. *Holistic Health Care and 'Positive Living'*

It is important to note that the concept of wellness for PLWHA, closely associated with the idea of 'living positively' with HIV, encompasses far more than medication alone. It also incorporates good nutrition, exercise, physical and mental relaxation, and a variety of psychosocial coping strategies and mind-body approaches that contribute towards overall quality of life. Nutritional supplements, taken as tablets, have been found to be useful in reducing the side effects of highly active antiretroviral therapy in the US (Kaiser *et al.*, 2004), while in developing countries, nutritional status can be improved at low cost by promoting the cultivation and use of vitamin- and mineral-rich indigenous fruits and vegetables. One example is *Moringa oleifera* leaf powder, a 'nutritional supplement' that provides a good source of protein, fat (Lockett *et al.*, 2000), calcium (Freiberger *et al.*, 1998), zinc (Barminas *et al.*, 1998) and vitamin A (Nambiar *et al.*, 2003).

The emerging discipline of psychoneuroimmunology, which addresses the connections between emotional states and the functioning of the immune system, underscores the importance of considering health in a holistic sense rather than focusing on a viral infection alone. In this context, traditional and complementary health systems have much to offer. Among the Maasai people of East Africa, for example, a holistic health care ritual known as *olpul* — which takes place at specially prepared forest or bushland sites — is often used as a response to chronic illness, including HIV-related illness. Alongside the sacrifice of an ox or goat and the preparation of medicinal soup from locally available barks and roots, the ritual incorporates traditional songs that praise the herbal medicines and the site itself, stories recounting the strength and courage of earlier generations of warriors, prayers, and relaxation. The overall effect is to create a strong expectation of recovery, which in turn contributes towards a sense of well-being (Burford *et al.*, 2001). Songs, dances and other healing rituals performed by charismatic practitioners, in a supportive community context, may have similar effects.

11.2. Pre-clinical (*In Vitro*) Studies on Natural Products in an HIV/AIDS Context

11.2.1. *Natural Products with Antiretroviral Properties*

Many substances derived from natural products such as plants, algae and fungi have been found to possess some type of antiretroviral activity *in vitro*, whether by direct action against a viral enzyme (e.g. HIV-1 protease, integrase or reverse transcriptase); by interfering with the adhesion of the HIV virus to lymphocytes; or by modulating cellular factors, such as NF-κB, that are involved in HIV replication. Cos *et al.* (2004) have summarised a large body of such research, arranged according to the putative mechanism of action of the substances, and conclude that several plant-derived antiretroviral agents should be further studied for their potential to contribute to the systemic therapy and/or prophylaxis of HIV infection. These compounds are described, however, in a purely biomedical context, as isolated 'active ingredients': some of them have already been chemically synthesised, and in many cases, the plants from which the compounds were originally isolated are not even named in the text. The approach is clearly one of identifying new candidate molecules for conventional pharmaceutical research, leading to the development of novel antiretroviral drugs to supplement (or perhaps ultimately replace) the existing HAART regimens. Table 11.1a lists some plant-derived compounds with activity against HIV-1; this is not intended to be an exhaustive list, but a brief overview of recent research findings.

In a number of other published studies, whole plant and alga extracts have been shown to have antiretroviral properties. Some of these are summarised in Table 11.1b. The focus on whole extracts is probably not, however, indicative of a more holistic approach to traditional medicine, nor of a desire to identify plant preparations that could be made and used locally by PLWHA in developing countries as inexpensive alternatives to HAART. Rather, it seems likely that most of these studies simply represent an earlier stage in the drug development process, whereby anti-HIV screening of whole extracts is followed up by attempts to characterise and purify single active ingredients (e.g. Bessong *et al.*, 2005). Even where this aim is not openly stated, the use of standard laboratory solvents such as methanol and acetone implies that the *in vitro* evaluation is limited to a conventional biomedical framework, rather than traditional preparations as they might be used in the field. The vast majority of these plants are unlikely to be subjected to any further research or development with regard to their potential in managing the HIV epidemic at a local level.

11.2.2. *Immunostimulants and Immunomodulators*

Many plants used in traditional medicine have immunomodulatory or immunostimulant properties, which can potentially contribute a great deal to the well-being of people living with HIV/AIDS. Even if the HIV-1 virus cannot be directly inactivated or killed, altering the activity of other components of the human immune system — such as the complement system, macrophages, dendritic cells, helper T cells, natural killer (NK) cells, polymorphonuclear (PMN) leukocytes, and B lymphocytes — may compensate to some extent for the loss of the CD4+ T-cells that are destroyed by the virus. It is beyond the scope of this chapter to consider the immunomodulatory effects of natural products in detail, but for the purpose of illustration, we will cite just three examples of well-known medicinal plants with such activities, from India, China and North America, respectively.

Table 11.1a.   Antiretroviral Properties of Compounds Derived from Natural Products.

Family	Plant Species	Type of Compound	Target(s)	Reference
Agaricaceae	*Agaricus bisporus*	Lectin	RT	Wang & Ng, 2001
Amaryllidaceae	*Hippeastrum* hybrid	Lectin	AD	Cos *et al.*, 2004
Araliaceae	*Panax notoginseng*	Protein (pananotin)	RT	Tewtrakul *et al.*, 2003
Asteraceae	*Erigeron breviscapus*	Flavonoid (scutellarin)	AD, FU, RT	Zhang *et al.*, 2005
Cannabaceae	*Humulus lupulus*	Flavonoid (xanthohumol)	REP	Wang *et al.*, 2004
Clusiaceae	*Calophyllum lanigerum*	Coumarin derivative (calanolide A)	RT	Cos *et al.*, 2004
Combretaceae	*Terminalia triflora*	Ellagitannin	RT	Martino *et al.*, 2004
Cucurbitaceae	*Momordica charantia*	Protein (MAP-30)	IN, RT	Lee-Huang *et al.*, 1990; Jiratchariyakul *et al.*, 2001
	Trichosanthes kirilowii	Protein (trichosanthin)	IN	Cos *et al.*, 2004
Cynomoriaceae	*Cynomorium songaricum*	Triterpene	PR	Nakamura, 2004
Euphorbiaceae	*Gelonium multiflorum*	Protein (GAP-31)	PR	Lee-Huang *et al.*, 1995
	Homolanthus nutans	Phorbol ester	REP	Cos *et al.*, 2004
	Ricinus communis	Lectin	RT	Wang & Ng, 2001

(*Continued*).

Table 11.1a. *(Continued)*

Family	Plant Species	Type of Compound	Target(s)	Reference
Fabaceae	*Glycine max*	Trypsin inhibitor	RT	Wang & Ng, 2001
	Glycine soja	Protein (glysojanin)	RT	Ngai & Ng, 2003
	Phaseolus coccineus cv. 'Major'	Peptide (coccinin)	RT	Ngai & Ng, 2004
	Phaseolus lunatus	Trypsin inhibitor	RT	Wang & Ng, 2001
	Phaseolus vulgaris	Lectin	RT	Wang & Ng, 2001
Fumariaceae	*Corydalis yanhusuo*	Alkaloid	RT	Wang & Ng, 2001
Ganodermataceae	*Ganoderma lucidum*	Various compounds	REP	el-Mekkawy *et al.*, 1998
Liliaceae	*Leucojum vernum*	Alkaloid	REP	Szlavik *et al.*, 2004
Menispermaceae	*Stephania cepharantha*	Alkaloid (cepharanthine)	GE	Cos *et al.*, 2004
Myrtaceae	*Eucalyptus globoidea*	Lignan (globoidnan A)	IN	Ovenden *et al.*, 2004
Orchidaceae	*Cymbidium* hybrid	Lectin	AD	Cos *et al.*, 2004
	Epipactis helleborine	Lectin	AD	Cos *et al.*, 2004
	Listera ovata	Lectin	AD	Cos *et al.*, 2004
Polyporaceae	*Coriolus versicolor*	Polysaccharo-peptide	RT	Wang & Ng, 2001
Rubiaceae	*Gardenia thailandica*	Cycloartane	REP, RT	Tuchinda *et al.*, 2004
Sapindaceae	*Xanthoceras sorbifolia*	Triterpene	PR	Nakamura, 2004
Urticaceae	*Urtica dioica*	Lectin	AD	Cos *et al.*, 2004
Zingiberaceae	*Curcuma longa*	Curcumin	GE	Cos *et al.*, 2004
Zygophyllaceae	*Larrea tridentata*	Lignin	GE	Cos *et al.*, 2004

AD = HIV-1 adhesion to CD4+ cells; FU = HIV-1 fusion with CD4+ cells; GE = HIV-1-driven gene expression; IN = HIV-1 integrase; PR = HIV-1 protease; REP = replication of HIV-1 (mechanism of inhibition unknown); RT = HIV-1 reverse transcriptase.

Table 11.1b. Antiretroviral Properties of Natural Product Extracts.

Family	Plant Species	Preparation	Target	Reference
Acanthaceae	*Justicia gendarussa*	Aqueous extract of aerial parts	RT	Woradulayapinij *et al.*, 2005
Blechnaceae	*Woodwardia unigemmata*	Methanol extract	PR	Lam *et al.*, 2000
Boraginaceae	*Lobostemon trigonus*	Aqueous extract of leaves	RT	Harnett *et al.*, 2005
Cannaceae	*Canna indica*	Aqueous extract of rhizome	RT	Woradulayapinij *et al.*, 2005
Clusiaceae	*Calophyllum brasiliense*	Extracts of leaves	RT	Huerta-Reyes *et al.*, 2004
Combretaceae	*Combretum molle*	Methanol extract of roots	RT	Bessong *et al.*, 2005
Combretaceae	*Combretum paniculatum*	Acetone extract of leaves	REP	Asres *et al.*, 2001
Convolvulaceae	*Ipomoea carnea* subsp. *fistulosa*	Aqueous extract of aerial parts	RT	Woradulayapinij *et al.*, 2005
Crassulaceae	*Rhodiola rosea*	Extract of roots	PR	Min *et al.*, 1999
Euphorbiaceae	*Croton tiglium*	Extract of seeds	REP	Nakamura, 2004
	Phyllanthus amarus	Aqueous/ethanol extract	AD, IN, PR, RT	Notka *et al.*, 2004
	Phyllanthus orbicularis	Aqueous extract	REP	Garcia *et al.*, 2003
Fabaceae	*Peltophorum africanum*	Methanol extract of stem bark	RT	Bessong *et al.*, 2005
	Spatholobus suberectus	Methanol extract	PR	Lam *et al.*, 2000
Lamiaceae	*Coleus parvifolius*	Ethanol extract of aerial parts	IN	Tewtrakul *et al.*, 2003
	Mentha longifolia	Ethyl acetate extract of aerial parts	REP, RT	Amzazi *et al.*, 2003
	Prunella vulgaris	Aqueous extract	PR	Lam *et al.*, 2000
	Scutellaria baicalensis	Aqueous extract	PR	Lam *et al.*, 2000

(Continued).

Table 11.1b. (*Continued*)

Family	Plant Species	Preparation	Target	Reference
Melianthaceae	*Bersama abyssinica*	Extract of root bark	REP	Asres *et al.*, 2001
Olacaceae	*Ximenia americana*	Extract of stem bark	REP	Asres *et al.*, 2001
Paeoniaceae	*Paeonia suffruticosa*	Methanol extract	PR	Lam *et al.*, 2000
Phaeophyaceae	*Dictyota pfaffii*	Extract of alga	RT	Barbosa *et al.*, 2004
Punicaceae	*Punica granatum*	Juice	AD	Neurath *et al.*, 2004
Rosaceae	*Prunus sargentii*	Extract of leaves	PR	Park *et al.*, 2005
	Rosa rugosa	Extract of roots	PR	Park *et al.*, 2005
Sapindaceae	*Dodonaea angustifolia*	Methanol extract of leaves	REP	Asres *et al.*, 2001
Simaroubaceae	*Ailanthus altissima*	Extract of stem bark	AD	Chang & Woo, 2003
Verbenaceae	*Vitex glabrata*	Aqueous extract of branches	RT	Woradulayapinij *et al.*, 2005
	Vitex negundo	Aqueous extract of aerial parts	RT	Woradulayapinij *et al.*, 2005
	Vitex trifolia	Aqueous extract of aerial parts	RT	Woradulayapinij *et al.*, 2005

AD = HIV-1 adhesion to CD4+ cells; IN = HIV-1 integrase; PR = HIV-1 protease; REP = replication of HIV-1 (mechanism of inhibition unknown); RT = HIV-1 reverse transcriptase.

Research has shown immunomodulatory activity in the leaves, bark, seeds and oil of the popular Indian medicinal tree neem (*Azadirachta indica*), including enhancement of *in vitro* production of interleukin-1, interferon, TNF and GM-CSF by human peripheral blood leukocytes (Upadhyay *et al.*, 1993) and modulation of cell-mediated immune responses in mice (Upadhyay *et al.* 1990; Ray *et al.*, 1996; Njiro & Kofi-Tsepo, 1999). This is of particular interest given that neem also appears to have antiretro-viral activity (Udeinya *et al.*, 2004), raising the possibility of synergistic interactions between different plant components.

A polysaccharide isolated from the root of the Chinese herbal medicine *Astragalus membranaceus* (Astragali radix), widely used in immune sup-plements, has been shown to activate macrophages and B cells, but not T cells, *in vitro* (Wang *et al.*, 2002; Shao *et al.*, 2004; Lee & Jeon, 2005). In patients with herpes simplex keratitis, extract of *A. membranaceus* can mod-ulate the imbalance state of Th1/Th2 cells, significantly improving serum cytokine concentrations — reducing elevated levels of IL-4 and IL-10, while raising the levels of IL-2 and gamma-interferon (Mao *et al.*, 2004). The saponin astragaloside IV, purified from *A. membranaceus*, completely abolishes both the TNF-alpha-stimulated nuclear translation of NF-κB and the DNA-binding activity of NF-κB in endothelial cells, thus blocking the expression of adhesion molecules and the adhesion of endothelial cells to leukocytes, a key process in the pathogenesis of inflammation (Zhang *et al.*, 2003). The inhibition of the NF-κB pathway may also be of importance in blocking HIV-1-directed gene expression, as discussed above.

Echinacea purpurea (purple coneflower), originally used by Native Americans, has become well known as an immune tonic in many indus-trialised countries. It is widely utilised in the prevention and treatment of upper respiratory infections, particularly the common cold (e.g. Schulten *et al.*, 2001; Barrett, 2003). *E. purpurea* has been shown to enhance both humoral immunity, via the IgM-specific antibody-forming cell response (Freier *et al.*, 2003) and non-specific cell-mediated immunity, by activa-tion of macrophages, PMN leukocytes and NK cells (reviewed by Barrett, 2003). It has been suggested that at least one mechanism of action of the herb is to stimulate new production of NK cells and monocytes in the bone marrow, as the first line of defence against virus-infected and transformed cells (Sun *et al.*, 1999). In an *in vitro* study of peripheral blood mononuclear cells (PBMC) from patients with normal immunity and patients with either AIDS or chronic fatigue syndrome, *E. purpurea* extract was found to significantly enhance both NK cell activity and antibody-dependent cellular cytotoxicity in all patient groups (See & Broumand, 1997).

In addition to their direct pharmacokinetic action, medicinal plants and traditional diets may contain nutrients that contribute to slowing the progression of HIV and enhancing an immune response to HIV. Many are rich in vitamins and flavonoids, which can serve as anti-infective agents and antioxidants and which may contribute to slowing disease progression. Building on observational studies that suggest that micronutrient status is a determinant of the progression of HIV status, researchers from the Harvard School of Public Health assessed the effects of multivitamins (vitamins A, B, C and E) on the health status of HIV-positive pregnant women in Tanzania. Using double blind randomised controlled clinical trial (RCT) methodology, they found a significantly lower rate of progression to Stage 4 AIDS and a significantly lower death rate in the multivitamin group as compared with the placebo group. Multivitamins also resulted in significantly higher CD4+ and CD8+ cell counts and significantly lower levels of viral load (Fawzi *et al.*, 2004). Other clinical trials suggesting a role for nutritional supplements in the management of HIV-related illness are discussed by Liu (Chapter 12 of this volume).

11.2.3. *Treatment of Opportunistic Infections*

Candida albicans, an opportunistic infection that causes significant impairment of quality of life in AIDS patients, is a popular target for ethnopharmacological studies because of the relative ease of assay. The ethnobotanical literature contains many hundreds of *in vitro* studies demonstrating antifungal activity against *C. albicans* in various natural products, including honey and propolis as well as plant extracts. Of these, few have been subjected to further research in the specific context of HIV/AIDS. A preliminary study conducted at Teikyo University School of Medicine in Japan in 1999 showed that oral administration of a Kampo medicine, Hochu-ekki-to, can prevent lethal *C. albicans* infection in immunosuppressed mice (Abe *et al.*, 1999); these findings were discussed by the authors in the context of glucocorticoid-induced immunosuppression, but also have important implications for avoiding opportunistic *Candida* infection associated with AIDS. We have identified one prospective open-label trial of *Melaleuca alternifolia* (tea tree oil) preparations, both with and without alcohol, in AIDS patients with fluconazole-refractory oropharyngeal *C. albicans* infection (Vazquez & Zawawi, 2002). The initial findings were promising: overall, using a modified intent-to-treat analysis, 60% of patients showed a clinical response, with seven patients cured and eight clinically improved.

(+)-Calanolide A, a pyranocoumarin HIV-1 reverse transcriptase inhibitor isolated from *Calophyllum lanigerum* (Cos *et al.*, 2004; see Table 11.1a) has been demonstrated to be consistently active against four drug-susceptible strains of *Mycobacterium tuberculosis*, together with strains resistant to isoniazid, rifampin, streptomycin and ethambutol, respectively. It also reduces intracellular replication of *M. tuberculosis* strains in murine and human monocytic cell lines, while maintaining cell viability above 75% in most cases. The intracellular activity is maintained at concentrations below the *in vitro* minimum inhibitory concentration (MIC), suggesting that (+)-calanolide A may somehow stimulate macrophages to be more bactericidal. These findings are of particular significance in the light of the fact that *M. tuberculosis* is one of the leading opportunistic infections associated with AIDS, and no other compound — whether synthetic or natural in origin — has yet been shown to possess activities against both TB and HIV simultaneously. Challenges in the conventional management of HIV-infected TB patients include the drug regimen itself, which consists of 30–32 tablets per day, and interactions between drugs, e.g. rifampin and protease inhibitors (Xu *et al.*, 2004).

11.3. Involving African Traditional Health Practitioners in HIV/AIDS Management

In Uganda, where there is only one doctor for every 20,000 people, there is one traditional health practitioner per 200–400 people (Green, 1994). In such settings, partnerships may be the only way that effective health care coverage can be achieved in managing the twin epidemics of AIDS and malaria. Clearly, such partnerships not only make good public health sense but, based on a growing body of pharmacological evidence, may also yield important preventative and treatment modalities.

In light of the widespread availability of traditional health care services and the reliance of the population on these services, it is inevitable that people suffering from AIDS will turn to traditional health care practitioners (THPs) for treatment. Collaborative AIDS programmes have been established in many African countries, including Malawi, Mozambique, Uganda, Senegal, South Africa, Swaziland, Zambia and Zimbabwe.

Information sharing and educational programmes in South Africa have resulted in THPs providing correct HIV/AIDS advice as well as demonstrations of condom use. One such programme trained 1510 THPs and it was calculated that during the first ten months of the programme, some 845,600 of their clients may have been reached with AIDS/STD prevention messages. In similar programmes in Mozambique, traditional healers learned that AIDS is transmitted by sexual contact, by blood and unsterile razor blades used in traditional practice. In a follow-up evaluation, 81% of those trained reported that they had promoted condom use with at least their STD patients (Green, 1997).

One of the challenges in such workshop situations is to move beyond 'training' to genuine information sharing. It has been noted that it is difficult to modify the manner in which health professionals teach about AIDS — a style that tends towards the didactic and use of scientific jargon. Removing communication barriers such as these is a necessary first step in ensuring that training is an effective tool in mobilising traditional health practitioners as partners in AIDS control. An important example of how this may be done was conducted in Brazil, where a face-to-face educational intervention by healers blended traditional healing — with its language, codes, symbols and images — with scientific medicine, and simultaneously addressed social injustices and discrimination. New information about HIV/AIDS transmission was conveyed using languages and concepts intimately familiar to traditional health practitioners. A controlled evaluation found significant increases in AIDS awareness, knowledge about risky HIV behaviour, information about correct condom use, and acceptance of lower-risk, alternative ritual blood practices among the 126 members of the trainee group compared to 100 untrained controls. There were significant decreases in prejudicial attitudes related to HIV transmission among the trainee group compared to controls (Nations and de Souza, 1997).

The Ugandan NGO, Traditional and Modern Health Practitioners Together Against AIDS (THETA), was established in 1992 to conduct research on potentially useful traditional medicines with HIV-related illness and to promote a mutually respectful collaboration between traditional and modern health workers in the fight against AIDS. THETA has conducted workshops to share knowledge on AIDS prevention and also treatment of opportunistic infections using local herbal remedies. Traditional healers participating in clinical observational studies of their herbal medicines have subsequently sought training in prevention, education, and counselling issues as well as in basic clinical diagnostic skills. A 1998 UNAIDS sponsored evaluation of THETA found that it had reached 125 THPs (44 women and 81 men) in five districts of Uganda. Fifty thousand people were found to have benefited from the improved services offered by traditional health practitioners over a period of two years (Kabatesi, 1998). In the box below, THETA director, Dr. Donna Kabatesi has outlined the challenges entailed in such partnership-building programmes (Kabatesi, 1998).

Challenges

- Many health workers expressed scepticism about this kind of collaboration, while healers feared losing their treatment secrets to scientists and researchers.
- Major questions remain to be researched on the identity and processing of useful herbs.
- Healers feared that doctors would not respect their rights and knowledge because of previous experience with other researchers.
- Medical doctors continued to misunderstand traditional medical practice by attempting to apply the scientific model of biomedicine to traditional medicine.
- Traditional healers feared talking about AIDS and discussing death with their patients because this would indicate failure and possibly also because they were not sure how to deal with the situation after that. Training them in counselling has since improved their skills in talking about AIDS.
- For those healers whose herbal treatments had no efficacy, THETA clinical study results were not so easily accepted.

(Continued)

> (*Continued*)
>
> - Traditional healer associations who initially agreed to work together have continued to have internal power wrangles, which have sometimes interfered with project activities.
> - The projects raised many unmet expectations, such as immediate official recognition by the Ministry of Health.
> - Methodological issues, including the consistency of herbal preparations used during the study; availability of sufficient herbs for study subjects; and non-compliance by patients of each study arm, were major concerns.

In addition to THETA, two other examples of ongoing collaborative projects to involve traditional healers in HIV/AIDS care and prevention in East Africa were described by UNAIDS (2002) in a case study of best practices. These are Women Fighting AIDS in Kenya (WOFAK) and the Tanga AIDS Working Group (TAWG), Tanzania. These initiatives have integrated a traditional medicine component into more comprehensive AIDS prevention and care programmes, and ongoing programmes of HIV/AIDS education via traditional healers are well established. In the WOFAK case, outreach programmes are focused on schools, religious groups, minibus (*matatu*) drivers, youth groups and other NGOs, and include a discussion of harmful traditional practices such as widow inheritance, early marriage and female genital cutting. TAWG takes a slightly different approach, working in association with theatre groups to conduct performances aimed at increasing HIV awareness and behavioural change in three target districts of Tanzania. There is also a Community Health Information and Care Centre that provides regular seminars. Biomedical health practitioners facilitate the training of healers on STI and AIDS, condom use and primary health care (UNAIDS, 2002; see also Mbindyo, Chapter 9 of this volume).

In South Africa, a follow-up of educational workshops found that some THPs reported that local medical staff had begun referring HIV-positive and STD patients to them for condom demonstrations and HIV counselling. All THPs reported having given condom demonstrations to not only clients but to any member of their communities with any potential interest.

Giving a perspective on the benefits from investment in this involvement of local traditional health practitioners in AIDS prevention exercises, Edward C. Green, an organiser of the workshops, reported:

'630 second generation healers had been trained in 12 workshops held in diverse parts of South Africa. The total direct cost of training these 630 was about $23.30 per healer, or $5.90 per day per healer. In addition to these 630 direct beneficiaries of training, up to 229,320 patients or clients of these healers may have benefited from AIDS education within seven months of the first generation training [calculated as 26 weeks times an average of 14 patients a week per healer (see below) times 630 healers trained]. Not all these healers specialise in STDs or AIDS, but most of them see a great number of at least STD patients. Finally, an inestimable number of friends, family members, and others in the local community (local associations, sports teams, youth groups, etc.) benefited from informal AIDS education'. (Green, 1994).

11.3.1. *Clinical Research on African Traditional Medicine*

Health care consumers and THPs want information on the safety and efficacy of local treatments, their effect on opportunistic infections, and how to test claims of cure in an efficient and cost-effective manner. Experience on HIV/AIDS from some African countries such as Burkina Faso, Ghana, Kenya, Nigeria, Senegal, South Africa, Uganda, the United Republic of Tanzania and Zimbabwe is that allopathic health care providers have been collaborating with traditional health care providers in research as well as in HIV/AIDS prevention activities. While 'gold standard' double-blind, placebo-controlled trials are few, a number of prospective open-label studies have been conducted. Researchers have observed reductions in viral load; increases in CD4:CD8 ratios; improvement of the clinical condition of patients; and in some cases, such as Burkina Faso, a weight increase of up to 20 kilograms (Kasilo *et al.*, 2005).

Specific examples of successful collaboration were provided by participants in an International Workshop on Traditional Medicine and HIV/AIDS, convened by the Uganda branch of the non-governmental organisation PROMETRA and held in Nairobi, Kenya, from 17–20 September 2003

                                        G. Bodeker et al.

(PROMETRA/TICAH/Twaweza, 2003). This was followed by an official satellite session to the 13th International Conference on AIDS and Sexually Transmitted Diseases in Africa (ICASA), also in Nairobi, on 21 September 2003. Some of the clinical studies presented during the workshop included the following:

- Trial of a four-plant mixture on 200 terminally ill HIV patients in South Africa over a period of two years (Dr. Gilbert Matsabisa, Head, Indigenous Knowledge Systems Health Division, South African Medical Research Council): in 62 of the patients, the mixture was effective in boosting CD4 counts by 199%, reducing viral loads by 79%, and enabling weight gain of 23%.
- Trial of a two-plant therapy on 268 patients in the Democratic Republic of the Congo, each with a CD4 count below 450 and at least one opportunistic infection, over a period of 180 days (Dr. Constantin Bashengezi, Senior Lecturer, University of Kinshasa, and Director, Research Centre for Physiotherapy and African Traditional Pharmacopoeia). Therapy succeeded in reducing fevers within five days in 95% of patients, curing diarrhoea within 10 days, enabling 76% of patients to gain weight, and increasing CD4 counts up to 400% in 75% of patients. The University of Chicago later studied patients' viral loads and found significant declines. This treatment has received an international and a United States patent.
- Trial of Metrafaids, a herbal medicine developed in Ivory Coast, on 62 patients in Fatik, Senegal, for a period of six months (Dr. Erick Gbodossou, President, PROMETRA International). Therapy found to be effective in reducing viral loads by more than 66% in 56% of the participants, and by as much as 99% in some cases; increasing CD4 counts more than 100% in 63% of the participants; and enabling more than 85% of participants to gain weight and obtain relief from opportunistic infections, e.g. diarrhoea, fever and anorexia.

In another example, a study conducted by the Blair Research Institute Clinic in Harare, Zimbabwe evaluated the impact of traditional medicine in persons with HIV infection and assessed their quality of life with respect to HIV disease progression. There were 105 HIV infected persons in the study, at various stages of HIV infection, of whom 79% were on traditional herbal medicine and 21% were on conventional medical care (CMC). Using the

WHO Quality of Life Scale, it was found that the proportions of scores on five domains measuring different aspects of quality of life for patients on traditional medicine were much lower than those on conventional therapy (p < 0.0001, for all variables). The research team concluded that the data supported the role of traditional medicine in improving the quality of life of HIV-I infected patients, although its pharmacological basis is unknown (Sebit *et al.*, 2000).

There has been little official response from governments on this front. However, in one of the more forward-looking national programmes, the Uganda AIDS Commission and the Joint Clinical Research Centre in Kampala have worked with traditional healers in evaluating several traditional treatments used locally for OIs. The research has found traditional medicine to be *'better suited to the treatment of some AIDS symptoms such as herpes zoster (HZ), chronic diarrhoea, shingles and weight loss'*. THETA has conducted controlled clinical trials on a Ugandan herbal treatment for herpes zoster. Comparing subjects with herbal treatments with controls using acyclovir, the conventional treatment for HZ, both groups were found to experience similar rates of resolution of HZ attacks. The traditional medicine group had less super-infection and showed less keloid formation than did subjects on acyclovir. HZ pain resolved significantly faster in the herbal group. The investigators concluded that herbal treatment is an important local and affordable alternative in managing HZ in HIV infected patients in Uganda (Homsy *et al.*, 2000).

A Traditional Medicine and AIDS in East and Southern Africa Task Force, established in Kampala in early 2000, aims to build a research programme which will identify, assess, and develop safe and effective local treatments for HIV-related illnesses. Coordinated by THETA in Uganda (Mbindyo, Chapter 9 of this volume), the programme favours use of simplified but controlled clinical protocols to conduct rapid evaluations of promising treatments (Bodeker *et al.*, 2000).

Nigeria has made an important commitment to evaluate traditional medicines for HIV. The programme was given momentum by increased government research funding in March 2000, when the Nigerian health minister announced that *'the Government has significantly increased its budget for verifying HIV/AIDS cure claims, after a recommendation by the World Bank and UNAIDS'* (Bodeker, 2003).

11.4. Asian Perspectives

While much of the international focus on AIDS in the developing world has focused on Africa, there has been growing awareness of the rapid spread of the disease in Asia. Reflecting the concerns now beginning to be addressed in many African countries, India's national AIDS policy states:

> *'In a scenario where antiretroviral drugs are extremely expensive, there is a great need to look into the indigenous systems of medicine (ISM), like Ayurveda, Unani and Siddha. Some of the medicines in these systems have the potential of reducing the viral load in the body of the patient thus ensuring a healthier and longer life with the infection. The Government has sponsored research projects in ISM and is receiving encouraging response. It will pursue a policy of sponsoring research in ISM for development of drugs which can serve the purpose of antiretrovirals'.*

The policy statement cautions about false claims of cures among unscrupulous practitioners, and makes the point that *'Any medicine or system of treatment which cannot stand the test of scrutiny by the professional organisations like the Ayurveda Council cannot be accepted as a drug or a system of treatment in the country'*. Clearly, drugs that are shown by rigorous research methods to have an effect can become part of a system of treatment in India (Indian Health Policy, Government of India, 1999).

Traditional Chinese medicine is also being used in HIV management, not only in China, but also in Africa and in other parts of Asia, where traditional Chinese medicines are exported. In one study, Tai Bao, a Chinese herbal medicine developed in Kenya by Dr. Li Chuan, was tested in 40 HIV-positive patients from the slum community of Kibera in Nairobi, all of whom had opportunistic infections. Patients were put on Tai Bao (three times daily, after meals) for a period of 18 months. The study found that Tai Bao was highly effective in treating opportunistic infections, particularly dermatological diseases and sarcomas; that CD4 counts increased over time to an average of 374 within 12 months; and viral loads declined for a majority of patients. Conversely, an open prospective trial of the Chinese herbal medicine Jin Huang in 21 asymptomatic HIV-infected volunteers in Thailand showed no significant changes in either viral load or CD4 count, although some patients reported better appetite and sleep (Maek-a-nantawat *et al.*, 2003).

In another study, Qian-kun-nin, a Chinese herbal formulation considered to have anti-infection, antitumour, antiretroviral and immunomodulatory properties, was evaluated for its anti-HIV effects. Eight HIV-positive subjects were given oral qian-kun-nin capsules for 24 consecutive weeks in a single blind design. Compared to baseline level, the plasma virus load decreased significantly at the end of week 12 ($p < 0.01$) and week 24 ($p < 0.01$), respectively. Four weeks after cessation of qian-kun-nin treatment, plasma virus load was still significantly lower compared to baseline ($p < 0.01$). Blood CD4 cell counts were increased significantly at the end of the 12th week compared to the baseline level ($p < 0.01$). No adverse effects were observed, and no significant side effects were recorded in any subjects (Zhan *et al.*, 2000).

This is one of many emerging studies that require adequate funding to ensure that the research methodology is sound. While these data appear to suggest that qian-kun-nin has therapeutic potential in the treatment of HIV positive patients, clearly the trial design and the sample size make it difficult to draw solid conclusions from the study. What this study does highlight is the potential for anti-HIV effects in traditional medicines, and the need for standard operating procedures for the clinical evaluation of these medicines. A meeting on Indian Systems of Medicine and the response to HIV/AIDS held in Delhi in November 2000 addressed research needs in this field, and a clinical protocol has subsequently been published for use in the clinical evaluation of herbal medicines with HIV-related illness (Chaudhury, 2001). The importance of reaching a consensus with regard to methodological issues in research, discussed in depth by Chaudhury *et al.* (Chapter 15 of this volume) is illustrated by the example of the Siddha medical system, given below.

11.4.1. *Siddha and the Management of HIV/AIDS in India*

It is widely acknowledged that the Siddha texts, written many centuries ago, contain formularies for the effective treatment of HIV/AIDS — treatment that can suppress the virus and prolong a patient's life — and possibly even a cure (TANSACS, 2005b). Specifically, the Siddha texts prescribe a combination therapy for HIV/AIDS that is termed RAN, an acronym for its three formulations: Rasagandhi mezhugu, Amukara churanam and Nellikai elagam. At the 2003 International Siddha Conference on HIV/AIDS, it was learnt that hundreds of vaidyas throughout Tamil Nadu are treating HIV/AIDS with the RAN preparations. The Government of India has published an official formulary for RAN therapy.

11.4.1.1. Government Research on Siddha in HIV/AIDS

One primary function of the Central Councils for Research in Ayurveda and Siddha (CCRAS), a body established by the Ministry of Health and Family Welfare in 1978, is to support research on Siddha HIV/AIDS treatments with the goal of finding a low-cost alternative to antiretrovirals (ARVs) which could be incorporated into national AIDS control policy. The CCRAS, in partnership with the Tamil Nadu State AIDS Control Society (TANSACS), has funded research on the efficacy of RAN therapy at the enormous Tambaram Government Hospital of Thoracic Medicine (Saraswathy, 2004; Tambaram, 2005; TANSACS, 2003; TANSACS, 2005a). Since 1992, Tambaram — one of Asia's largest in-patient AIDS treatment centres (Cohen, 2004) — has treated over 35,000 patients with standard RAN therapy as prescribed in the government formulary (Tambaram, 2005).

TANSACS's website describes the results as 'encouraging', and states that 'a 40-day trail [sic] with RAN has proved to suppress the viral load and raise the immune status of the patients for a period of up to three months' (TANSACS, 2005a). Interviews with TANSACS's Deputy Director, Dr. Palanichamy confirmed that TANSACS's own scientific subcommittees have established that RAN treatment is an effective alternative to antiretrovirals. He stated, 'Whatever allopathy is doing, the same thing is achieved through Siddha — equality in outcomes exists between these two systems. Both can only control the multiplication of the virus' (Palanichamy, 2003).

While the research at Tambaram seemed initially promising, the findings have been contested over issues of methodology. Specifically, many in the biomedical establishment do not accept the results. Thus, the CCRAS is leading a new pilot study at Tambaram, which will employ rigorous methodology (according to WHO guidelines) and address many of the previous concerns. Particular attention will be focused on drug standardisation.

It is not only the Government of India (GOI) that supports research on Siddha medicine through a biomedical framework. International donors also have expressed a willingness to fund scientific research into Siddha treatments for HIV/AIDS (International Siddha Conference, 2003). However, critics assert that conducting research of TRM through a biomedical lens may lead to its biomedicalisation — a process in which the practice of traditional medicine, and the patient experience with TRM, may more closely resemble that of biomedicine. While biomedicine is generally characterised as reductionist, impersonal, and objectifying, proponents of TRM contrast those qualities with the philosophy and practice of TRM which is portrayed as just the opposite — holistic, highly personal (often offering individualised treatments), and empowering.

Several studies have revealed that patients prefer traditional medicine on account of their distrust for biomedicine — a distrust that has arisen both from the memory of poor experiences with government clinics, and also from the association they have drawn between biomedicine and the very processes of modernisation that they blame for their ailment (Basi, 2003; Nichter, 1989). Petersen & Swartz (2002) have shown that reductionism and objectification of the patient in the context of HIV/AIDS can leave patients feeling disempowered — a state of reduced human development (Petersen & Swartz, 2002) and reduced psychological well-being (Seedat & Nell, 1992). This is of particular concern in the light of the finding in Africa that psychological well-being is correlated with a delay in the onset of full-blown AIDS (Mayhew, 1996).

It is difficult, however, to reconcile criticisms of biomedicalisation with the need for standardisation and safety that are incumbent upon any government-supported health care system. Given the fact that unqualified practitioners do exist and can cause harm (UNAIDS, 2000; Srinivasan, 1995), and that they may in fact see economic opportunity in the provision of 'cures' for HIV/AIDS within a loosely regulated treatment environment (Bourdier, 1998; NACO, 2002; Solomon and Ganesh, 2002), increased government regulation of TRM, with all the standardisation of practice *and* knowledge that regulation supports, is widely considered by the public health literature to be a critical prerequisite for its incorporation into national health policy (WHO, 2002; UNAIDS, 2000; Bodeker, 2003). Thus, the harm associated with its objectification and reductionism must be balanced against the positive impact that biomedicalisation has on safety and the efficiency of administration. Given this, it would seem that incorporating traditional medicine into the fight against HIV/AIDS will require complex manoeurves by, and negotiation between, the government, and India's traditional and biomedical systems of medicine.

11.4.1.2. Experiences of Gandeepam with AIDS Control Using Siddha Medicines

Nammakkal in Tamil Nadu is recognised by the state government and the United Nations Development Programme (UNDP) as a high-prevalence district: the official UNDP estimate is 6.5% (UNDP, 2005). Nammakkal is India's major truck building and transportation hub, from which truckers distribute the goods from local industries and India's southern ports all over India. As a result, over 60,000 individuals migrate in and out of Nammakkal every day (Shreedharr, 1995; FRLHT Consultant, 2003) and its highly mobile population is widely recognised as a high-risk community. The state's only government in-patient facility for HIV/AIDS outside of Tambaram is located here, at the Nammakkal Government Hospital. Treatments for HIV/AIDS are free, and many poor families who cannot travel to Tambaram, 400 km from Nammakkal, have sought treatment here (Manorama, 2003).

Ten miles away, an NGO named Gandeepam has established a Siddha hospital whose primary mission is to stem the spread of AIDS in this epicentre of the epidemic: 90% of its patients are treated for HIV/AIDS and related illnesses. Other NGOs in the Nammakkal area also provide Siddha treatments for HIV/AIDS, yet Gandeepam's programme is, by many estimates, ten times larger than any others (Ramani, 2003; Nammakkal Doctor, 2003; FRLHT Consultant, 2003). Since opening in September 2003, Gandeepam has treated over 250 patients for HIV/AIDS, tested several hundreds using the ELISA test, and engaged in significant education, awareness building and prevention campaigns. The majority of patients treated are in stages I and II of AIDS; only a few are being treated in the chronic stage. Gandeepam has facilities for in-patients and out-patients, and it treats critical patients in their homes.

All HIV patients at the Nammakkal clinic are treated free and have agreed to participate in Gandeepam's research programme. This programme has been funded primarily by revenue generated from the sale of non-HIV/AIDS medicines, family savings and more recently, international donor support from the National Institute of Health (NIH) in America, which is supporting preparation for clinical trials.

Community outreach has been critical to the development of Gandeepam's HIV programme. At the Nammakkal clinic, there are five field staff members who are responsible for covering specific geographic zones within the district. Every day, these five employees spend at least six hours in the field, building relationships with their communities so that they can effectively raise awareness of HIV. By forging trust, which has deepened over time as positive word has spread throughout the community about Gandeepam's treatments for HIV/AIDS, the Nammakkal field staff have found their communities increasingly receptive to messages about HIV education and prevention. All of this has allowed Gandeepam's field staff to engage in conversations normally considered taboo, particularly in regard to sexual behaviour and infidelity. Community outreach is also a key mechanism through which community members are motivated to be tested for HIV.

Gandeepam's treatment for HIV/AIDS, as with all other Siddha treatments, is adapted to the patient's constitution, or 'prakriti' as it is known in Siddha and Ayurveda. An individual's prakriti can be predominantly *Vatha* (air and ether), *Pitta* (fire) or *Kapha* (water and earth) (Leslie, 1976). An individual's prakriti informs the diagnosis and determines the most effective treatment. Thus, recognising HIV manifestations specific to each prakriti is required for proper diagnosis and treatment. This is especially important in determining the course of treatment for opportunistic infections (OIs). The failure to distinguish one prakriti from another — for example, providing *pitta* patients with asthma medication prepared for a *kapha* patient — can produce undesirable side-effects (Chaudury & Thatte, 2003).

Like RAN, Gandeepam's Siddha HIV treatment is a combination therapy. It includes three components: immuno-stimulation, antiviral treatment, and treatment for OIs. Immuno-stimulation medicine is provided for the first three days of treatment, and up to seven days for more acute cases. It is a natural liquid extract made from 27 medicinal plants and which is to be consumed orally every morning on an empty stomach. The antiviral medicines, typically started on day four, raise the haemoglobin and continue to strengthen the immune system. This medication is given in the form of capsules, containing 10–15 medicinal plants. This medicine is taken for three months, and four different OI treatments are given concurrently during this time. These medicines treat infection, build stamina and increase weight. Throughout the treatment course, patients must return for checkups every seven to ten days. The total duration of treatment is three months, after which time Gandeepam considers most patients to have achieved a full return to health. Siddha treatment is accompanied by strict dietary guidelines and restrictions.

Gandeepam is also treating psychological conditions associated with HIV, such as depression, anxiety, and suicidal tendencies. This treatment includes Siddha medicines, as well as psychological counseling oriented to both the patient and his/her family. This counselling includes education on the nature of HIV/AIDS, how to treat and manage opportunistic infections and a regular flow of information on the patient's conditions and improvements. This, too, is important in empowering patients and increasing the sense of control they have in their lives (Petersen & Swartz, 2002) — factors which have been shown to improve patient compliance with their treatment regimen (Conrad, 1985), and reduce unsafe sexual practices (Campbell & Williams, 1999).

Since October 2003, 60 HIV/AIDS patients from Nammakkal's research programme have been systematically tracked. Semi-structured interviews with 21 of these 60 patients found that Gandeepam serves an overwhelmingly poor client base. Most families report a monthly income of less than 1083 rupees per month, or 36 rupees per day — not even one dollar a day for the entire family. Moreover, most patients are significantly indebted — three-quarters of Gandeepam's patients reported owing an average debt of 16,700 rupees — and nearly half of the patients take less than three meals a day due to financial constraints. An analysis of the socio-economic impact of HIV/AIDS found that meeting the cost of treatment often required a reduction in expenditures on food (Gupta, 1998: 111). Thus, low cost is the most cited reason given by patients asked to explain why they chose Gandeepam's HIV/AIDS treatment course. Sixty-two per cent of patients indicate that they seek treatment at Gandeepam because its medicines and consultations are free.

HIV-positive patients commonly reported symptoms of cough, fever and body pain. In nearly every case, all symptoms were completely alleviated within two weeks of beginning treatment. Patients also reported significant weight gain (more than three kilograms) and a corresponding increase in energy and strength by the end of the first month's treatment course. More-over, the data show that more than half of the patients also present symptoms of at least one STD. There are four commonly presented STDs, and Gan-deepam's treatments have arrested the symptoms of three of these STDs in less one week, while control of the fourth STD is achieved in under two weeks. This syndromic approach to STDs is considered to be an effective method of STD control, one that may significantly reduce the transmission of HIV, and it is a recommended alternative for poor countries whose scarce resources need not be spent on laboratory tests for STDs (Nagelkerke & De Vlas, 2003). However, as Section 11.4.1 detailed, by the standards of science and Indian official policy, the medicine's efficacy against HIV itself cannot be determined on the basis of the qualitative data assembled.

11.5. Future Directions

TCAM is clearly part of the health care choice of the majority of PLWHA today. Given this widespread use, it is perhaps surprising that relatively little research funding and scholarly attention has gone into this trend and the effectiveness of the treatments being used.

Some future directions in this arena would include prioritisation and support for both biomedical and social science research; policy develop-ment; and partnerships leading to team approaches to containing HIV/AIDS rather than a segmented approach with power resting in the hands of a few highly qualified biomedical professionals and the vast majority of commu-nity healthcare providers being excluded from a significant professional contribution to containing and managing HIV/AIDS.

11.5.1. *Research Agenda: Biomedical Evaluation of TCAM*

Some important areas for inclusion in the biomedical evaluation of TCAM approaches to the management of HIV/AIDS include:

- Documentation and evaluation of traditional methods used in the preven-tion of STIs and their possible effects in preventing HIV transmission.
- Cohort studies and controlled clinical evaluation of traditional treatments for STIs.

- A similar approach to the evaluation of traditional treatments for opportunistic infections associated with HIV.
- Experimental and clinical evaluation of the antiviral effects of TCAM preparations.
- Experimental and clinical evaluation of immunomodulatory effects of TCAM preparations.
- Studies into the effects of traditional medicines in preventing mother to child transmission (MTCT).
- Evaluation of the effects of traditional strategies of diet and nutrition in managing HIV-related illness.
- Evaluation of the effects of traditional counselling and other psychosocial interventions, including holistic treatments that address emotional and spiritual dimensions of well-being, in managing HIV-related illness.

11.5.2. *Research Agenda: Social Science*

Social science research is needed to assess the extent of use, differential choices of various communities and ethnic groups, and also gender differences in traditional medicine use with HIV. Some important areas for investigation would include:

- The practitioners — identifying precisely where they are located within areas known to have high HIV prevalence, in comparison with modern medical personnel.
- The knowledge, attitudes and practices of THPs regarding HIV: what they know; their attitudes about HIV; what they are doing with respect to prevention, treatment, support, and client and community HIV education.
- The social and educational effects of their interventions. To what extent are they giving an effective HIV prevention message — before formal training, after formal training? How are clients rating this message and what behaviour changes are these messages producing?
- Documentation and evaluation of traditional means of psycho-social support.
- Utilisation — documenting and understanding who, in the context of HIV, uses the services of THPs and why.
- Identification of gender differences in patterns and frequency of use as well as in outcomes.

- Cost: research into the economic dimensions of THP services for HIV/AIDS, including cost savings and impact of TCAM use on disability-adjusted life years.

11.5.3. *Policy: Framework for a National Strategy*

Some of the key ingredients of national policy development in this context would include:

- Decentralisation of service delivery so that national AIDS coordination is addressed at local levels and draws on local resources for public education and disease control and management.
- Training for both THPs and mainstream health personnel on the basics of a partnership for HIV/AIDS control.
- Increasing national capacity for research on TCAM and HIV/AIDS.
- Ensuring the establishment of a viable legal framework for protection of indigenous intellectual property rights pertaining to useful traditional medicines.
- A gender perspective in both policy and research, recognising potential gender differences in social behaviours with respect to risk, treatment seeking, disease progression, response to treatment and the psycho-social dimensions of HIV/AIDS.
- Economic policy: recognition of the potential for medicinal plant-based and traditional medicine production micro enterprise projects for income generation and national, bilateral and multilateral support for such projects.
- Medicinal plant sustainability: this global issue of concern (see Chapter 6 of this volume) pertains equally to HIV as to other diseases. The depletion of wild stocks of the African potato, *Hypoxis rooperii*, as it has come to be seen as an anti-HIV medicine in southern Africa, serves to illustrate the point that high use must be matched by a shift from wild harvesting to high-yield production of priority species and corresponding investment to achieve this.

11.5.4. *Partnerships*

Scientists, THPs, PLWHA, the public sector, the NGO community and others all have diverse perspectives, each of which, while different, is valid.

Forging partnerships requires political will, and a perceived benefit to the partnership. This in turn will need to be grounded in education about the contribution that each partner can bring to the multidisciplinary partnership. In setting priorities for identifying and monitoring desirable outcomes of such partnerships, some areas for inclusion would be:

- Levels of community use of the various partners and community assessment of their respective contributions and quality of treatment and care.
- The extent of cross-referral between traditional and biomedical practitioners.
- Monitoring of outcomes.
- A clear R&D agenda.
- A commitment to action and provision of financial resources.

11.6. Challenges

Historic mistrust, resource constraints and the absence of a clear agenda for collaboration and inclusion of THPs within the national AIDS control programme, are all barriers to be overcome in planning partnerships and a formal role for the traditional health care services and treatments already used by the majority of PLWHA. Some of the major challenges to be identified and addressed include:

- False claims of the effectiveness or safety of TCAM medicines against HIV.
- Lower priority in funding for TCAM activities.
- Resistance by mainstream health workers and researchers to a role for, or partnership with, TCAM.
- Difficulty in reaching the informal component of this sector, as there is no central system of communication.
- Resistance by some in the TCAM sector to participating in HIV prevention education if this is dissonant with their cultural and religious values.
- Uncertainty on how to integrate these plans into existing state and national programmes.

• Threat to local and national intellectual property rights from patenting challenges on traditional knowledge.

There will be many other challenges. But excluding the traditional sector from HIV control is to exclude the largest and often the most familiar and trusted health care resource available in most developing countries. Including the sector is clearly needed as a means to ensure widespread AIDS prevention messages, affordable means of managing HIV-related illness, and locally available and culturally relevant means of managing and containing HIV in the areas of the world most severely afflicted by this disease.

References

Abes *et al.* Protection of immunosuppressed mice from lethal *Candida* infection by oral administration of a kampo medicine, hochu-ekki-to. *Immunopharmacol Immunotoxicol* 1999;21(2):331–342.

ALERT. *Summary of HIV/AIDS Statistics from India and South-East Asia.* http://www.alert.org (accessed 12 July 2005 at 14:32).

Amzazi S, Ghoulami S, Bakri Y, Il Idrissi A, Fkih-Tetouani S, Benjouad A. Human immunodeficiency virus type 1 inhibitory activity of *Mentha longifolia. Therapie* 2003;58(6):531–534.

Anastasi JK, McMahon DJ. Testing strategies to reduce diarrhea in persons with HIV using traditional Chinese medicine: acupuncture and moxibustion. *J Assoc Nurses AIDS Care* 2003;14(3):28–40.

Anonymous. China urges caution in herbal cures for AIDS. *AIDS Wkly Plus* 1996;23–30:10 11.

Asres K, Bucar F, Kartnig T, Witvrouw M, Pannecouque C, De Clercq E. Antiviral activity against human immunodeficiency virus type 1 (HIV-1) and type 2 (HIV-2) of ethnobotanically selected Ethiopian medicinal plants. *Phytother Res* 2001;15(1):62–69.

Barbosa JP, Pereira RC, Abrantes JL, Cirne dos Santos CC, Rebello MA, Frugulhetti IC, Texeira VL. *In vitro* antiviral diterpenes from the Brazilian brown alga *Dictyota pfaffii. Planta Med* 2004;70(9):856–860.

Barminas JT, Charles M, Emmanuel D. Mineral composition of non-conventional leafy vegetables. *Plant Foods Hum Nutr* 1998;53(1):29–36.

Barnett T, Whiteside A. *AIDS in the 21st Century: Disease and Globalization.* Basingstoke: Palgrave Macmillan, 2002.

Barrett B. Medicinal properties of Echinacea: a critical review. *Phytomedicine* 2003;10(1):66–86.

Basi M. *Biomedicine as a Health Option in Contemporary Rural Punjab*, Discussion Paper 103. Montreal: Centre for Developing-Area Studies, McGill University, 2003.

Beal MW, Nield-Anderson L. Acupuncture for symptom relief in HIV-positive adults: lessons learned from a pilot study. *Altern Ther Health Med* 2000;6:33–42.

Bessong PO, Obi CL, Andreola ML, Rojas LB, Pouysegu L, Igumbor E, Meyer JJ, Quideau S, Litvak S. Evaluation of selected South African medicinal plants for inhibitory properties against human immunodeficiency virus type 1 reverse transcriptase and integrase. *J Ethnopharmacol* 2005;99(1):83–91.

Bodeker G. Traditional medicine. In: Cook GC, Zumla A (eds.) *Manson's Tropical Diseases*, 21st edn. Philadelphia: W. B. Saunders, 2003.

Bodeker G, Kabatesi D, Homsy J, King R. A regional task force on traditional medicine and AIDS in East and Southern Africa. *Lancet* 2000; 355:1284.

Bourdier F. Ethno-epidemiology of AIDS and responses of Tamil medical science. In: Bourdier F (ed.) *Of Research and Action — Contribution of Non-governmental Organization and Social Scientists in the Fight Against the HIV/AIDS Epidemic in India*. Pondicherry: Societes, Sante, Developpement, 1998, pp. 116–119.

Burack JH, Cohen MR, Hahn JA, Abrams DI. Pilot randomised controlled trial of Chinese herbal treatment for HIV-associated symptoms. *J Acquir Immune Defic Syndr Hum Retrovirol* 1996;12(4):386–393.

Burford G, Rafiki MY, Ngila LO. The forest retreat of *orpul*, a holistic system of health care practised by the Maasai tribe of northern Tanzania. *J Altern Complem Med* 2001;7(4):547–551.

Campbell C, Williams B. Beyond the biomedical and the behavioural: towards an integrated approach to HIV prevention in the Southern African mining industry. *Soc Sci Med* 1999;48:1625–1639.

Chang YS, Woo ER. Korean medicinal plants inhibiting to human immunodeficiency virus type 1 (HIV-1) fusion. *Phytother Res* 2003;17(4):426–429.

Chaudhury RR. A clinical protocol for the study of traditional medicine and human immunodeficiency virus-related illness. *J Altern Complement Med* 2001;7(5):553–566.

Chaudhury RR, Thatte U. Beyond Dots: avenues ahead in the management of tuberculosis: *Nat Med J India* 2003;16:321–327.

Cohen J. HIV/AIDS in Asia. *Sci Mag* 2004;304:504–509.

Conrad P. The meaning of medications: another look at compliance. *Soc Sci Med* 1985;20(1):29–37.

Cos P, Maes L, Vanden Berghe D, Hermans N, Pieters L, Vlietinck A. Plant substances as anti-HIV agents selected according to their putative mechanism of action. *J Nat Prod* 2004;67:284–293.

el-Mekkawy *et al.* Anti-HIV-1 and anti-HIV-1-protease substances from *Ganoderma lucidum. Phytochemistry* 1998;49(6):1651–1657.

Fawzi WW, Msamanga GI, Spiegelman D, Wei R, Kapiga S, Villamor E *et al.* A randomised trial of multivitamin supplements and HIV disease progression and mortality. *N Engl J Med* 2004;351:23–32.

Freiberger CE, Vanderjagt DJ, Pastuszyn A, Glew RS, Mounkaila G, Millson M, Glew RH. Nutrient content of the edible leaves of seven wild plants from Niger. *Plant Foods Hum Nutr* 1998;53(1):57–69.

Freier DO, Wright K, Klein K, Voll D, Dabiri K, Cosulich K, George R. Enhancement of the humoral immune response by *Echinacea purpurea* in female Swiss mice. *Immunopharmacol Immunotoxicol* 2003;25(4):551–560.

FRLHT Consultant. *Field Interview* Foundation for the Revitalization of Local Health Traditions, Consultant, Mr. Hari Ram Murthy, 2003 (www.frlht-india.org).

Garcia SV, del Barrio Alonso G, Gaiten YG, Diaz LM. Preliminary evaluation of the antiviral activity of the aqueous extract of *Phyllanthus orbicularis* versus HIV-1 infection. *Rev Cubana Med Trop* 2003;55(3):169–173 article in Spanish.

Green EC. *AIDS and STDs in Africa: Bridging the Gap Between Traditional Healers and Modern Medicine.* Boulder, Co. and Oxford, UK: Westview Press, 1994.

Green EC. The participation of African traditional healers in AIDS/STD prevention programmes. *Trop Doct* 1997;27(Suppl 1):56–59.

Gupta I. Planning for the socio-economic impact of the epidemic: the costs of being ill. In Godwin P (ed.) *The Looming Epidemic: The Impact of HIV and AIDS in India.* London: Hurst and Company, 1998, pp. 94–125.

Harnett SM, Oosthuizen V, van de Venter M. Anti-HIV activities of organic and aqueous extracts of *Sutherlandia frutescens* and *Lobostemon trigonus. J Ethnopharmacol* 2005;96(1–2):113–119.

Homsy J, Katabira E, Kabatesi D, Mubiru F, Kwamya L, Tusaba C, Kasolo S, Mwebe D, Ssentamu L, Okello M, King R. Evaluating herbal medicine for the management of Herpes zoster in human immunodeficiency virus-infected patients in Kampala, Uganda. *J Altern Complement Med* 2000;6(1):1–2.

288   *G. Bodeker et al.*

Hsieh PW, Chang FR, Lee KH, Hwang TL, Chang SM, Wu YC. A new anti-HIV alkaloid, drymaritin, and a new C-glycoside flavonoid, diandraflavone, from *Drymaria diandra. J Nat Prod* 2004;67(7):1175–1177.

Huerta-Reyes M, Basualdo M del C, Abe F, Jimenez-Estrada M, Soler C, Reyes-Chilpa R. HIV-1 inhibitory compounds from *Calophyllum brasiliense* leaves. *Biol Pharm Bull* 2004;27(9):1471–1475.

Independent Living. *World Health Organization — Facts About Traditional Medicine* (http://www.independentliving.co.uk/tradmed.html).

International Siddha Conference. *International Meet on Prevention, Care and Control of HIV/AIDS Under Time Tested Indian Medical System — Siddha*, 4–6 December 2003, organized by the Gandeepam Siddha Hospital and Research Center (www.gandeepam.org).

Jiratchariyakul W *et al.* HIV inhibitor from Thai bitter gourd. *Planta Med* 2001;67(4):350–353.

Kabatesi D. Use of traditional treatments for AIDS-associated diseases in resource-constrained settings. In: Robertson L, Bell K, Laypang L, Blake B (eds.) *Health in the Commonwealth: Challenges and Solutions 1998/99*. London: Kensington Publications, 1998.

Kaiser J, Ondercin J, Santos G, Leoung G, Brown S, Mass M, Baum M. Broad-spectrum micronutrient supplementation in HIV-infected patients with dideoxynucleoside-related peripheral neuropathy: a prospective, double-blind, placebo controlled trial. Presented as an abstract at the *Conference on Retroviruses and Opportunistic Infections*, 8–12 February 2004, San Francisco, California.

Kasilo OMJ, Soumbey-Alley E, Wambebe C, Chatora W. Regional overview: African region. In: Bodeker G, Ong C-K, Grundy C, Burford G, Shein K (eds.) *WHO Global Atlas of Traditional, Complementary and Alternative Medicine*. Geneva: World Health Organization, 2005.

La Trobe University. *HIV Futures Community Report*. Centre for the Study of Sexually Transmissible Disease, La Trobe University, 1998.

Labadie RP *et al.* An ethnopharmacognostic approach to the search for immunomodulators of plant origin. *Planta Med* 1989;55(4):339–348.

Lam TL *et al.* A comparison of human immunodeficiency virus type-1 protease inhibition activities by the aqueous and methanol extracts of Chinese medicinal herbs. *Life Sci* 2000;67(23):2889–2896.

Lavekar GS, Sharma SK. Republic of India. In: Bodeker G, Ong C-K, Grundy C, Burford G, Maehira Y (eds.) *WHO Global Atlas on Traditional, Complementary and Alternative Medicine*. Geneva: WHO, 2005, pp. 89–96.

Lee KY, Jeon YJ. Macrophage activation by polysaccharide isolated from *Astragalus membranaceus*. *Int Immunopharmacol* 2005;5(7–8):1225–1233.

Lee-Huang S *et al*. MAP 30: a new inhibitor of HIV-1 infection and replication. *FEBS Lett* 1990;272(1–2):12–18.

Lee-Huang S *et al*. Inhibition of the integrase of human immunodeficiency virus (HIV) type 1 by anti-HIV plant proteins MAP30 and GAP31. *Proc Natl Acad Sci USA* 1995;92(19):8818–8822.

Leslie C. Ambiguities of revivalism in Modern India. In: Leslie C (ed.) *Asian Medical Systems — A Comparative Study*. Berkeley, CA: University of California Press, 1976, pp. 356–367.

Lockett CT, Calvert CC, Grivetti LE. Energy and micronutrient composition of dietary and medicinal wild plants consumed during drought. Study of rural Fulani, northeastern Nigeria. *Int J Food Sci Nutr* 2000;51(3):195–208.

Maek-a-nantawat W *et al*. Six-month evaluation of JinHuang Chinese herbal medicine study in asymptomatic HIV infected Thais. *Southeast Asian J Trop Med Public Health* 2003;34(2):379–384.

Manorama P. In support of T.N. doctors. *Yahoo: AIDS INDIA eFORUM*, 14 March 2003, <http://health.groups.yahoo.com/group/AIDS-INDIA/message/2288> (accessed 15 April 2005).

Mao SP, Cheng KL, Zhou YF. Modulatory effect of *Astragalus membranaceus* on Th1/Th2 cytokine in patients with herpes simplex keratitis. *Zhongguo Zhong Xi Yi Jie He Za Zhi* 2004;24(2):121–123 (article in Chinese).

Martino V, Morales J, Martinez-Irujo JJ, Font M, Monge A, Coussio J. Two ellagitannins from the leaves of *Terminalia triflora* with inhibitory activity on HIV-1 reverse transcriptase. *Phytother Res* 2004;18(8):667–669.

Mayhew S. Integrating MCH/FP and STD/HIV services: current debates and future directions. *Health Policy Plan* 1996;11:339–353.

Mills E, Cooper C, Seely D, Kanfer I. African herbal medicines in the treatment of HIV: Hypoxis and Sutherlandia. An overview of evidence and pharmacology. *Nutr J* 2005;4(1):19.

Min BS *et al*. Screening of Korean plants against human immunodeficiency virus type 1 protease. *Phytother Res* 1999;13(8):680–682.

NACO. *National AIDS Prevention and Control Policy*. New Delhi: Ministry of Health and Family Welfare, National AIDS Control Organisation, Government of India, 2002.

Nagelkerke NJD, De Vlas SJ. *The Epidemiological Impact of an HIV Vaccine on the HIV/AIDS Epidemic in Southern India*. World Bank, Working Paper 2978. Washington DC: World Bank Development Research Group, 2003.

Nakamura N. Inhibitory effects of some traditional medicines on proliferation of HIV-1 and its protease. *Yakugaku Zasshi* 2004;124(8):519–529 (article in Japanese).

Nambiar VS, Bhadalkar K, Daxini M. Drumstick leaves as source of vitamin A in ICDS-SFP. *Indian J Pediatr* 2003;70(5):383–387.

Nammakkal Doctor. *Field Interview.* Gandeepam Siddha Hospital and Research Centre, Siddha Doctor at Nammakkal Clinic, Dr. Buneveshwari, 2003.

Nations MK, de Souza MA. Umbanda healers as effective AIDS educators: case-control study in Brazilian urban slums (*favelas*). *Trop Doct* 1997; 27(Suppl 1):60–66.

Neurath AR, Strick N, Li YY, Debnath AK. *Punica granatum* (Pomegranate) juice provides an HIV-1 entry inhibitor and candidate topical microbicide. *BMC Infect Dis* 2004;4(1):41.

Ngai PH, Ng TB. Purification of glysojanin, an antifungal protein, from the black soybean *Glycine soja. Biochem Cell Biol* 2003;81(6):387–394.

Ngai PH, Ng TB. Coccinin, an antifungal peptide with antiproliferative and HIV-1 reverse transcriptase inhibitory activities from large scarlet runner beans. *Peptides* 2004;25(12):2063–2068.

Nichter M. *Anthopology and International Health: South Asian Case Studies.* Amsterdam: Gordon and Breach, 1989.

Njiro SM, Kofi-Tsepo WM. Effect of an aqueous extract of stem bark of *Azadirachta indica* on the immune response in mice. *Onderstepoort J Vet Res* 1999;66:59–62.

Notka F, Meier G, Wagner R. Concerted inhibitory activities of *Phyllanthus amarus* on HIV replication *in vitro* and *ex vivo. Antiviral Res* 2004; 64(2):93–102.

Ovenden SP, Yu J, Wan SS, Sberna G, Tait RM, Rhodes D, Cox S, Coates J, Walsh NG, Meurer-Grimes BM. Globoidnan A: a lignan from *Eucalyptus globoidea* inhibits HIV integrase. *Phytochemistry* 2004;65(24):3255–3259.

Palanichamy K. *Field Interview.* Tamil Nadu State AIDS Control Society, Deputy Director, Dr. K. Palanichamy, 2003.

Park JC, Kim SC, Choi MR, Song SH, Yoo EJ, Kim SH, Miyashiro H, Hattori M. Anti-HIV protease activity from Rosa family plant extracts and rosamultin from *Rosa rugosa. J Med Food* 2005;8(1):107–109.

Petersen I, Swartz L. Primary health care in the era of HIV/AIDS. Some implications for health system reform. *Soc Sci Med.* 2002;55:1005–1013.

PROMETRA/TICAH/Twaweza. *A Journey of Connectedness: Workshop on Traditional Medicine and HIV/AIDS,* 17–20 September 2003, Brackenhurst Conference Centre, Nairobi, Kenya. *13th International Conference on AIDS and*

Sexually Transmitted Diseases in Africa (ICASA), 21–26 September 2003, Nairobi, Kenya. Nairobi: PROMETRA, TICAH (Trust for Indigenous Culture and Health) and Twaweza Communications.

Ramani V. *Field Interview*. Gandeepam Siddha Hospital and Research Centre, Director and Founder, Dr. V. Ramani, 2003.

Ray A, Bannerjee BD, Sen P. Modulation of cell-mediated immune responses by *Azadirachta indica* in mice. *Indian J Exp Biol* 1996;34:698–701.

Saraswathy. *Field Interview*. Central Councils for Research in Ayurveda and Siddha, Chennai, Deputy Director in Charge, Dr. Saraswathy, 2004.

Schulten B, Bulitta M, Ballering-Bruhl B, Koster U, Schafer M. Efficacy of *Echinacea purpurea* in patients with a common cold. A placebo-controlled, randomised, double-blind clinical trial. *Arzneimittelforschung* 2001;51(7): 563–568.

Sebit MB, Chandiwana SK, Latif AS, Gomo E, Acuda SW, Makoni F, Vushe J. Quality of life evaluation in patients with HIV-I infection: the impact of traditional medicine in Zimbabwe. *Cent Afr J Med* 2000;46(8):208–213.

See DM, Broumand N. *In vitro* effects of echinacea and ginseng on natural killer and antibody-dependent cell cytotoxicity in healthy subjects and chronic fatigue syndrome or acquired immunodeficiency syndrome patients. *Immunopharmacology* 1997;35(3):229–235.

Seedat M, Nell V. Authoritarianism and autonomy. Conflicting value systems in the introduction of psychological services in a South African primary care system. *S Af J Psychol* 1992;22:185–193.

Shao BM, Xu W, Dai H, Tu P, Li Z, Gao XM. A study on the immune receptors for polysaccharides from the roots of *Astragalus membranaceus*, a Chinese medicinal herb. *Biochem Biophys Res Commun* 2004;320(4): 1103–1111.

Shreedharr J. *Passage Through India Maps a Deadly Course*. Cambridge, MA: Harvard AIDS Review, Fall, 1995.

Solomon S, Ganesh AK. HIV in India. *Topics HIV Med* 2002;10(3):19–24.

Sparber A, Wootton JC, Bauer L, Curt G, Eisenberg D, Levin T, Steinberg SM. Use of complementary medicine by adult patients participating in HIV/AIDS clinical trials. *J Altern Complement Med* 2000;6(5):415–422.

Srinivasan P. National health policy for traditional medicine in india. *World Health Forum* 1995;16(2):190.

Sun LZ, Currier NL, Miller SC. The American coneflower: a prophylactic role involving nonspecific immunity. *J Altern Complement Med* 1999; 5(5):437–446.

Sun Y *et al.* Anti-HIV agent MAP30 modulates the expression profile of viral and cellular genes for proliferation and apoptosis in AIDS-related lymphoma cells infected with Kaposi's sarcoma-associated virus. *Biochem Biophys Res Commun* 2001;287(4):983–994.

Szlavik L, Gyuris A, Minarovits J, Forgo P, Molnar J, Hohmann J. Alkaloids from *Leucojum vernum* and antiretroviral activity of Amaryllidaceae alkaloids. *Planta Med* 2004;70(9):871–873.

Tambaram. *Tambaram Government Hospital of Thoracic Medicine Website*, http://education.vsnl.com/thoracic/sidupd.html (accessed 28 March 2005).

TANSACS. *Tamil Nadu State AIDS Control Society Website*, http://www. aidsfreetn.com/understandingaids/treatment.html (accessed 28 March 2005a).

TANSACS. Siddha Page, *Tamail Nadu State AIDS Control Society Website*, http://www.aidsfreetn.com/tnsacs/siddhapage.html (accessed 25 April 2005b).

TANSACS. *TANSACS Annual Report*. Chennai: TANSACS, 2003.

Tewtrakul S *et al.* HIV-1 integrase inhibitory substances from *Coleus parvifolius*. *Phytother Res* 2003;17(3):232–239.

Tuchinda P, Saiai A, Pohmakotr M, Yoosook C, Kasisit J, Napaswat C, Santisuk T, Reutrakul V. Anti-HIV-1 cycloartanes from leaves and twigs of *Gardenia thailandica*. *Planta Med* 2004;70(4):366–370.

Udeinya IJ, Mbah AU, Chijioke CP, Shu EN. An antimalarial extract from neem leaves is antiretroviral. *Trans R Soc Trop Med Hyg* 2004;98(7): 435–437.

UNAIDS. *Ancient Remedies, New Disease: Involving Traditional Healers in Increasing Access to AIDS Care and Prevention in East Africa*, UNAIDS/02.16E. Geneva: UNAIDS, 2002.

UNAIDS. *Collaboration with Traditional Healers in HIV/AIDS Prevention and Care in Subsaharan Africa*. Geneva: UNAIDS, 2000.

UNDP. *Regional Update — India*, http://www.hivandevelopment.org/ regionalupdate/india/index.asp (accessed 15 April 2005).

Upadhyay S, Kaushic C, Talwar GP. Antifertility effects of neem (*Azadirachta indica*) oil by intrauterine administration: a novel method for contraception. *Proc R Soc Lond* 1990;242:175–179.

Upadhyay SN, Dhawan S, Garg S, Wali N, Tucker L, Anderson DJ. Immunomodulatory properties of neem (*Azadirachta indica*). *Proceedings of the World Neem Conference*, Bangalore, India, 24–28 February 1993.

Vazquez JA, Zawawi AA. Efficacy of alcohol-based and alcohol-free melaleuca oral solution for the treatment of fluconazole-refractory oropharyngeal candidiasis in patients with AIDS. *HIV Clin Trials* 2002;3(5):379–385.

Wang HX, Ng TB. Examination of lectins, polysaccharopeptide, polysaccharide, alkaloid, coumarin and trypsin inhibitors for inhibitory activity against human immunodeficiency virus reverse transcriptase and glycohydrolases. *Planta Med* 2001;67(7):669–672.

Wang RT, Shan BE, Li QX. Extracorporeal experimental study on immuno-modulatory activity of *Astragalus membranaceus* extract. Zhongguo Zhong Xi Yi Jie He Za Zhi 2002;22(6):453–456 (article in Chinese).

Wang Q, Ding ZH, Liu JK, Zheng YT. Xanthohumol, a novel anti-HIV-1 agent purified from Hops, *Humulus lupulus. Antiviral Res* 2004;64(3):189–194.

Weber R, Christen L, Loy M, Schaller S, Christen S, Joyce CR *et al.* Randomised, placebo-controlled trial of Chinese herb therapy for HIV-infected individuals. *J Acquir Immune Defic Syndr* 1999;22(1):56–64.

WHO. *WHO Traditional Medicine Strategy 2002–2005*. Geneva: World Health Organization, 2002.

Woradulayapinij W, Soonthornchareonnon N, Wiwat C. *In vitro* HIV type 1 reverse transcriptase inhibitory activities of Thai medicinal plants and *Canna indica* L. rhizomes. *J Ethnopharmacol*, 2005 (Epub ahead of print).

Xu Z-Q, Barrow WW, Suling WJ, Westbrook L, Barrow E, Lina Y-M, Flavin MT. Anti-HIV natural product (+)-calanolide A is active against both drug-susceptible and drug-resistant strains of Mycobacterium tuberculosis. *Bioorg Med Chem* 2004;12:1199–1207.

Xu Z-Q, Flavin MT, Jenta TR. Calanolides, the naturally occurring anti-HIV agents. *Curr Opin Drug Disc Dev* 2000;3:155–166.

Zhan L, Yue ST, Xue YX, Attele AS, Yuan CS. Effects of qian-kun-nin, a Chinese herbal medicine formulation, on HIV positive subjects: a pilot study. *Am J Chin Med* 2000;28(3–4):305–312.

Zhang GH, Wang Q, Chen JJ, Zhang XM, Tam SC, Zheng YT. The anti-HIV-1 effect of scutellarin. *Biochem Biophys Res Commun* 2005;334(3):812–816.

Zhang WJ, Hufnagl P, Binder BR, Wojta J. Antiinflammatory activity of astragalo-side IV is mediated by inhibition of NF-κB activation and adhesion molecule expression. *Thromb Haemost* 2003;90(5):904–914.

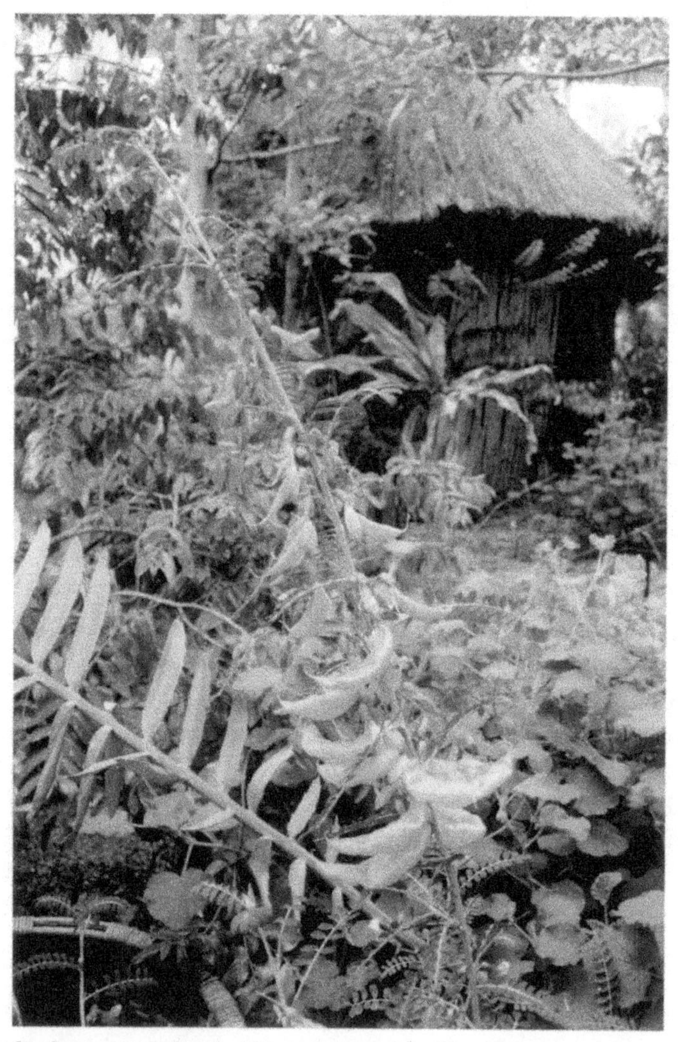

Sutherlandia frutescens, a South Africa plant used in the management of AIDS. (*Photo courtesy of M. L. Wilcox.*)

CHAPTER 12

AN OVERVIEW OF CLINICAL STUDIES ON COMPLEMENTARY AND ALTERNATIVE MEDICINE IN HIV INFECTION AND AIDS

Jianping Liu

12.1. Background

The introduction of highly active anti-retroviral therapy (HAART) into clinical practice in 1996 has dramatically changed the development of HIV-related diseases in industrialised countries (Bonfanti *et al.*, 1999; Shafer & Vuitton, 1999; Vella & Palmisano, 2000; Tirelli & Bernardi, 2001). Although they cannot cure HIV infection and AIDS, anti-retrovirals have an impact on reducing morbidity and mortality, prolonging lives, and improving the quality of life of many people living with HIV/AIDS (WHO, 2002). However, many people with HIV/AIDS in developing countries cannot afford the high costs of HAART. Moreover, HAART has a limited response in some patients, includes a complicated dosage regimen, and is associated with some drug toxicities. In addition, there is a problem with cross-resistance among anti-retroviral drugs of the same class (Bonfanti *et al.*, 1999; Vella & Palmisano, 2000). The therapeutic options of treating HIV/AIDS are currently still limited, and alternative approaches are needed.

Complementary and alternative medicine (CAM) has been defined as diagnosis, treatment and/or prevention that complements mainstream medicine by contributing to a common whole, by satisfying a demand not met by orthodoxy, or by diversifying the conceptual frameworks of medicine (Ernst, 1995). Complementary therapies are increasingly being used (Eisenberg *et al.*, 1998; Vickers, 2000; Bodeker *et al.*, 2005). The number of randomised trials of complementary treatments has doubled every five years (Vickers, 2000). Many people turn to this therapy when conventional medicine fails them or because they believe strongly in the effectiveness of complementary medicine. Complementary therapies vary from herbal medicine, homeopathy, acupuncture, massage, aromatherapy, therapeutic exercise, dietary supplements, to meditation. Because of the chronic course and the impact of the HIV-related diseases on quality of life and the possibility of severe complications and death, patients with HIV/AIDS are very likely to seek CAM therapies (Ernst, 1997, Ozsoy & Ernst, 1999; Faragon *et al.*, 2002), particularly in the areas of the world where HAART is not available or not economically feasible. A survey by telephone in the United States found that HIV-infected persons used CAM at a high rate, made frequent visits to CAM providers, incurred substantial expenditures, and reported considerable improvement with these treatments (Fairfield *et al.*, 1998). Generally, people with HIV/AIDS use complementary therapies for three main reasons: the enhancement of their immune function, treatment of HIV-related symptoms, and management of medication-related side effects.

12.2. Herbal Medicine in HIV and AIDS

A previous systematic review published in 1999 identified two randomised trials on herbal medicines for HIV infection (Ozsoy & Ernst, 1999). A recent Cochrane systematic review assessed the beneficial and harmful effects of herbal medicines in patients with HIV infection and AIDS (Liu *et al.*, 2004). This review used a comprehensive approach to search both electronic databases and handsearch relevant journals to include randomised clinical trials and quasi-randomised trials that compared herbal medicines with no intervention, placebo, or anti-retroviral drugs in patients with HIV infection, HIV-related disease, or AIDS. The outcome measurements included mortality, HIV disease progression, new AIDS-defining events, adverse events, CD4 cell counts, viral loads, psychological status and health-related quality of life, and health economics.

The review identified eight randomised clinical trials that tested seven different herbal medicines involving 473 HIV infected individuals or AIDS patients compared with placebo (Table 12.1). Methodological quality was assessed as generally adequate in studies as full publication. The reported outcomes included progress to AIDS-related events, symptoms, health-related quality of life, viral loads, CD4 cell counts, and adverse effects.

A randomised trial enrolled 30 symptomatic people with HIV, with CD4 cell counts between 200 and 499 in the United States, to receive a 12-week course of 31 Chinese herbs (IGM-1) or placebo (Burack *et al.*, 1996). The study found significantly better effect in improvement of health-related quality of life than placebo. However, there was no significant difference in overall health perception, symptom severity, CD4 cell counts, anxiety or depression.

In a Swiss study, 68 people with HIV were randomised to receive a six-month course of treatment with 35 herbs Chinese herbal medicine, or placebo (Weber *et al.*, 1999). All participants had CD4 cell counts below 500, and were comparable regarding previous anti-retroviral use, viral loads and CD4 cell counts at entry. After six months, there was no significant difference in CD4 cell counts, HIV-1 RNA loads, new AIDS-defining events, number of reported symptoms, psychosocial measurements, and quality of life between arms. Gastrointestinal discomforts were more common amongst herb recipients (79% versus 38%).

SPV-30 is a natural herb preparation extracted from an evergreen tree called the Boxwood (*Buxus sempervirens* L.). This plant was listed in the *French Pharmacopoeia* 10th edition (Durant *et al.*, 1998). A pilot randomised double-blind trial was conducted in 1992 in France (Durant & Dellamonica, 1997), and 43 asymptomatic HIV patients with CD4 cell counts between 250 and 500 $\times$ 10^6/l were included in the SPV-30 group (n = 22) and placebo group (n = 21). SPV-30 (or placebo) was administered at a dose of 330 mg three times a day for 30 weeks. The results showed that patients receiving SPV-30 had a lower risk for progressing to AIDS-related complications and decrease of CD4 cell counts below 200 $\times$ 10^6/l. Based on this study, 145 previously untreated patients with asymptomatic

Table 12.1.　Summary of Seven Included Randomised Trials on Herbal Medicines for HIV/AIDS.

Study ID (Country)	Design	Participants (No.)	Treatment	Control	Outcome Measures	Findings
Burack *et al.*, 1996 (USA)	Parallel, two arms, double-blind trial	Symptomatic HIV-infected people with decreased CD4 cells (30)	Chinese herbal preparation (IGM-1) for 12 weeks	Placebo	Symptoms, CD4 cell counts, quality of life, adverse effects	Overall life satisfaction improved in patients treated with herbs, no difference in CD4 cell counts and symptom severity
Durant and Dellamonica, 1997 (France)	Parallel, two arms, double-blind trial	Asymptomatic, HIV-infected people with decreased CD4 cells (43)	SPV30 (*Buxus sempervirens* L. Preparations), 990 mg/day, for 30 weeks	Placebo	AIDS-related events, CD4 cell counts, adverse effects	Patients treated with SPV-30 had a lower risk for progressing to AIDS-related events, and decrease of CD4 cell counts
Durant *et al.*, 1998 (France)	Multi-centre, parallel, three arms, double-blind trial	Asymptomatic, HIV-infected people with decreased CD4 cells (145)	SPV30 (*Buxus sempervirens* L. Preparations), 990 mg/day, 1980 mg/day, for 37 weeks	Placebo	AIDS-related events, CD4 cell counts, viral loads, adverse effects	A tendency toward less AIDS-related events in herb group (RR 0.12, 95% CI 0.01–1.08; p = 0.06); no difference in CD4 cell counts and viral loads between groups
Hellinger *et al.*, 1996 (USA)	Parallel, two arms, dose finding trial	HIV-positive people (40)	Oral curcumin (extract of spice turmeric) for eight weeks	Different dosage	HIV viral loads, CD4 cell counts	No difference in decreases of viral loads and change of CD4 cell counts

Table 12.1. (*Continued*)

Study ID (Country)	Design	Participants (No.)	Treatment	Control	Outcome Measures	Findings
Holodniy *et al.*, 1999 (USA)	Multi-centre, parallel, two arms, double-blind trial	AIDS patients with diarrhoea (51)	SP-303 (herbal extract from *Croton lechleri*) for two days	Placebo	Symptom of diarrhoea, adverse effects	Improvement of symptom of diarrhoea in herb group
Sangkitporn *et al.*, 2004 (Thailand)	Multi-centre, double-blind, placebo controlled trial	Adults with HIV-1 infection (60)	Chinese herbal compound-SH (five herbs) for 24 weeks	Placebo	HIV RNA, CD4 cell counts, adverse effects	Significant decrease in HIV RNA in SH group vs placebo, without serious adverse events
Shi and Peng, 2003 (China)	Parallel, two arms, double-blind trial	HIV-infected male adults and AIDS patients (36)	Qiankunning (extracts from 14 herbs) for seven months	Placebo	CD4 cell counts, viral loads, adverse effects	No significant difference in HIV-1 RNA levels between groups
Weber *et al.*, 1999 (Switzerland)	Parallel, two arms, double-blind trial	HIV-infected adults with decreased CD4 cells (68)	Chinese herbs (35 herbs) for six months	Placebo	AIDS-related events, CD4 cell counts, viral loads, quality of life, adverse effects	No positive findings for the outcomes, and herbs associated with adverse effects

HIV infection and decreased CD4 cell counts were randomised to SPV30 (990 mg/day, n = 48), SPV30 (1980 mg/day, n = 49), or placebo (n = 48) for treatment of 37 weeks (Durant *et al.*, 1998). There was an insignificant tendency that the occurrence of AIDS-related complications was less frequent in the SPV30 group than in the placebo group. SPV30 was not more effective than placebo in CD4 cell counts or viral loads. Both trials did not report severe adverse effects.

Chinese herbal medicine Qiankunning is composed of 14 herbs (Shi & Peng, 2003). Thirty-six male adults with HIV infection or AIDS were randomised to receive Qiankunning (n = 18) or placebo (n = 18) (Shi & Peng, 2003). Among the outcomes reported, data of HIV-1 RNA levels were available. Both intention-to-treat analysis and computer data analysis showed that there was no significant difference in HIV-1 RNA levels between Qiankunning and placebo after the end of seven months' treatment. In this trial, the use of medicinal herbs was related to gastroenterological adverse effects (Shi & Peng, 2003).

SP-303, a South American herb preparation, was evaluated in 51 patients with AIDS and diarrhoea who were randomised to receive SP-303 (n = 26) or placebo (n = 25) (Holodniy *et al.*, 1999). According to an analysis of the treatment effect over four days based on daily measurements by random regression models, patients treated with SP-303 experienced a statistically significant reduction in stool weight (p = 0.008) and in abnormal stool frequency (p = 0.04) when compared with placebo. The trial also reported outcome of stool chloride concentration. No other relevant outcomes were reported. The trial reported that treatment with SP-303 was well tolerated, with no major difference between SP-303 and placebo in the occurrence of adverse events or in laboratory abnormalities.

A randomised clinical trial enrolled 40 HIV-positive people treated by two doses of oral curcumin (extract from spice turmeric) (4800 mg/day versus 2700 mg/day) (Hellinger *et al.*, 1996). There was no significant difference in decrease of viral loads or change of CD4 cell counts during eight weeks of therapy. A Chinese herbal compound-SH containing five herbs were combined with zidovudine and zalcitabine in the treatment of 60 HIV-infected Thai patients in a randomised trial (Sangkitporn *et al.*, 2004). The trial found that adding SH herbs to the two nucleoside reverse transcriptase inhibitors has greater antiviral activity than anti-retrovirals alone. However, the above benefits need to be accounted for with care because the number of patients in these trials is small and the size of effects is moderate.

The review concluded that no compelling evidence exists to support the use of herbal medicines for HIV infection and AIDS. Further studies should be large, and rigorous controlled designs are needed to assess the safety and efficacy of such interventions. Attention to possible harmful interactions between herbal medicines and conventional drugs should be paid (Izzo & Ernst, 2001).

12.3. Acupuncture and Massage in HIV Infection and AIDS

Although acupuncture is used by people with HIV disease as a complementary treatment to western medicine, research studies resulted in different findings. A prospective pilot study was conducted using low-voltage non-invasive electroacupuncture in 11 HIV/AIDS patients who had anti-retroviral drug-induced neuropathy (Galantino *et al.*, 1999). The study showed that low-voltage electroacupuncture improved the condition of neuropathy, but the positive finding was based on data from seven patients who completed the treatment. However, a randomised controlled trial showed that neither a standardised acupuncture regimen nor amitriptyline was more effective than placebo in relieving pain caused by HIV-related peripheral neuropathy (Shlay *et al.*, 1998). Another pilot randomised trial with small numbers of participants demonstrated trends toward improvement in symptoms and quality of life in HIV-infected patients (Beal & Nield-Anderson, 2000).

A randomised trial compared massage therapy with progressive muscle relaxation twice per week for 12 weeks in 24 HIV positive adolescents with CD4 cell counts less than 500 (Diego *et al.*, 2001). The participants from both groups reported feeling less anxious and less depressed, and showed enhanced immune function by the end of the study. CD4/CD8 ratio and CD4 cell counts showed increase only in the massage group. Twenty-eight neonates born to HIV-positive mothers were assigned randomly to a massage therapy (15 minutes daily for ten days) or control group (Scafidi & Field, 1996). The trial showed better performance on newborn score and a greater daily weight gain favouring massage therapy. A multi-centre, randomised controlled pilot trial compared therapeutic touch with mimic therapeutic touch in 20 HIV-infected children (Ireland, 1998). Therapeutic touch resulted in lower overall mean anxiety scores compared with mimic touch. Thus, it provides preliminary support for the use of therapeutic touch in reducing the state anxiety of children with HIV infection.

12.4. Homeopathy in HIV Infection and AIDS

A literature review identified five controlled clinical trials evaluating homeopathic treatment for HIV-positive or AIDS patients (Ullman, 2003). A randomised, double-blinded, placebo-controlled study was conducted on 50 asymptomatic HIV-positive subjects (stage II) and 50 subjects with persistent generalised lymphadenopathy (stage III) in whom individualised single-remedy homeopathic treatment was provided. Based on patients' symptoms, a total of 25 different homeopathic medicines were prescribed. The study found no statistically significant improvement in CD4 T-lymphocytes, but in AIDS subjects at stage III, there was statistically significant change in CD4 cell counts ($p = 0.008$) and an elevation of CD8 cell counts ($p = 0.04$).

Two preliminary randomised double-blinded, placebo-controlled studies were conducted with a total of 77 people with AIDS who used only natural therapies over an eight- to 16-week period without use of antivirals or steroids. Two other follow-up studies in an open-label format were conducted over a 2.5-year period with 27 subjects to evaluate the long-term effects of these homeopathic medicines. One of these follow-up studies compared natural approaches with and without homeopathic growth factors to antivirals drug therapies. Seven subjects received homeopathic growth factors plus natural therapies, six subjects were given natural therapies without homeopathic growth factors, and 14 subjects were given antiviral drugs. These studies found physical, immunologic, neurological, metabolic, and quality-of-life benefits from the homeopathic growth factors. However, since the studies were quite small and preliminary, one cannot determine the association of specific benefits with the homeopathic growth factors. Further large studies are needed. The review concluded that homeopathic medicine may play a useful role as an adjunctive and/or alternative therapy.

12.5. Vitamins and Other Supplements for HIV/AIDS

A randomised, double-blind, placebo-controlled trial was conducted in pregnant women infected with HIV in Tanzania (Fawzi *et al.*, 2004). Sixty-seven out of 271 women who received multivitamins had disease progression to WHO stage IV disease or died, compared with 83 of 267 women who received placebo. Multivitamins also resulted in significantly higher CD4 and CD8 cell counts and significantly lower viral loads. The study concludes that multivitamin supplements delay the progression of HIV disease and provide an effective, low-cost means of delaying the initiation of anti-retroviral therapy in HIV-infected women. A randomised placebo-controlled trial tested multiple micronutrient supplementation for 48 weeks in 481 HIV-infected individuals with CD4 cell counts ranging from 50–550 in Thailand (Jiamton *et al.*, 2003). Multiple micronutrient may enhance the survival of HIV-infected individuals with CD4 cell counts less than 200. The authors suggest positive finding to be reproduced in other setting.

A randomised, double-blind, placebo-controlled pilot study found a promising effect of arginine supplementation on immune function in persons with HIV/AIDS, which warrants further study with larger sample and longer periods (Swanson *et al.*, 2002). A randomised, double-blind, placebo-controlled trial evaluated the impact of selenium chemoprevention on hospitalisations in HIV-positive individuals (Burbano *et al.*, 2002). Selenium supplementation appears to be a beneficial adjunct treatment to decrease hospitalisations as well as the cost of caring for HIV-1-infected patients. L-glutamine supplementation was tested in a randomised, double-blind, placebo-controlled crossover study in HIV-infected patients with nelfinavir-associated diarrhoea for more than one month (Huffman & Walgren, 2003). L-glutamine 30 g/day significantly reduced the severity of nelfinavir-associated diarrhoea and improved quality of life in HIV-infected participants. Nutritional supplements combined with dietary counselling diminish whole body protein catabolism in HIV-infected patients compared with no supplements or nutritional advice in a randomised trial (Berneis *et al.*, 2000). But the nutritional intervention had no significant effect on CD4 cell counts and on quality of life.

12.6. Mind-Body Therapy in HIV/AIDS

There is no controlled study on mind-body therapy in HIV and AIDS. A prospective observational cohort investigated one-year change in self-reported quality of life by use of 13 mind-body interventions including psychological, spiritual and energy therapies among HIV-1-positive individuals (Standish *et al.*, 2004). Evidence from this longitudinal study shows that participation in spiritual activities may improve mental health status for HIV-positive individuals.

12.7. Aromatherapy in HIV/AIDS

Aromatherapy is defined as the use of essential oils from aromatic plants for treatment of diseases or conditions especially related to stress. It has been used as part of nursing care in Switzerland, Germany, Australia, Canada, the United Kingdom, and more recently, in the United States. As antimicrobial agents, essential oils may have potential in HIV/AIDS for specific opportunistic infections such as *Cryptococcus neoformans*, *Candida albicans*, methicillin-resistant *Staphylococcus aureus*, and herpes simplex types I and II (Buckle, 2002). Methods of application vary depending on the site of infection and the psychological profile of the patient and can include inhalation, compresses, baths, massage, and the 'm' technique. However, aromatherapy needs to be evaluated in clinical trials in HIV/AIDS.

12.8. Clinical Research Priorities in CAM for HIV/AIDS

The objectives of CAM research in the treatment of HIV/AIDS are to identify safe and effective CAM therapies that have potential roles in treating HIV/AIDS and its complications, or to ameliorate medication side effects; to establish possible synergistic combinations of CAM and conventional treatments for HIV; and to understand mechanisms of action of CAM therapies. According to a research funding initiative by the National Center for Complementary and Alternative Medicine, USA (NCCAM, 2002), the following is a list of the possible types of studies that might be undertaken:

- The use of CAM interventions to decrease symptoms of HIV infection or medication side effects.
- Clinical studies of herbs shown to have anti-HIV activity *in vitro*.
- Studies of the effects of herbs or other CAM interventions, alone or in combination with anti-retroviral therapy, on progression of HIV infection or on patient adherence.
- Projects to characterise and investigate the safety and efficacy of traditional medicine treatments in widespread use.
- Studies of the potential benefits to persons with HIV infection of dietary supplements such as vitamins A, C, E, selenium, and natural substances.
- Studies of the impact of massage therapy and other manual therapies on objective and subjective measures of symptoms and HIV infection.
- The use of CAM interventions to improve the well-being or enhance quality of life for patients with HIV infection.
- Studies of the benefits of using homeopathic remedies in HIV-infected patients.
- Studies on the potential role for energy therapies including therapeutic touch, Qi gong, or magnets in treating symptoms or slowing the progression of HIV infection.
- Studies to assess the impact, using objective or subjective measures, of using meditation and other mind-body interventions on patients with HIV infection.
- Outcomes research investigating the use of a single CAM modality, a combination of CAM modalities, or traditional medicine approaches, alone or in association with conventional treatment for HIV/AIDS.

References

Beal MW, Nield-Anderson L. Acupuncture for symptom relief in HIV-positive adults: lessons learned from a pilot study. *Altern Ther Health Med* 2000; 6:33–42.

Berneis K, Battegay M, Bassetti S, Nuesch R, Leisibach A, Bilz S *et al.* Nutritional supplements combined with dietary counselling diminish whole body protein catabolism in HIV-infected patients. *Eur J Clin Invest* 2000; 30:87–94.

Bodeker G, Ong C-K, Grundy C, Burford G, Maehira Y (eds.) *WHO Global Atlas of Traditional, Complementary and Alternative Medicine*. Kobe, Japan: WHO Centre for Health Development, 2005.

Bonfanti P, Capetti A, Rizzardini G. HIV disease treatment in the era of HAART. *Biomed Pharmacother* 1999;53:93–105.

Buckle J. Clinical aromatherapy and AIDS. *J Assoc Nurses AIDS Care* 2002; 13:81–89.

Burack JH, Cohen MR, Hahn JA, Abrams DI. Pilot randomised controlled trial of Chinese herbal treatment for HIV-associated symptoms. *J Acquir Immune Defic Syndr Hum Retrovirol* 1996;12(4):386–393.

Burbano X, Miguez-Burbano MJ, McCollister K, Zhang G, Rodrigues A, Ruiz P *et al.* Impact of a selenium chemoprevention clinical trial on hospital admissions of HIV-infected participants. *HIV Clin Trials* 2002;3:483–491.

Diego MA, Field T, Hernandez-Reif M, Shaw K, Friedman L, Ironson G. HIV adolescents show improved immune function following massage therapy. *Intern J Neurosci* 2001;106:35–45.

Durant J, Chantre PH, Gonzalez G, Vandermander J, Halfon PH, Rousse B. Efficacy and safety of *Buxus semperirens* L. preparations (SPV 30) in HIV-infected asymptomatic patients: a multicentre, randomised, double-blind, placebo-controlled trial. *Phytomedicine* 1998;5(1):1–10.

Durant J, Dellamonica P. Efficacy of SPV on asymptomatic patients with HIV-positive: a randomised double-blind placebo controlled trial. *IV Congress of the Mediterranean Society of Infectious and Parasitic Diseases*, 1997, pp. 30–59.

Eisenberg DM, Davis RB, Ettner SL, Appel S, Wilkey S, Rompay MV *et al.* Trends in alternative medicine use in the United States, 1990–1997. Results of a follow-up national survey. *JAMA* 1998;280:1569–1575.

Ernst E. Complementary AIDS therapies: the good, the bad and the ugly. *Int J STD AIDS* 1997;8:281–285.

Ernst E. Complementary medicine: common misconceptions. *J R Soc Med* 1995;88:244–247.

Fairfield KM, Eisenberg DM, Davis RB, Libman H, Philips RS. Patterns of use, expenditures, and perceived efficacy of complementary and alternative therapies in HIV-infected patients. *Arch Intern Med* 1998;158:2257–2264.

Faragon JJ, Purdy BD, Piliero PJ. An assessment of herbal therapy use, adherence and utilization of pharmacy services in HIV clinics. *J Herbal Pharmacother* 2002;2:27–37.

Fawzi WW, Msamanga GI, Spiegelman D, Wei R, Kapiga S, Villamor E *et al.* A randomised trial of multivitamin supplements and HIV disease progression and mortality. *N Engl J Med* 2004;351:23–32.

Galantino ML, Eke-Okoro ST, Findley TW, Condoluci D. Use of non-invasive eletroacupuncture for the treatment of HIV-related peripheral neuropathy: a pilot study. *J Altern Complement Med* 1999;5:135–142.

Hellinger JA *et al.* Phase I/II randomised, open-label study of oral curcumin safety, and antiviral effects on HIV-RT PCR in HIV+ individuals? *Third Conference on Retroviruses and Opportunistic Infections*, Washington, 1996, Abstract 140.

Holodniy M, Koch J, Mistal M, Schmidt JM, Khandwala A, Pennington JE *et al.* A double-blind, randomised, placebo-controlled phase II study to assess the safety and efficacy of orally administered SP-303 for the symptomatic treatment of diarrhea in patients with AIDS. *Am J Gastroenterol* 1999;94(11):3267–3273.

Huffman FG, Walgren ME. L-glutamine supplementation improves nelfinavir-associated diarrhea in HIV-infected individuals. *HIV Clin Trials* 2003; 4:324–329.

Ireland M. Therapeutic touch with HIV-infected children: a pilot study. *J Assoc Nurses AIDS Care* 1998;9:68–77.

Izzo AA, Ernst E. Interactions between herbal medicines and prescribed drugs: a systematic review. *Drugs* 2001;61:2163–2175.

Jiamton S, Pepin J, Suttent R, Filteau S, Mahakkanukrauh B, Hanshaoworakul W *et al.* A randomised trial of the impact of multiple micronutrient supplementation on mortality among HIV-infected individuals living in Bangkok. *AIDS* 2003;17:2461–2469.

Liu JP, Manheimer E, Yang M. Herbal medicines for treating HIV infection and AIDS (Cochrane Review). *The Cochrane Library*, 2004 (in press).

NCCAM. *Complementary and Alternative Medicine Therapy in the Treatment of HIV/AIDS*. http://grants1.nih.gov/grants/guide/rfa-files/RFA-AT-03-001.html. Accessed by 25 October 2002.

Ozsoy M, Ernst E. How effective are complementary therapies for HIV and AIDS? — a systematic review. *Int J STD AIDS* 1999;10:629–635.

Sangkitporn DR, Luo SD, Klinbuayaem DR, Leenasirimakul DR, Wirayutwatthana DR, Leechanachai DR *et al.* Efficacy and safety of Zidovudine and Zalcitabine combined with combination of herbs in the treatment of HIV-infected Thai patients. *Abstract of XV International AIDS Conference*, Bangkok, Thailand, July 2004:B10233.

Scafidi F, Field T. Massage therapy improves behavior in neonates born to HIV-positive mothers. *J Pediatr Psychol* 1996;21:889–897.

Shafer RW, Vuitton DA. Highly active antiretroviral therapy (HAART) for the treatment of infection with human immunodeficiency virus type 1. *Biomed Pharmacother* 1999;53:73–86.

Shi D, Peng ZL. Randomised, double-blind, placebo-controlled clinical study on Qiankunning for HIV/AIDS. *J Tradit Chin Med Res* 2003;21(9): 1472–1474.

Shlay JC, Chaloner K, Max MB, Flaws B, Reichelderfer P, Wentworth D *et al.* Acupuncture and amitriptyline for pain due to HIV-related peripheral neuropathy: a randomised controlled trial. *JAMA* 1998;280:1590–1595.

Standish LJ, Fitzpatrick AL, Berger J, Kim JG, Sanders F, Polissar N *et al.* Mind-body therapies and quality of life in HIV-1+ individuals. *Int J Naturopath Med* 2004;1:23–31.

Swanson B, Keithley JK, Zeller JM, Sha BE. A pilot study of the safety and efficacy of supplemental arginine to enhance immune function in persons with HIV/AIDS. *Nutrition* 2002;18:688–690.

Tirelli U, Bernardi D. Impact of HAART on the clinical management of AIDS-related cancers. *Eur J Cancer* 2001;37:1320–1324.

Ullman D. Controlled clinical trials evaluating the homeopathic treatment of people with human immunodeficiency virus or acquired immune deficiency syndrome. *J Altern Complement Med* 2003;9:133–141.

Vella S, Palmisano L. Antiretroviral therapy: state of the HAART. *Antiviral Res* 2000;45:1–7.

Vickers A. Recent advances: complementary medicine. *Br Med J* 2000; 321:683–686.

Weber R, Christen L, Loy M, Schaller S, Christen S, Joyce CR *et al.* Randomised, placebo-controlled trial of Chinese herb therapy for HIV-infected individuals. *J Acquir Immune Defic Syndr* 1999;22(1):56–64.

World Health Organization (WHO). *Scaling Up Antiretroviral Therapy in Resource-Limited Settings.* http://www.who.int/HIV_AIDS/first.html. (2002). Accessed by July 2003.

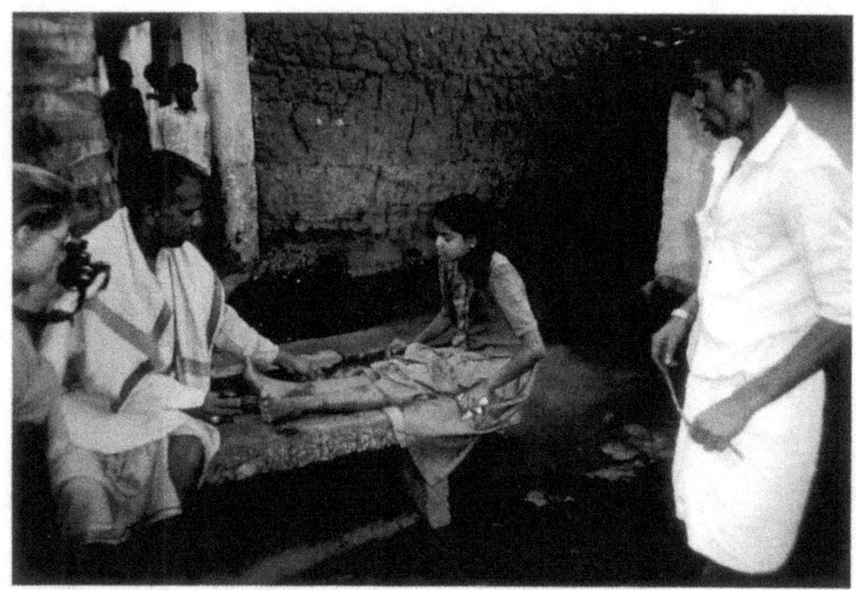

A village herbalist in Karnataka, India, treats a chronic skin condition. (*Photo courtesy of G. Bodeker.*)

CHAPTER 13

SKIN AND WOUND CARE: TRADITIONAL, COMPLEMENTARY AND ALTERNATIVE MEDICINE IN PUBLIC HEALTH DERMATOLOGY[1]

Gemma Burford, Gerard Bodeker and Terence J. Ryan

13.1. Introduction

The skin is the body's largest organ, and its failure to function correctly —
whether as a result of wounds, infections, cancer or inherited disorders —
is a major cause of morbidity and disability. Skin disease is very common,
affecting around one-quarter to one-third of the population (Williams,
1997). The social impact of skin failure is compounded by its visibility:
unsightly skin diseases such as eczema or psoriasis, and other conditions
such as albinism, can lead to social rejection and a lack of confidence in
one's appearance. Thus, relatively minor skin complaints often cause more
anguish to people than other, more serious medical conditions. The loss of
the so-called 'look good/feel good' factor has been described by Ong &
Ryan (1994) as 'the greatest disability of all'.

---

[1] This chapter builds on work originally published as: Burford G, Bodeker G, Ryan TJ. Traditional,
complementary and alternative medicine. In Skin and Wound Care. *Int J Dermatol* (in press).

Biomedical health care systems have tended to assign a relatively low priority to the skin, as illustrated by the fact that treatments for skin conditions and wounds comprise only 1–3% of all pharmaceuticals, most of which are either antibiotics or steroids. In the traditional health care sector, by contrast, skin and wound treatments are estimated to account for approximately a third of all traditional medicines (Balick & Cox, 1996). This figure may not include the natural products applied regularly to healthy skin in many parts of the world to promote hygiene, such as 'soap plants' (Section 13.4, below) and emollients (Section 13.5). Other traditional/complementary interventions that do not involve topical application, such as Tai Chi Chuan, acupuncture and music therapy, can also have a beneficial effect on skin health, as discussed in Section 13.2.1.

The distinction between skin disease and 'cosmetic' skin problems is unclear in biomedicine, but even more blurred in traditional systems of health care such as Ayurveda, which seek to nurture natural outer and inner beauty. Ayurveda aims to preserve youth and delay ageing, and recognises the importance of confidence in one's presentation to others. It finds skin lustre and radiance desirable, and uses emollients and massage as a means to achieve this healthy state. Such a system of medicine seeks equilibrium and wholeness of the body, and places much less value on the recognition of pattern and naming of physical signs that are so much a feature of the biomedical practice of dermatology. With its emphasis on purging and the removal of toxins by obtaining flow through various channels, as well as dietary regimens and behavioural advice, Ayurveda may have more in common with the cosmetic industry in industrialised countries than with 'conventional' dermatology.

13.1.1. *Epidemiology*

There have been few studies of the epidemiology of complementary and alternative medicine (CAM) use for skin conditions, and even fewer for traditional medicine. A systematic review of CAM utilisation surveys among dermatological patients in industrialised countries (Ernst, 2000) identified seven studies that met the inclusion criteria: lifetime prevalence of CAM utilisation was high but variable, ranging from 35% to 69%. More recent studies are summarised in Table 13.1, and continue to illustrate a high prevalence of utilisation, typically 40–50%. An analysis of data from the

Table 13.1. Prevalence of TCAM Utilisation for Skin Conditions: New Research Conducted Since 2000.

Country	Study Details	Major Findings	Reference
Taiwan	CAM utilisation questionnaire: 198 patients recruited from Dermatology Clinic, Show Chwan Memorial Hospital, Changhua City.	41% had used some form of TCAM for their skin conditions. Popular therapies included not only traditional Chinese medicine, but also 'Western' CAM.	Chen & Chang, 2003
United Kingdom	CAM utilisation questionnaire: 100 children with atopic dermatitis in secondary care in Leicester.	46% had used, or were currently using, some form of CAM. A further 17% intended to try CAM in the future.	Johnston *et al.*, 2003
United Kingdom	CAM utilisation survey questionnaire: 100 contact dermatitis patients in secondary care in Leicester.	30% of patients, and 62% of the Indo-Asian subgroup, had used some form of CAM for their condition.	Nicolaou & Johnston, 2004
United States	CAM utilisation questionnaire: 70 consecutive patients diagnosed with atopic dermatitis at a university clinic in Portland, Oregon.	50.4% used some form of CAM for their condition. Vitamin supplements and herbal creams were most popular.	Simpson *et al.*, 2003

Oxford Healthy Lifestyle Survey (Ong *et al.*, 2002) showed that about one in ten (9.8%) of respondents with a chronic skin condition had visited a complementary practitioner within three months of the survey. The study by Johnston *et al.* (2003) found a strong association ($P < 0.01$) between CAM utilisation and ethnicity among children with atopic dermatitis in the United Kingdom, and a follow-up study (Nicolaou & Johnston, 2004) of contact dermatitis patients at the same hospital showed the CAM utilisation rate for Indo-Asian patients to be more than twice the rate for the group as a whole.

We have identified only one study relating specifically to the utilisation of traditional medicine for skin conditions, with the exclusion of 'Western' CAM (Satimia *et al.*, 1998). In this study, face-to-face interviews and dermatological examinations were conducted among 800 villagers in a rural area of south-western Tanzania, to determine the prevalence of skin diseases and utilisation of health care facilities. The authors found that 37.4% of villagers had one or more skin diseases, and that modern and traditional health care facilities were equally used. Heads of households older than 55 years, and individuals who were not Christians, were found to prefer traditional medicine.

The high utilisation of TCAM services by dermatology patients in industrialised countries, as well as their ongoing use as the first and last resort for skin care in rural areas of many developing countries, illustrates the need for health care providers worldwide to gain an adequate understanding of these approaches. As in other fields of TCAM, the focus of most research to date has been scientific evaluation of individual treatments — often *in vitro*, in animals, or in small and poorly designed clinical trials — and, to a lesser extent, self-reporting of utilisation by patients attending conventional healthcare facilities. While there have been some promising developments in terms of evaluation at the formulation level, the majority of pre-clinical studies still follow similar protocols to those employed for the evaluation of pharmaceuticals, with little acknowledgement of the unique features of TCAM. Reports of serious side effects from Chinese herbal treatment are also a matter of concern.

This review cannot attempt to be comprehensive, for many reasons. A search of dermatological literature will tend to exclude nursing literature, or the literature on burns and wounds. We have concentrated on English language journals, especially those listed on MEDLINE. In the field of skin care, the majority of TCAM research reported in such journals relates to traditional Chinese medicine, which is popular in many other countries of the world. Healing modalities from the Indian subcontinent are underrepresented, and the situation is even worse in the case of traditional health care approaches from Africa, Latin America and the Middle East, for which only a small number of ethnobotanical and pre-clinical studies are available. There is also an evident literature bias in favour of treatments for chronic inflammatory skin conditions, which affect large numbers of patients in Europe and the United States, with relatively less attention paid to the infectious and parasitic conditions that continue to plague the developing world. The topic of preventative skin care is barely mentioned: Voegeli (2005) highlights the fact that in spite of the considerable time invested by nursing staff in washing patients suffering from chronic skin inflammation or at risk of skin breakdown, or assisting them to wash, there has been little scientific appraisal of these activities to date.

The literature on the skin for lay readers is often written by, and read by, the medical profession. This literature is huge in most nations, and many of the dermatological diagnostic categories cater for those affected through their societies and associations with substantial newsletters and guidelines. For example, the Dystrophic Epidermolysis Bullosa Research Association, DEBRA, has long had notable manuals on best management of the skin of child sufferers, and no such literature is indifferent to traditional practices.

This review underscores the importance of systematic research into the safety and cost-effectiveness of TCAM therapies, and the demographics of utilisation, as well as high-quality clinical studies for the assessment of efficacy. This applies not only to those non-biomedical interventions that are popular in the industrialised world, but also particularly to the traditional approaches that constitute the mainstay of skin care in the tropics. There is a need to translate research findings into practical action, without compromising the livelihoods of the rural poor.

13.2. TCAM Therapies for the Treatment of Skin Diseases

13.2.1. *Clinical Trials*

Reviews of the literature on TCAM treatments for inflammatory skin conditions such as eczema, psoriasis and atopic dermatitis indicate promising initial results, but a disappointing lack of 'gold standard' research. Many of the published clinical trials are very small, and/or methodologically flawed, and the diversity of TCAM treatments leads to difficulties in comparison. This is well illustrated by a systematic review of both biomedical and TCAM treatments for atopic eczema (Hoare *et al.*, 2000), which identified a total of 1165 possible randomised controlled trials. Of these, 893 (77%) were eliminated because of a lack of appropriate data, leaving 272 trials that covered at least 47 different interventions, broadly categorised into ten main groups. Of the TCAM treatments, only psychological approaches were classed as having 'reasonable RCT evidence to support use'. There was insufficient evidence to make recommendations on Chinese herbs, homeopathy, massage therapy, hypnotherapy or evening primrose oil.

A recent Cochrane review focusing specifically on randomised controlled trials of Chinese herbal preparations for treating atopic eczema (Zhang *et al.*, 2004) identified only four small, poorly reported trials of the same product, Zemaphyte, which met the inclusion criteria. In two out of the three placebo-controlled two-phase crossover trials, the reduction in erythema and surface damage was greater on Zemaphyte than on placebo, and participants slept better and itched less and expressed a preference for Zemaphyte. The reviewers recommended larger, well-designed trials of the product, but Zemaphyte is no longer being manufactured.

While we have not identified any systematic reviews, isolated RCTs have been conducted on polyherbal preparations for the treatment of other skin conditions. Zerehsaz *et al.* (1999) carried out a double blind randomised clinical trial of a topical herbal preparation, containing extract of *Althaea rosa*, *Althaea officinalis* and a number of other plants, versus systemic meglumine antimoniate for the treatment of cutaneous leishmaniasis in 171 patients in Iran. It was found that the herbal preparation achieved a 74% cure rate, compared with only 24% for the conventional treatment. Beltrami *et al.* (2001) conducted a clinical trial on a topical herbal formulation for the treatment of acne vulgaris, incorporating a lipophilic extract of *Krameria trianda* (anti-bacterial), *Serenoa repens* (which inhibits 5-α' reductase) and *Centella asiatica* (which stimulates collagen production). The findings included a significant increase in skin hydration, decreased transepidermal water loss and decreased sebum production in comparison with placebo.

Due to the magnitude of placebo effects — often comparable with treatment effects, but significantly higher than non-treatment protocols (Wampold *et al.*, 2005; Eisenberg, 1997) — and the nature of certain non-herbal therapies, it is evident that placebo-controlled RCTs are not necessarily the only valid means of evaluating the clinical efficacy of TCAM treatments. To cite just a few examples, case reports for acupuncture in the treatment of psoriasis (Liao & Liao, 1992) and facial skin diseases (Dai, 1997; Xu, 1990) have shown good results; regular practice of Tai Chi Chuan has been associated with improved endothelial function in the skin vasculature of older men (Wang *et al.*, 2002); and even listening to music by Mozart has been shown to reduce allergic skin wheal responses in atopic dermatitis patients with latex allergy (Kimata, 2003). Mind-body therapies may be helpful in treating melanoma, warts and psoriasis (Eisenberg, 1997).

There have been various efforts to develop protocols for sham acupuncture (Goddard *et al.*, 2005; Park *et al.*, 2002; Jerner *et al.*, 1997) and acupuncture at non-specific points (e.g. Joos *et al.*, 2004), but it is difficult to imagine how a double-blind methodology could meaningfully be employed for bodywork- or music-based therapies. In the light of this — and given that most TCAM practices are already in regular use in non-industrialised countries — there is clearly an argument for expanding the role of clinical observational studies, including case series, to follow basic toxicological research and perhaps a minimal pre-clinical assessment of efficacy.

Because there is a good response of the majority of skin-impaired patients to any care, it is the sub-groups of recalcitrant disease that, if they are not excluded at the beginning, may show a better response with traditional medicine (Henz *et al.*, 1999; Tjioe *et al.*, 2002). Titrating treatment to the needs of the patient, changing therapy from day to day, is a feature of TCAM that is incompatible with RCTs. It is, however, the way in which many patients use even their biomedical topical prescriptions, and they are consequently labelled non-concordant or non-compliant.

13.2.2. *Toxicological Studies*

It is often assumed that toxicological studies are unnecessary for traditional health care regimens, which have evolved over hundreds or even thousands of years and would have been discontinued if they were associated with serious side effects. However, this assumption does not necessarily hold true in every case. A medicine that is safely used in one setting may bring about an increased incidence of side effects when transferred to another population with a different genetic make-up, or when stored under different conditions. There is also a higher risk of problems with crude drug identification or labelling, and practitioner error in general, due to varying educational standards in different countries. The *Aristolochia* disaster in Belgium, in which over 100 women developed kidney failure and some died after consuming a Chinese herbal slimming preparation in which *Aristolochia fangchi* had been accidentally substituted for *Stephania* sp. (Vanherweghem, 1998) is probably the most extreme example, but even in the case of skin treatments, various side effects have been reported among users of Chinese medicines in industrialised countries. The most common is contact dermatitis (Lin-Feng, 1995; Lee & Lam, 1988), but more serious reactions have also been reported, such as cardiomyopathy (Ferguson *et al.*, 1997) and liver damage (Perharic *et al.*, 1995; Eisenberg, 1997).

Thus, there is an urgent need for improved standards of toxicological assessment, quality control and post-market surveillance for all TCAM therapies and practices, but particularly those that are widely used outside the communities in which they evolved. These issues are discussed in more depth by Shia *et al.* (Chapter 4 of this volume). Research into toxicology may also include ways of mitigating or abolishing the side effects of TCAM therapies, as in the example of *Gingko biloba* seed pulp, which induces severe contact dermatitis: some causative constituents can be removed, and the protective effects against sunburn enhanced by chemical manipulation (Kim, 2001).

13.2.3. *Pre-clinical Research*

In recent years, dermatologists have developed a number of distinctive pre-clinical research methodologies for studying the skin, many of which are useful in the evaluation of TCAM therapies. Trans-epidermal water loss is often used as a tool for studying barrier function (e.g. Darmstadt *et al.*, 2002). The blood supply of the skin has been especially well studied in China, using non-invasive techniques such as nailfold video microscopy and laser Doppler flowmetry (e.g. Ryan, 1996; Sander *et al.*, 2001). These seek to distinguish a healthy system from a disordered system, and restore the latter to health using oral Chinese herbal medicines, acupuncture and other Chinese traditional systems.

Standard protocols for the evaluation of pharmaceuticals *in vitro* or in animals often need to be modified for traditional preparations, in order to make them as relevant as possible to the real contexts of utilisation (c.f. Yuan & Lin, 2000). Scientific convention demands evaluation at the level of the single 'active ingredient', but in pre-clinical studies of traditional health care there is now a growing appreciation of the importance of synergism — both between compounds within a single plant, and between different plants in a mixture. A study by Tatsumi *et al.* (2001) illustrates this point well.

Oral administration of *Byakko-ka-ninjin-to* (Bai-Hu-Jia-Ren-Sheng-Tang), a traditional Japanese herbal formula, inhibits the IgE-mediated triphasic skin reaction in mice. It has been shown, however, that variant formulas missing one of the crude drugs are less effective than the complete formulation, and in HPLC profiles, some peaks could be detected only when all five crude drugs were simultaneously present during the preparation phase. Other examples of pre-clinical research conducted on Oriental medicines for skin diseases at the formulation level include studies by Lin *et al.* (2000), Tahara *et al.* (1999), Matsumoto *et al.* (1997) and Higaki *et al.* (1997). The synergistic interaction of different components within a single plant is discussed by Dattner (2003) with reference to the anti-bacterial, anti-inflammatory, and bile-stimulating properties of Oregon grape root (*Mahonia aquifolium*), making the crude extract useful in acne.

13.3. Traditional Medicine in the Treatment of Wounds and Burns

13.3.1. *'First Aid' for Acute Wounds*

Traditional systems of health care can be useful in administering immediate 'first aid' for wounds, by preventing excessive blood loss, microbial infection and oxidative damage. Many local communities worldwide have recognised the importance of haemostatic compounds in plants: almost all ethnobotanical inventories contain some reference to leaves (and occasionally other plant parts) that can be applied to wounds to halt bleeding. Informants can often name several common plants useful for this purpose, since awareness of a number of different haemostats increases the likelihood that one will be close at hand in an emergency. Bhattarai (1997) lists 42 plant species used in wound treatment in Nepal, and of these, eight are listed as haemostats.

A great many traditional wound treatments have antimicrobial properties. Indeed, the very existence of secondary metabolites in plants is an adaptive response to microbial attack: as Ryan (1997) points out, *'plants have learned to deal with bacteria and viruses probably long before the human being did so'*. The antiseptic properties of plant preparations can be studied very easily without the use of sophisticated equipment, and there is a wide literature on the subject. Watt & Breyer-Brandwijk (1962), Kokwaro (1993) and Hutchings *et al.* (1996) have provided comprehensive overviews of primary literature on the anti-microbial properties of plants in Southern and Eastern Africa. Indian and Chinese journals, in particular, continue to publish many such studies, together with international journals such as the *Journal of Ethnopharmacology*. Biswas & Mukherjee (2003) have reviewed 164 plant medicines of Indian origin that are utilised for wound healing. In a commentary on this paper in the same journal, Ryan (2003) highlights the difficult terminology of both botany and dermatology: 1613 plants in India have 12,699 names (Kareem, 1997) and every ethnic group also has its own terminology for wounds.

One specific example of a plant product now marketed internationally as a topical anti-microbial is *Melaleuca alternifolia* (tea tree) oil, which has been found to be 13 times stronger than phenol as an antiseptic (Altman, 1989; see also Williams *et al.*, 1988, and Carson *et al.*, 1998).

Both honey (reviewed by Molan, 1999 and 2001, and Bodeker *et al.*, 1999) and propolis (Ugur & Arslan, 2004; Stepanovic *et al.*, 2003) are also effective anti-microbial agents. In particular, honey may be useful in the treatment of methicillin-resistant strains of *Staphylococcus aureus* (MRSA), which are often difficult to eradicate by conventional means (Cooper *et al.*, 2002; Bonn, 2003). Propolis has been shown to work in synergy with conventional anti-microbials (Stepanovic *et al.*, 2003). However, the spores of gas gangrene and of tetanus have long been a risk factor in traditional practices using honey, as they have been for the use of dung on wounds.

In addition to preventing blood loss and bacterial infection, a third important aspect of 'first aid' for wounds is to neutralise reactive oxygen species such as superoxide radicals and hydrogen peroxide, which can cause significant tissue damage and delay healing (Cheatle, 1991; Martin, 1996). Thus, the antioxidant properties of plant constituents, such as polyphenols, may be as important as their antiseptic activity. Van Hien *et al.* (1997) have demonstrated that leaf extracts from the Vietnamese medicinal plant *Cudrania cochinchinensis* (Moraceae) can protect both fibroblasts and endothelial cells *in vitro* against oxidative damage induced by hydrogen peroxide. It is likely that many other plants used traditionally in wound treatment have similar properties.

13.3.2. *Longer-Term Wound Care: Debridement, Dressings and Tissue Repair*

Debridement is the removal of necrotic tissue and eschar from an older wound, in order to promote healing. Certain plants, such as papaya (*Carica papaya*) and some Australian spurges, are useful for this purpose (Ryan, 1997). However, other types of living organisms can also be used. Fly larvae (maggots) were traditionally used in wound healing in China, Burma, Australia and Central America (Grossmann, 1994), and the infestation of battlefield wounds during World War I drew attention to their beneficial effects. Larvae were abandoned as modern medicine gained in popularity, but in recent years there has been a resurgence of interest in their application, sometimes referred to as 'biosurgery' (Courtenay *et al.*, 2000). They have been demonstrated to be more effective than surgical debridement, as they are capable of removing all dead tissue — even under overhanging wound edges — with no damage to healthy tissue (Church, 1996; Bodeker *et al.*, 1999; Courtenay *et al.*, 2000). A certain species of fish, *Macropodus cupanus*, is similarly used in Trivandrum, Kerala State, India, where patients with leg wounds, infections and infestations often stand in 'holy pools' for debridement (Cohen, 2000). This method is said to be especially useful for wounds with high moisture content, which larvae are unable to debride.

Another important application of traditional health systems in chronic wound management is the provision of moist, non-adherent dressings that can keep wounds clean while promoting healing. The concept of natural dressings has a long history, particularly in India; references to the use of banana leaves and cabbage leaves for this purpose have been found in ancient Ayurvedic texts. Frog skin, a known anti-microbial, was traditionally used in India as a wound dressing, and gained popularity during the Vietnam War for the treatment of napalm burns (Bodeker *et al.*, 1999). More recently, the Burns Association of India has promoted boiled potato peel as a painless dressing that does not adhere to wounds (Patil, 1990). In a study in which potato peel was compared with plain gauze dressings, the application of the potato peel dressing reduced or eliminated dessication, permitted the survival of superficial skin cells and hastened epithelial regeneration, although it had no intrinsic anti-bacterial activity (Keswani *et al.*, 1990). It has been suggested that the steroidal glycoalkaloids in the peel may contribute to the favourable results (Dattatreya *et al.*, 1991). In a subsequent open controlled trial by Gore and Akolekar (2003), banana leaf dressing and boiled potato peel were found to have equal efficacy in protecting partial thickness burns and aiding healing. The authors recommend the use of banana leaf in the Indian context because it is cheaper, readily available throughout the year, and easy to grow.

There is evidence from *in vitro* and *in vivo* experiments that several of the traditional preparations applied to wounds play an active role in tissue repair. A wide variety of mechanisms have been cited, including the stimulation of fibroblast proliferation, protein precipitation (as part of the process of crusting), granulation tissue formation and re-epithelialisation. Bodeker *et al.* (1999) have reviewed many of these, and the findings are summarised in Table 13.2a. There are also several more recent studies demonstrating active tissue repair on application of natural products (many of them complex formulations) to experimental wounds in animals, using incision, excision and burn wound models (Table 13.2b).

As in the case of traditional preparations for inflammatory skin conditions, wound treatments often rely on synergism between different components, with important implications for research design. Chen *et al.* (1994) have demonstrated that the efficacy of the South American wound treatment 'dragon's blood' — sap from the bark of various *Croton* species (Euphorbiaceae) — cannot be attributed to a single constituent. Attempts to isolate an 'active ingredient' resulted in a decrease, rather than an increase, in the efficacy of healing. Their conclusion was that the sap acts as a natural dressing, forming an occlusive layer with an anti-microbial environment and cell proliferative effects, to which several compounds contribute.

13.4. TCAM Therapies and Practices for the Maintenance of Skin Health

13.4.1. *'Soap Plants' and Skin Hygiene*

Since ancient times, plants have been used throughout the world as affordable and readily available soap substitutes for washing the skin, hair and clothes. Bark, fruit, leaves, roots and seeds are variously utilised for this purpose in different societies. While some plants provide one of two

Table 13.2(a). Early Experimental Findings Demonstrating an Active Role for Traditional Preparations in Tissue Repair.

Plant Species	Experimental Findings	Reference(s)
Aloe barbadensis (Liliaceae): 'aloe vera'	In addition to anti-microbial properties, dilates capillaries to increase blood flow; inhibits thromboxane A2, a mediator of progressive tissue damage in burn injuries; local anaesthetic; maintains homeostasis in vascular endothelium.	Grindlay & Reynolds (1986); Robson *et al.* (1982)
Chromolaena odorata (Asteraceae)	Enhances haemostasis, stimulates granulation tissue and re-epithelialisation, and inhibits hydrated collagen lattice contraction by dermal fibroblasts.	Phan *et al.* (1996)
Croton spp. (Euphorbiaceae): 'dragon's blood'	Contains proanthocyanins, which promote wound contracture and protein precipitation; stimulates collagen formation and epithelial regeneration.	Pieters *et al.* (1995)
Cudrania cochinchinensis (Moraceae)	Stimulates fibroblast proliferation, in addition to protecting fibroblasts and endothelial cells against oxidative damage.	Van Hien *et al.* (1997)
Justica pectoralis (Acanthaceae)	Contains coumarin, which reduces inflammation and enhances wound healing *in vivo* in rats.	Mills *et al.* (1986)

(Adapted from Bodeker *et al.*, 1999).

substances — oil and ash — which are mixed together to produce the soap, others can be applied directly to the skin as 'traditional soaps'. Many of those in the latter category contain saponins, compounds whose characteristic property is the formation of lather when added to water.

Although researchers have thus far paid little attention to this context of plant utilisation, with the exception of one systematic ethnobotanical study conducted in Angola (Bossard, 1993), the importance of good skin hygiene and preventative health care is increasingly being recognised in tropical medicine. It is by now widely accepted that regular hand-washing with soap — especially after using the toilet and before preparing food — can bring about a significant decrease in the incidence of diarrhoea and other gastrointestinal disorders, and a reduction in childhood deaths, by removing pathogenic bacteria from hands. A recent systematic review of the relevant literature (Curtis & Cairncross, 2003) estimates the risk reduction at 47%,

Table 13.2(b). Recent Experimental Findings Demonstrating an Active Role for Traditional Formulations in Tissue Repair, Using *in Vivo* Wound Healing Models (MEDLINE Search, 2002–2005).

Methodology	Experimental Findings	Reference
Shiunko, a traditional Chinese formula, applied as ointment to sterilised and *Pseudomonas aeruginosa*-contaminated incision wounds in rats; controls treated with Povidone-iodine or saline.	Incidence of wound infection following *P. aeruginosa* inoculation lower in treated group than controls ($p < 0.01$). Higher percentage of complete epithelialisation on day 7 in treated group (100% in sterilised wounds, 90% in contaminated wounds) than control groups ($p < 0.01$).	Huang *et al.* (2004)
Extract of *Punica granulatum* peel as 10% (w/w) water-soluble gel and applied to excision wounds in rats; controls treated with commercial topical anti-bacterial gel.	Wound healing measured by percentage contraction in skin and measurement of hydroxyproline content. Group treated with 5.0% gel showed 59.5% and 44.5% healing compared with negative and positive controls, respectively. Complete healing observed on day 10 for 5.0% gel and after 16–18 days in positive controls.	Murthy *et al.* (2004)
10% (w/w) ethanolic extract of *Celosia argentea*, as ointment, applied to burn wounds in rats.	Wound closure occurred earlier in the treated rats (15 days vs. 30 in the untreated group; $p < 0.05$). Granulation tissue collected on every fifth day of healing showed an increase in collagen and hexosamine content at a faster rate in the treated wounds.	Priya *et al.* (2004)
10% and 5% (w/w) extracts of *Hamelia patens*, as ointment, applied to double incision wound model in rats. In Group I, left side treated with 5% *H. patens* and right with petroleum jelly (PJ); Group II, left treated with 10% *H. patens* and right with PJ; Group III, left treated with PJ and right untreated.	Breaking strength of incisions measured on days 7 and 12. No significant difference between *H. patens*-treated and PJ-treated incisions on day 7. Significant difference between *H. patens*-treated and PJ-treated incisions for Groups I and II on day 12. No significant difference between PJ-treated and untreated incisions for Group III on either day 7 or day 12.	Gomez-Beloz *et al.* (2003)

Table 13.2(b). *(Continued)*

Methodology	Experimental Findings	Reference
Ointment and lotion containing *Terminalia arjuna* extract applied to incision and excision wounds in rats; controls treated with nitrofurazone.	In both wound models, results with herbal formulations were comparable to controls in terms of wound contracting ability, epithelisation period, tensile strength and regeneration of tissues at the wound area.	Mukherjee *et al.* (2003)
10% (w/w) ethanolic extract of *Datura alba* Nees. applied to burn wounds in rats; controls untreated.	Effects of ointment, in terms of wound contracting ability, wound closure time, tissue regeneration at the wound site and histopathological characteristics were significant in treated rats. Collagen, hexosamine and gelatinase expressions correlated with observed healing pattern.	Priya *et al.* (2002)

and suggests that over a million deaths from diarrhoea could be averted every year by hand washing with soap. Washing with soap, together with the subsequent application of emollients to the skin, has also been cited as a useful morbidity control measure in global programmes for the elimination of lymphatic filariasis. The literature suggests strongly that what matters is the 'entry points' to the skin for bacteria: care of the skin to maintain barrier function is the most important management point to prevent cellulitis, and that no penicillin is needed if washing and emollients are well used (Ryan, 2004; Vaqas & Ryan, 2003).

The potential public health importance of effective traditional soaps is underscored by a hand washing study conducted in Bangladesh (Hoque *et al.*, 1995; Hoque, 2003) in which 75% of rural women claimed that they could not afford to buy commercial soap. In Burkina Faso, the total cost to households associated with the implementation of a hand-washing programme was $7.30 per year, or 1.3% of annual household income (Borghi *et al.*, 2002). Even where the cost of commercial soap is not prohibitive, traditional plant-based soaps have a significant advantage in terms of economic and environmental sustainability. They do not need to be imported or transported from urban centres, but can be produced exactly where they are needed, on a renewable basis.

In a preliminary search of published ethnobotanical literature and Internet sources (Burford *et al.*, in preparation), we identified 135 traditional soaps derived directly from plants — i.e. excluding those made from combinations of plant-based ashes and oils — representing 74 genera and 42 families. The families Agavaceae (13 species), Caryophyllaceae (12 species), Fabaceae (21 species) and Sapindaceae (7 species) were all well represented in the list. In some cases, the botanical names of the plants themselves reflect their widespread usage as soaps, based on the Latin root *sapon* — meaning soap, as in the case of *Aloe saponaria* (Asphodelaceae) and *Quillaja saponaria* (Rosaceae) as well as the genus *Saponaria* (Caryophyllaceae). The name of the family Sapindaceae is derived from a Latin term meaning 'soap of the Indes' (Oklahoma Biological Survey, 1999). Other plants have a common English name that provides the clue to usage, such as 'soap tree' (*Dracaena* sp., Dracaenaceae), 'soap berry' (*Shepherdia canadensis*, Elaeagnaceae), 'soap pod' (*Acacia concinna*, Fabaceae) or 'Ethiopian soap berry vine' (*Phytolacca dodecandra*, Phytolaccaceae). The plant *Chlorogalum pomeridianum*, whose bulb was traditionally dried and grated as soap flakes in California, has as many as five common names of this nature: soap plant, soap apple, soap weed, soap bulb and soap root. Several of the listed plants also have vernacular names that translate as some variation of 'soap plant'.

In several cases, there is scientific evidence to support traditional claims that these plants are 'good for the skin', as detailed in Table 13.3. Antimicrobial activity is perhaps the most obvious example, since the lather-generating saponins themselves are often toxic to bacteria, fungi, viruses and parasites. Additionally, some soap plants have been shown to possess anti-inflammatory, analgesic and/or immunomodulatory properties. The plant part generating the soap is not always the part that has been subjected to scientific analysis, as in the example of *Withania somnifera*, whose saponin-rich fruit can be used as soap (Emboden, 1979), but roots and bark, widely used in Indian traditional medicine, have both been extensively analysed for anti-bacterial activities (Owais *et al.*, 2005; Arora *et al.*, 2004) and a wide variety of other medicinal properties (reviewed by Mishra *et al.*, 2000).

Use of soap plants, like many other folk practices with preventative health benefits, has already declined throughout the industrialised world.

Table 13.3. Experimental Findings Relating to Selected Plants Currently or Historically Used as Soap Substitutes.

Plant Species	Ethnobotanical Use	Saponins	Effects
Aesculus hippocastanum, horse chestnut (Hippocastanaceae)	Seed historically used as soap in Europe	(A)escin(e), a mixture of triterpene saponins (Karuza & Blekic, 1995; Derkach *et al.*, 1999; Cristoni and Di Pierro, 1998)	Increases cAMP concentration, stimulating lipolysis and blood microcirculation: may be useful in managing cellulite (Cristoni and Di Pierro, 1998).
Agave americana, maguey or century plant (Agavaceae)	Flower used as soap in Central America	Agavasaponin, chlorogenin and others (Duke, 1992); spirostanol saponin and others (Yokosuka *et al.*, 2000)	Aqueous extract, and genins isolated from it, showed anti-inflammatory effects in a carrageenan-induced oedema model (Peana *et al.*, 1997).
Aloe saponaria, soap aloe (Aloeaceae)	Leaf pulp used as soap in Transkei, South Africa; also for treating wounds and ringworm	None cited	Anti-bacterial activity against three Gram-negative and two Gram-positive bacteria (Tian *et al.*, 2003).
Dracaena mannii, West African soap tree (Dracaenaceae)	Used as soap and antiseptic in West Africa (no further details)	Spiroconazole A and other saponins (Okunji *et al.*, 1996)	Fungicidal/fungistatic against 17 species of fungi; bacteriostatic against four species of bacteria; anti-leishmanial (Okunji *et al.*, 1996).

(Continued).

In 1934, Saunders (reprinted 1976) remarked, 'Before the white traders introduced the sale of commercial soap, *amole* [*Yucca* sp.] was universally used by Mexicans and Indians [Native Americans] for washing purposes, and the practice is not yet obsolete by any means'. Saunders also commented

Table 13.3. *(Continued)*

Plant Species	Ethnobotanical Use	Saponins	Effects
Guaiacum officinale Linn., soapbush (Zygophyllaceae)	Leaves historically used as soap in southern USA and Caribbean	Guaianin R and other saponins from bark (Ahmad *et al.*, 2004); guaianin M (Ahmad *et al.*, 1992)	Anti-inflammatory in carrageenan-induced oedema model in rats (Duwiejua *et al.*, 1994); anti-bacterial against *Shigella flexneiri, Klebsiella ozaenae* and *Corynebacterium xerosis* (Ahmad *et al.*, 1992).
Sapindus saponaria, Western soap berry (Sapindaceaé)	Fruit used as soap in Mexico and South America	Saponins present (Lemos *et al.*, 1992 and 1994)	Anti-bacterial against *Pseudomonas aeruginosa, Bacillus subtilis* and *Cryptococcus neoformans* (Lemos *et al.*, 1992).

on the pleasant effect of *amole* on the skin, 'leaving it soft and comfortable'. Today, however, soap plants have largely fallen out of use throughout Europe and North America. A similar trend can be observed in developing countries, as noted by Esser & Gundersen (1999) with reference to the use of *Phytolacca dodecandra* (*endod*) for soap in Ethiopia. Due to the low social status of *endod* soap, preference for commercial soap and clearance of land for cultivation of other crops, the plant itself is now disappearing from many areas. This particular example has wider public health implications than skin care alone: in 1964, the Ethiopian scientist Aklilu Lemma observed dead schistosomal vector snails in a river immediately downstream from where local people were washing clothes with *endod*, while live snails were found upstream and further downstream. Subsequent research (e.g. Goll *et al.*, 1983; Erko *et al.*, 2002) has shown the plant to be an effective molluscicide, useful in schistosomiasis control programmes.

In the light of the increasing erosion of traditional knowledge, there is clearly a need for a systematic research agenda relating to soap plants: ethnobotanical studies to document current and historical utilisation; pre-clinical studies to characterise saponins, identify anti-microbial or anti-inflammatory properties, and assess the risk of dermatological or systemic side-effects; epidemiological studies, in areas where soap plants are still widely used, to assess their role (if any) in maintaining skin health; and clinical trials to determine their efficacy against specific dermatological conditions.

13.4.2. *Emollients*

Emollients (moisturisers) are widely used throughout the developing world, often on a daily basis, to promote skin health and suppleness. Ryan (2004) states that 'in dermatology, the first commandment is the use of emollients', and they have been emphasised as a low cost management tool for morbidity control in lymphatic filariasis patients (Vaqas & Ryan, 2003).

Jones & Gruger (2003) made a cross-sectional study of hospitalisation data in the US for the year 2001, covering ten million people. Erysipelas and cellulitis of the leg and foot accounted for 0.6% of all admissions. Toe-web intertrigo is a major risk factor (Dupuy *et al.*, 1999). Recently completed studies of several European nations by the same group have shown that in shoe-wearing countries, a majority of the population will have skin problems affecting the feet. Similarly, cracks in the skin are present in 100% of the barefoot population in rural areas of the tropics, and where there is clear pathology — as in those affected by leprosy — washing and emollients have long been regarded as essential preventative therapy. The impending threat of a global epidemic of foot ulcers in the diabetic and obese population is creating similar programmes of foot care to that long established in the field of leprosy, thus broadening the potential role for emollients.

Around the world, coconut oil is often favoured as an emollient. Coconut oil, unlike olive oil and animal fats, consists of short chained and saturated fatty acids and therefore it is not easily oxidised to become rancid. It can be used to preserve medicinal plants (Sachs *et al.*, 2002). Other popular traditional emollients include shea butter (*Butyrospermum parkii*), mustard oil and sunflower seed oil. In many societies, skin massage with emollients is considered particularly important during the later stages of pregnancy, during the postpartum period, and for newborn infants. In Nigeria, it is believed that rubbing a paste of kola nuts on the abdomen of a pregnant woman helps to prevent skin infections and thrush in the neonate (Iweze, 1983).

The practice of oil massage of neonates is extremely widespread throughout the Indian subcontinent. A study in Bangladesh (Darmstadt & Saha, 2002) showed that oil massage was practised by over 96% of surveyed caretakers of newborns (340/352), irrespective of socio-economic status or place of residence. Mustard oil was used alone or in combination by 95% of respondents, over the infant's entire body, one to three times daily (96%), starting in the first three days of life (72%) in both term and preterm neonates. The most common reason given for the practice was prevention of infections (69%). Similarly, in Karachi, Pakistan, neonatal oil massage was universally practised by 387 surveyed women, with mustard oil (75.9%) being the most frequently used emollient (Fikree *et al.*, 2005). In the Sarlahi district of rural Nepal, a questionnaire administered to the caretakers of over 8000 newborns revealed that approximately 99% of the infants were massaged at least once with mustard oil in the first two weeks after birth, and 80% were massaged at least twice daily (Mullany *et al.*, 2005).

Darmstadt *et al.* (2002) have studied the impact of topical oils on mouse epidermal barrier function (rate of trans-epidermal water loss over time following acute barrier disruption by tape-stripping) and ultrastructure. It was found that a single application of sunflower seed oil significantly accelerated skin barrier recovery within one hour, and the effect was sustained for five hours after application. In contrast, the other vegetable oils tested (mustard, olive and soybean oils) all significantly delayed recovery of barrier function, in comparison with untreated controls and with a commercial preparation containing mineral oil. Adverse ultrastructural changes were observed under transmission electron microscopy in keratin intermediate filament, mitochondrial, nuclear, and nuclear envelope structure following a single application of mustard oil. A randomised controlled trial of sunflower seed oil massage for premature infants was recently conducted at Dhaka Shishu Hospital, Bangladesh (Darmstadt & Saha, 2002) and found that infants treated with sunflower seed oil were 41% less likely to develop nosocomial infections than untreated controls. In the light of these results,

Mullany *et al.* (2005) carried out focus group interviews in Nepal to explore the potential for introducing sunflower oil or other beneficial oils, such as sesame or safflower, as an alternative to mustard oil. Caretakers were found to be willing to consider adaptation of traditional practices for positive health outcomes, provided that essential contextual criteria — relating to factors such as smell, oiliness, mode of preparation and absorptive potential on the skin — are met.

There has been relatively little research on traditional emollients in a wider dermatological context. Agero and Verallo-Rowell (2004) conducted a randomised controlled study of extra virgin coconut oil and mineral oil as moisturisers for mild to moderate xerosis, and found the effects to be comparable, with both oils showing efficacy through significant improvement in skin hydration and increase in skin surface lipid levels. Shea butter has been shown to be an effective excipient for conventional topical medications, releasing the active ingredient at a faster rate than either petroleum jelly or lanolin (Thioune *et al.*, 2003), but its effects on the skin as an emollient in its own right have not yet been systematically studied.

13.4.3. *Prevention of Skin Carcinogenesis*

Another area in which TCAM may play an important role in the maintenance of skin health is in the prevention of carcinogenesis. In mouse and rat models, extracts of several plants used in traditional medicine have been shown to inhibit skin tumour formation induced by the application of 7,12-dimethylbenz(a)anthracene (DMBA) and other carcinogens. These include *Caesalpinia ferrea*, a Brazilian folk medicine (Nakamura *et al.*, 2002); *Azadirachta indica*, commonly known as neem (Dasgupta *et al.*, 2004); *Boerhaavia diffusa* (Bharali *et al.*, 2003a); *Phyllanthus urinaria* (Bharali *et al.*, 2003b) and *Withania somnifera* (Mathur *et al.*, 2004). Betulinic acid, a pentacyclic triterpene extracted from the bark of white birch (*Betula* sp.) has been identified as a selective inhibitor of human melanoma in athymic mice, which works by induction of apoptosis (Pisha *et al.*, 1995). A Japanese formulation, *Juzen-taiho-to*, has been shown to inhibit the growth of primarily developed melanocytic tumours, through potentiation of T-cell-mediated anti-tumour cytotoxic immunity, when administered orally to RET transgenic mice (Yan *et al.*, 2001).

It is unclear whether or not the above plants are already being utilised for skin care, and to what extent the laboratory findings can be extrapolated to the field. The high incidence of skin cancer in certain susceptible populations, such as Australians of Celtic descent (Hollis & Scheibner, 1988) and patients with albinism living in tropical countries (Kromberg *et al.*, 1989; Lookingbill *et al.*, 1995) illustrates the potential importance of further research in this area.

13.5. Towards Integrated Public Health Dermatology

13.5.1. *Incorporation of Traditional Medicine into Skin Care in Developing Countries*

The care of the skin is an ideal arena for attempting to integrate appropriate traditional preparations into 'modern' pharmacopoeias, in accordance with the guidance issued by the African Union and other intergovernmental organisations, for two reasons. Firstly, substances applied to the skin may be less likely to induce systemic side-effects than those taken internally, and are thus regarded as safer. Secondly, the use of local *materia medica* for cleaning the skin and treating wounds may be less context-bound than other TCAM modalities.

In African traditional medicine, in particular, therapy for internal illnesses (and in some cases disfiguring skin conditions) often includes elements such as divination, ritual sacrifice, music and dance, and/or requires close attention to the social context of the affliction. Wounds and burns, however, are often categorised as problems with a 'natural' or 'physical', as opposed to a 'supernatural' origin (e.g. Glick, 1967; Helman, 1994; Florey & Wolff, 1998) because their immediate causes are clearly visible and tangible — such as fires, knives and thorns. As a consequence, wound treatment in non-industrial societies often exemplifies the most empirical level of health care, involving only the bare minimum of ritual, and sometimes none at all. Biomedical treatment may be well accepted if it is readily available at an affordable price, and known to be effective. Likewise, plant-derived or animal-derived substances may be applied, on the same basis of efficacy demonstrated through prior practical experience. Even where the choice of plants for wound treatment appears to be entirely symbolic, some empirical basis may be present. In Native American medicine, for example, the red colour of many plants used to treat wounds — at first sight a straight-forward example of the 'doctrine of signatures', in which the appearance of plants somehow symbolises the affliction being treated — denotes the presence of red quinones, which have haemostatic and anti-microbial properties (Delaveau, 1981; cited in Etkin, 1996). As Etkin (1996) suggests: *'those physiologic actions may be the primary criteria for selection, with red color being simply the mnemonic tool'*.

While music and rituals are likely to be unwelcome in a hospital or clinic — and may even be ineffective in those settings — traditional soaps, ointments and other wound treatments are easily transferable between the domestic context and formal health care facilities. Some examples of institutions working primarily within the biomedical sector that are already practising an integrated approach to skin and wound care are the Regional Dermatology Training Centres (RDTCs) in Tanzania, Guatemala (Ong & Ryan, 1994) and China (Hay & Marks, 2004), established by the International Foundation for Dermatology, and the Le Huu Trac Institute of Burns in Hanoi, Vietnam, in collaboration with the Oxford Wound Healing Institute (Phan *et al.*, 1996). Also in Tanzania, the Tanga AIDS Working Group, based at the Tanga Regional Hospital, incorporates the treatment of skin manifestations of HIV/AIDS (such as rashes and herpes zoster) into its programme of collaboration with traditional healers (UNAIDS, 2002).

The Regional Dermatology Training Centres are distinctive in trying to change the image of dermatology from a primarily urban-based, elite profession to a more broadly accessible field with a focus on low-cost medications, traditional where appropriate. They focus on training Dermatology Officers, nurses and 'barefoot dermatologists', rather than postgraduate specialist physicians. At the Tanzanian RDTC, there is an ongoing partnership with the Association of Traditional Doctors (ATDO), which includes joint seminars and workshops, documentation of local ethnobotanical and ethnomedical knowledge relating to the skin, and small-scale clinical trials of promising topical medications. The centre has its own medicinal plant garden, with a particular focus on *Aloe* species, and a beekeeping project to produce honey and propolis. Its students and graduates have carried out epidemiological and ethnobotanical research in their home communities, to document the incidence of skin diseases and the utilisation of TCAM.

The newly established Chinese Regional Dermatology Training Centre project, coordinated by the Institute of Dermatology of the Chinese Academy of Medical Sciences (IDCAMS) in Nanjing, will adopt a similar approach to the training of Chinese doctors. In particular, it will focus on researching the traditional systems of medicine utilised by some 56 ethnic minorities in China, which, while having much in common with the 'standard' Traditional Chinese Medicine, also possess distinctive features. In particular, the centre will teach a policy of monitoring utilisation, safety and efficacy, with the aim of providing affordable skin care to the majority of the Chinese population.

In promoting greater collaboration between the biomedical and traditional health care sectors in developing countries, a note of caution is required to ensure that substances applied to the skin, and particularly to wounds, do not increase rather than decreasing the risk of infection. It may be necessary in some cases to provide traditional health practitioners (or, in particular, local communities practising self-medication) with training in hygiene. Education about preventing transmission of infectious agents such as HIV and hepatitis is also essential for those dealing with open wounds. Less severe side effects resulting from topical application of traditional preparations, such as contact dermatitis (Lin-Feng, 1995) may be difficult to predict or prevent, highlighting the importance of adequate post-treatment surveillance and documentation of side effects with a view to determining risk factors.

13.5.2. *Learning from TCAM in 'Western' Dermatology*

The high utilisation of TCAM for skin conditions by patients in Europe and the United States is forcing the dermatology profession and health policy-makers to consider the possibility of collaboration with, or at least referral to, specialised complementary providers. The personalised and patient-centred approach of many TCAM practitioners may also hold lessons for dermatologists in conventional practice: in common with other biomedical health care providers, they are often turning increasingly to technological solutions, at the expense of pastoral care and the 'healing art' (Gibbs, 2000). Psychosomatic dimensions of treatment are of particular importance in dermatology, in the light of the role of emotional factors in eliciting or worsening skin conditions, and the secondary stress associated with visible skin pathology (Augustin, 1999). In the Oxford Healthy Lifestyle Survey, users of CAM who had chronic skin problems and were also anxious or depressed were greatly helped by the CAM treatment, reporting greatly elevated energy, better mental health, less pain and higher physical functioning levels (Ong *et al.*, 2002).

There are isolated examples of genuinely integrated dermatology, usually at the level of individual dermatologists choosing to integrate TCAM therapies and holistic approaches into their practice (e.g. Dattner, 2003 and 2004). At the British Association of Dermatology annual meeting in 2005, Dr. Anthony Bewly advocated the employment of herbalists, based on his experience at Whipps Cross University Hospital where two herbalists are active in his dermatology clinic. In Iceland, the Ministry of Health has recognised the Blue Lagoon Dermatology Clinic, which offers therapies based on geothermal seawater, as an official treatment centre for psoriasis, and the Icelandic Social Insurance reimburses the cost of treatment. This treatment is also formally recognised in Denmark and the Faroe Islands (Alfredsdottir, 2005).

Chairello (2004) has argued for an even broader approach, which he calls 'functional or integrative dermatology', incorporating other disciplines such as psychology, sociology and exercise physiology alongside TCAM and conventional treatments, with a view to addressing the underlying causes of skin pathology rather than merely relieving the symptoms. He suggests that dermatology nurses may have a better mindset than physicians, in embracing and implementing this concept.

In general, though, integration of TCAM therapies with biomedicine is still carried out by the consumer rather than the provider. A study conducted by Stanford University (Pelletier, 1998) showed that among users of TCAM in the United States, over 95% also use conventional medicine, with less than 5% using TCAM methods exclusively.

In parallel with the broader trend towards incorporating TCAM modules into mainstream medical education (e.g. Highfield *et al.*, 2005; Owen & Lewith, 2004; Kligler *et al.*, 2004; Forjuoh *et al.*, 2003; Brokaw *et al.*, 2002), a specialised training programme has been developed in Israel with the aim of educating dermatologists and dermatology nurses about TCAM. The course objective is to expose participants to common methods in TCAM, emphasising the role of an evidence-based approach and the importance of communication between medical staff and patients about TCAM utilisation. Course evaluation revealed that participants acknowledged the existence of evidence-based research as an important consideration before referring patients to TCAM providers (Ben-Arye *et al.*, 2004).

13.6. Conclusion: Defining a Research Agenda

The evaluation of TCAM methodologies relevant to the care of the skin, particularly in the arena of disease prevention and general health maintenance, requires a flexible and inter-disciplinary approach to research. The studies by Darmstadt *et al.*, relating to traditional oil massage of neonates (see Section 13.4.2 above) provide a good illustration of the interdependence of laboratory research, clinical trials and anthropological methodologies in evaluating popular traditional skin care practices, and determining the potential for replacing harmful interventions with beneficial ones. This could serve as a model for future research protocols on 'soap plants' and other aspects of preventative skin care. The research by Etkin (1996) on the presence of red quinones in Native American wound treatments (discussed in Section 13.5.1) exemplifies another way in which the social and natural sciences can work together, this time in evaluating treatment rather than prevention: the former in identifying promising candidate species for further research, and the latter in assessing safety and efficacy.

As in other fields of ethnomedicine, the rapid pace of social change in developing countries threatens to bring about the disappearance of traditional understandings of skin health and hygiene, and of the *materia medica* used by practitioners. There is an urgent need for both documentation and active conservation measures, relating not only to the plants themselves that are utilised for soap and medicine, but also to specific indigenous knowledge and the language used to express it. Active conservation implies ongoing practice, and praxis-based education, to ensure that all relevant details are retained: younger members of a community may know in theory that certain plant species can be combined in an ointment to treat burns or skin infections, for example, but have no idea how to prepare and use the ointment. The assumption that a single 'active' compound, isolated under laboratory conditions, will have the same effect as the traditional preparation has already been demonstrated to be false in many cases.

As this review has demonstrated, there have been many positive developments within the profession of dermatology (and dermatology nursing) throughout the world, with respect to the integration of TCAM into mainstream care, and an increased willingness to collaborate with TCAM providers or to refer patients for TCAM treatment. These developments are the rational response to patient demand: given the high prevalence of utilisation in all settings studied to date, TCAM is a reality that neither dermatologists nor nurses can afford to ignore. The challenge that remains is for this high level of interest to be translated into a systematic research agenda, enabling skin care providers at all levels — from the rural mother in Bangladesh, massaging her newborn infant, to the consultant dermatologist practising in a private clinic in London or New York — to maintain or adopt beneficial traditional practices, and to modify or eliminate potentially harmful ones.

References

Agero AL, Verallo-Rowell VM. A randomized double-blind controlled trial comparing extra virgin coconut oil with mineral oil as a moisturizer for mild to moderate xerosis. *Dermatitis* 2004;15(3):109–116.

Ahmad VU, Saba N, Khan KM. Triterpenoid saponin from the bark of *Guaiacum officinale* L. *Nat Prod Res* 2004;18(2):111–116.

Ahmad VU, Saba N, Perveen S. Structure of guaianin M from *Guaiacum officinale*. *Fitoterapia* 1992;63(3):226–229.

Alfredsdottir R. Natural geothermal treatment of psoriasis at the Blue Lagoon Dermatology Clinic in Iceland. *International Skin-Care Nursing Group Newsletter*, February 2005, pp. 3–4. Published on the Internet and accessed 18.05.2005 at 08:55: http://www.isng.soton.ac.uk/newsletter/0205newsletter%20.pdf.

Altman PM. Australian Tea Tree oil — a natural antiseptic. *Aust J Biotechnol* 1989;3:247–418.

Arora S, Dhillon S, Rani G, Nagpal A. The *in vitro* antibacterial/synergistic activities of *Withania somnifera* extracts. *Fitoterapia* 2004;75(3–4):385–388.

Augustin M. Alternative medicine therapy in dermatology: dimensions, chances and approaches to an integrative understanding. *Forsch Komplementarmed* 1999;6(Suppl 2):1–4 (article in German).

Balick MJ, Cox P. *Plants, People and Culture: The Science of Ethnobotany*. New York: Scientific American Library, 1996.

Beltrami B, Vassallo C, Berardesca E, Borroni G. Anti-inflammatory, antimicrobial and comedolytic effects of a topical plant complex treatment in acne vulgaris: a clinical trial. *J Appl Cosmetol* 2001;19:11–20.

Ben-Arye E, Frenkel M, Ziv M. An approach to teaching dermatologists about complementary medicine. *J Altern Complement Med* 2004;10(5): 899–904.

Bharali R, Azad MR, Tabassum J. Chemopreventive action of *Boerhaavia diffusa* on DMBA-induced skin carcinogenesis in mice. *Indian J Physiol Pharmacol* 2003a;47(4):459–464.

Bharali R, Tabassum J, Azad MR. Chemopreventive action of *Phyllanthus urinaria* Linn. on DMBA-induced skin carcinogenesis in mice. *Indian J Exp Biol* 2003b;41(11):1325–1328.

Bhattarai NK. Traditional herbal medicines used to treat wounds and injuries in Nepal. *Trop Doct* 1997;27(Suppl 1):43–47.

Biswas TK, Mukherjee B. Plant medicines of Indian origin for wound healing activity: a review. *Low Extrem Wounds* 2003;2:25–39.

Bodeker GC, Ryan TJ, Ong C-K. Traditional approaches to wound healing. *Clin Dermatol* 1999;17:93–98.

Bonn D. Sweet solution to superbug infections? *Lancet Infect Dis* 2003;3(10):608.

Borghi J, Guinness L, Ouedraogo J, Curtis V. Is hygiene promotion cost-effective? A case study in Burkina Faso. *Trop Med Int Health* 2002;7(11):960–969.

Bossard E. Angolan medicinal plants used as piscicides and/or soaps. *J Ethnopharmacol* 1993;40:1–19.

Brokaw JJ, Tunnicliff G, Raess BU, Saxon DW. The teaching of complementary and alternative medicine in U.S. medical schools: a survey of course directors. *Acad Med* 2002;77(9):876–881.

Carson CF, Riley TV, Cookson BD. Efficacy and safety of tea tree oil as a topical antimicrobial agent. *J Hosp Infect* 1998;40:175–178.

Chairello SE. Functional or integrative dermatologic nursing for the 21st century. *Dermatol Nurs* 2004;16(3):275–276.

Cheatle T. Venous ulceration and free radicals [letter]. *Br J Dermatol* 1991;124:508.

Chen YF, Chang JS. Complementary and alternative medicine use among patients attending a hospital dermatology clinic in Taiwan. *Int J Dermatol* 2003;42(8):616–621.

Chen ZP, Cai Y, Phillipson JD. Studies on the antitumor, antibacterial and wound healing properties of dragon's blood. *Planta Med* 1994;60:541–545.

Choi S. Epidermis proliferative effect of the *Panax ginseng* ginsenoside Rb2. *Arch Pharm Res* 2002;25(1):71–76.

Church JCT. The traditional use of maggots in wound healing, and the development of larva therapy (biosurgery) in wound healing. *J Altern Complement Med* 1996;2:525–527.

Cohen J. Feeding the fish: an unusual treatment. *Br Med J* 2000;320:181.

Cooper RA, Molan PC, Harding KG. The sensitivity to honey of Gram-positive cocci of clinical significance isolated from wounds. *J Appl Microbiol* 2002;93(5):857–863.

Courtenay M, Church J, Ryan T. Larva therapy in wound management. *J R Soc Med* 2000;93:72–74.

Cristoni A, Di Pierro F. Management of local adiposity with botanicals. *Chim Oggi* 1998;16:11–14.

Curtis V, Cairncross S. Effect of washing hands with soap on diarrhoea risk in the community: a systematic review. *Lancet Infect Dis* 2003;3(5): 275–281.

Dai G. Advances in the acupuncture treatment of acne. *J Tradit Chin Med* 1997;17(1):65–72.

Darmstadt GL, Mao-Qiang M, Chi E, Saha SK, Ziboh VA, Black RE, Santosham M, Elias PM. Impact of topical oils on the skin barrier: possible implications for neonatal health in developing countries. *Acta Paediatr* 2002;91(5): 546–554.

Darmstadt GL, Saha SK. Traditional practice of oil massage of neonates in Bangladesh. *J Health Popul Nutr* 2002;20(2):184–188.

Dasgupta T, Banerjee S, Yadava PK, Rao AR. Chemopreventive potential of *Azadirachta indica* (Neem) leaf extract in murine carcinogenesis model systems. *J Ethnopharmacol* 2004;92(1):23–26.

Dattatreya RM, Nuijen S, van Swaaij AC, Klopper PJ. Evaluation of boiled potato peel as a wound dressing. *Burns* 1991;17(4):323–328.

Dattner AM. From medical herbalism to phytotherapy in dermatology: back to the future. *Dermatol Ther* 2003;16(2):106–113.

Dattner AM. Herbal and complementary medicine in dermatology. *Dermatol Clin* 2004;22(3):325–332, vii.

Davidson JR, Ortiz de Montellano B. The antibacterial properties of an Aztec wound remedy. *J Ethnopharmacol* 1983;8:149–161.

Delaveau P. Evaluation of traditional pharmacopoeias. In: Beal JL, Reinhard ER (eds.) *Natural Products as Medical Agents*. Stuttgart: Hippokrates Verlag, 1981, pp. 395–404.

Derkach AI, Kotov AG, Komissarenko SN, Komissarenko NF, Chermenyova GV, Spiridonov VN. Flavonoids, cumarins and triterpenes of *Aesculus hippocastanum* L. seeds. *Rastitel'nye Resursy* 1999;35:81–85.

Duke JA. *Handbook of Phytochemical Constituents of GRAS Herbs and Other Economic Plants.* Boca Raton, FL: CRC Press, 1992.

Dupuy A, Benchikhui H, Roujeau JC *et al. Br Med J* 1999;318:1591–1594.

Duwiejua M, Zeitlin IJ, Waterman PG, Gray AI. Anti-inflammatory activity of *Polygonum bistorta, Guaiacum officinale* and *Hamamelis virginiana* in rats. *J Pharm Pharmacol* 1994;46(4):286–290.

Eisenberg D. Alternative therapies for cutaneous disorders. *Arch Dermatol* 1997;133(3):379–380.

Emboden W. *Narcotic Plants*, 2nd edn. New York: MacMillan Publishing Co., 1979.

Erko B, Abebe F, Berhe N, Medhin G, Gebre-Michael T, Gemetchu T, Gundersen SG. Control of *Schistosoma mansoni* by the soapberry Endod (*Phytolacca dodecandra*) in Wollo, northeastern Ethiopia: post-intervention prevalence. *East Afr Med J* 2002;79(4):198–201.

Ernst E. The usage of complementary therapies by dermatological patients: a systematic review. *Br J Dermatol* 2000;142(5):857–861.

Esser KB, Gundersen SG. Control of schistosomiasis using berries from *Phytolacca dodecandra (endod)*. In: *Noragric BRIEF No. 8/99*, January 1999. Noragric, Centre for International Environment and Development Studies, Agriculture University of Norway (NLH). Also published on the Internet, accessed 17.05.2005 at 16:42: http://www.iastate.edu/~anthr_info/cikard/harvest/archive.htm.

Etkin NL. Ethnopharmacology: the conjunction of medical ethnography and the biology of therapeutic action. In: Sargent CF, Johnson TM (eds.) *Medical Anthropology: Contemporary Theory and Method*, revised edn., Westport, Connecticut & London: Praeger, 1996, pp. 151–164.

Ferguson JE, Chalmers RJ, Rowlands DJ. Reversible dilated cardiomyopathy following treatment of atopic eczema with Chinese herbal medicine. *Br J Dermatol* 1997;136(4):592–593.

Fikree FF, Ali TS, Durocher JM, Rahbar MH. Newborn care practices in low socioeconomic settlements of Karachi, Pakistan. *Soc Sci Med* 2005;60(5): 911–921.

Florey MJ, Wolff XY. Incantations and herbal medicines: Alune ethnobotanical knowledge in a context of change. *J Ethnobiol* 1998;18(1):39–67.

Forjuoh SN, Rascoe TG, Symm B, Edwards JC. Teaching medical students complementary and alternative medicine using evidence-based principles. *J Altern Complement Med* 2003;9(3):429–439.

Gibbs S. Losing touch with the healing art: dermatology and the decline of pastoral doctoring. *J Am Acad Dermatol* 2000;43(5 Pt 1):875–878.

Glick LB. Medicine as an ethnographic category: the Gimi of the New Guinea Highlands. *Ethnology* 1967;6:31–56.

Goddard G, Shen Y, Steele B, Springer N. A controlled trial of placebo versus real acupuncture. *J Pain* 2005;6(4):237–242.

Goll PH, Lemma A, Duncan J, Mazengia B. Control of schistosomiasis in Adwa, Ethiopia, using the plant molluscicide endod (*Phytolacca dodecandra*). *Tropenmed Parasitol* 1983;34(3):177–183.

Gomez-Beloz A, Rucinski JC, Balick MJ, Tipton C. Double incision wound healing bioassay using *Hamelia patens* from El Salvador. *J Ethnopharmacol* 2003;88(2–3):169–173.

Gore MA, Akokekar D. Evaluation of banana leaf dressing for partial thickness burn wounds. *Burns* 2003;29(5):487–492.

Grindlay D, Reynolds T. The *Aloe vera* phenomenon; a review of the properties and modern uses. *J Ethnopharmacol* 1986;16:117–131.

Grossmann J. Flies as medical allies. *The World and I*, October 1994, pp. 187–193.

Hay R, Marks R. The International foundation for Dermatology: an exemplar of the increasingly diverse activities of the International League of Dermatological Societies. *Br J Derm* 2004;150:747–749.

Helman CG. *Culture, Health and Illness*, 4th edn. Oxford: Butterworth-Heinemann, 1994.

Henz *et al.*, *Br J Dermatol* 1999;40:685–688.

Higaki S, Morimatsu S, Morohashi M, Yamagishi T, Hasegawa Y. Susceptibility of *Propionibacterium acnes*, *Staphylococcus aureus* and *Staphylococcus epidermidis* to 10 Kampo formulations. *J Int Med Res* 1997; 25(6): 318–324.

Highfield ES, McLellan MC, Kemper KJ, Risko W, Woolf AD. Integration of complementary and alternative medicine in a major pediatric teaching hospital: an initial overview. *J Altern Complement Med* 2005;11(2):373–380.

Hoare C, Li Wan Po A, Williams H. Systematic review of treatments for atopic eczema. *Health Technol Assess* 2000;4(37):1–191.

Hollis DE, Scheibner A. Ultrastructural changes in epidermal Langerhans cells and melanocytes in response to ultraviolet irradiation, in Australians of Aboriginal and Celtic descent. *Br J Dermatol* 1988;119(1):21–31.

Hoque BA. Handwashing practices and challenges in Bangladesh. *Int J Environ Health Res* 2003;13(Suppl 1):S81–87.

Hoque BA, Mahalanabis D, Pelto B, Alam MJ. Research methodology for developing efficient handwashing options: an example from Bangladesh. *J Trop Med Hyg* 1995;98(6):469–475.

Huang KF, Hsu YC, Lin CN, Tzeng JI, Chen YW, Wang JJ. Shiunko promotes epithelization of wounded skin. *Am J Chin Med* 2004;32(3):389–396.

Hutchings A, Haxton Scott A, Lewis G, Cunningham A. *Zulu Medicinal Plants*. Natal: University of Natal Press, 1996.

Iweze FA. Taboos of childbearing and child-rearing in Bendel state of Nigeria. *J Nurse Midwifery* 1983;28(3):31–33.

Jensen P. Use of alternative medicine by patients with atopic dermatitis and psoriasis. *Acta Derm Venereol* 1990;70(5):421–424.

Jerner B, Skogh M, Vahlquist A. A controlled trial of acupuncture in psoriasis: no convincing effect. *Acta Derm Venereol* 1997;77(2):154–156.

Johnston GA, Bilbao RM, Graham-Brown RA. The use of complementary medicine in children with atopic dermatitis in secondary care in Leicester. *Br J Dermatol* 2003;149(3):566–571.

Jones P, Gruger J. Cost of hospitalization for erysipelas and bacterial cellulitis of the leg and foot in the USA. *Europ Acad Derm Vener* 2003;17(Suppl 3):305.

Joos S, Brinkhaus B, Maluche C, Maupai N, Kohnen R, Kraehmer N, Hahn EG, Schuppan D. Acupuncture and moxibustion in the treatment of active Crohn's disease: a randomized controlled study. *Digestion* 2004;69(3): 131–139.

Kareem M. *Plants in Ayurveda: A Compendium of Botanical and Sanskrit Names*. Bangalore: Foundation for Revitalisation of Local Health Traditions, 1997, p. 244.

Karuza L, Blekic J. Standardization of aescin-based herbal drug preparations. *Acta Pharmaceutica Zagreb* 1995;45:495–498.

Keswani MH, Vartak AM, Patil A, Davies JW. Histological and bacteriological studies of burn wounds treated with boiled potato peel dressings. *Burns* 1990;16(2):137–143.

Kim SJ. Effect of biflavones of *Gingko biloba* against UVB induced cytotoxicity *in vitro*. *J Dermatol* 2001;28:193–199.

Kimata H. Listening to Mozart reduces allergic skin wheal responses and *in vitro* allergen-specific IgE production in atopic dermatitis patients with latex allergy. *Behav Med* 2003;29(1):15–19.

Kligler B, Maizes V, Schachter S, Park CM, Gaudet T, Benn R, Lee R, Remen RN. Core competencies in integrative medicine for medical school curricula: a proposal. *Acad Med* 2004;79(6):521–531.

Kokwaro JO. *Medicinal Plants of East Africa*, 2nd edn. Nairobi: Kenya Literature Bureau, 1993.

Kromberg JG, Castle D, Zwane EM, Jenkins T. Albinism and skin cancer in Southern Africa. *Clin Genet* 1989;36(1):43–52.

Lee TY, Lam TH. Irritant contact dermatitis due to a Chinese herbal medicine *lu-shen-wan*. *Contact Derm* 1988;18(4):213–218.

Lemos TLG, Mendes AL, Sousa MP, Braz Filho R. New saponin from *Sapindus saponaria*. *Fitoterapia* 1992;63(6):515–517.

Lemos TLG, Sousa MP, Mendes AL, Braz Filho R. Saponin from *Sapindus saponaria*. *Fitoterapia* 1994;65(6):557.

Liao SJ, Liao TA. Acupuncture treatment for psoriasis: a retrospective case report. *Acupunct Electrother Res* 1992;17(3):195–208.

Lin X, Tu C, Yang C. Study on treatment of eczema by Chinese herbal medicine with anti-type IV allergic activity. *Zhongguo Zhong Xi Yi Jie He Za Zhi* 2000;20(4):258–260 (article in Chinese).

Lin-Feng L. A clinical and patch test study of contact dermatitis from traditional Chinese medical materials. *Contact Derm* 1995;33:392–395.

Lookingbill DP, Lookingbill GL, Leppard B. Actinic damage and skin cancer in albinos in northern Tanzania: findings in 164 patients enrolled in an outreach skin care program. *J Am Acad Derm* 1995;32(4):653–658.

Martin A. The use of antioxidants in healing. *Dermatol Surg* 1996;22:156–160.

Mathur S *et al*. The treatment of skin carcinoma, induced by UVB radiation, using 1-oxo-5beta, 6beta-epoxy-witha-2-enolide, isolated from the roots of *Withania somnifera*, in a rat model. *Phytomedicine* 2004;11(5):452–460.

Matsumoto Y, Kato M, Tamada Y, Mori H, Ohashi M. Enhancement of interleukin-1 alpha mediated autocrine growth of cultured human keratinocytes by sho-saiko-to. *Jpn J Pharmacol* 1997;73(4):333–336.

Mills J, Pascoe KO, Chambers J, Melville GN. Preliminary investigations of the wound-healing properties of a Jamaican folk medicinal plant (*Justica pectoralis*). *West Indian Med J* 1986;34:190–193.

Mishra LC, Singh BB, Dagenais S. Scientific basis for the therapeutic use of *Withania somnifera* (ashwagandha): a review. *Altern Med Rev* 2000;5(4):334–346.

Molan P. The role of Honey in the management of wounds. *J Wound Care* 1999;8:415–418.

Molan PC. Potential of honey in the treatment of wounds and burns. *Am J Clin Dermatol* 2001;2(1):13–19.

Mukherjee PK, Mukherjee K, Rajesh Kumar M, Pal M, Saha BP. Evaluation of wound healing activity of some herbal formulations. *Phytother Res* 2003;17(3):265–268.

Mullany LC, Darmstadt GL, Khatry SK, Tielsch JM. Traditional massage of newborns in Nepal: implications for trials of improved practice. *J Trop Pediatr* 2005;51(2):82–86.

Murthy KN, Reddy VK, Veigas JM, Murthy UD. Study on wound healing activity of *Punica granatum* peel. *J Med Food* 2004;7(2):256–259.

Nakamura ES *et al.* Cancer chemopreventive effects of a Brazilian folk medicine, Juca, on *in vivo* two-stage skin carcinogenesis. *J Ethnopharmacol* 2002; 81(1):135–137.

Nicolaou N, Johnston GA. The use of complementary medicine by patients referred to a contact dermatitis clinic. *Contact Derm* 2004;51(1): 30–33.

Oklahoma Biological Survey. Published on the Internet and available at: http://www.biosurvey.ou.edu/shrub/sasad.htm. Last updated 20 September 1999, accessed 15 May 2005 at 15:17.

Okunji CO, Iwu MM, Jackson JE, Tally JD. Biological activity of saponins from two *Dracaena* species. *Adv Exp Med Biol* 1996;404:415–428.

Ong C-K, Petersen S, Bodeker GC, Stewart-Brown S. Health status of people using complementary and alternative medical practitioner services in four English counties. *Am J Public Health* 2002;92(10):1653–1656.

Ong C-K, Ryan T. *Healthy Skin For All.* Oxford: International Foundation for Dermatology, 1994.

Orafidiya LO, Agbani EO, Abereoje OA, Awe T, Abudu A, Fakoya FA. An investigation into the wound-healing properties of essential oil of *Ocimum gratissimum* Linn. *J Wound Care* 2003;12(9):331–334.

Owais M, Sharad KS, Shehbaz A, Saleemuddin M. Antibacterial efficacy of *Withania somnifera* (*ashwagandha*), an indigenous medicinal plant, against experimental murine salmonellosis. *Phytomedicine* 2005;12(3):229–235.

Owen D, Lewith GT. Teaching integrated care: CAM familiarisation courses. *Med J Aust* 2004;181(5):276–278.

Park J, White A, Stevinson C, Ernst E, James M. Validating a new non-penetrating sham acupuncture device: two randomised controlled trials. *Acupunct Med* 2002;20(4):168–174.

Patil AK. The emergence of boiled potato peel as a burn wound dressing. *AgniVarta: the quarterly publication of the Burns Association of India* 1990;10(3):2–3.

Peana AT, Moretti MDL, Manconi V, Desole G, Pippia P. Anti-inflammatory activity of aqueous extracts and steroidal saponins of *Agave americana. Planta Med* 1997;63:199–202.

Pelletier KR. Life with the new roommate: alternative medicine moves in with conventional medicine. *Health Forum J* 1998;41(6):35–37, 41.

Perharic L, Shaw D, Leon C, De Smet PA, Murray VS. Possible association of liver damage with the use of Chinese herbal medicine for skin disease. *Vet Hum Toxicol* 1995;37(6):562–566.

Phan TT, Hughes MA, Cherry GW *et al.* An aqueous extract of the leaves of *Chromolaena odorata* (formerly *Eupatorium odoratum*) inhibits hydrated collagen lattice contraction by normal human dermal fibroblasts. *J Altern Complement Med* 1996;2:335–344.

Phan TT, Wang L, See P, Grayer RJ, Chan SY, Lee ST. Phenolic compounds of *Chromolaena odorata* protect cultured skin cells from oxidative damage: implication for cutaneous wound healing. *Biol Pharm Bull* 2001;24(12):1373–1379.

Pieters L, de Bruyne T, van Poel B *et al. In vivo* wound healing of Dragon's blood (*Croton* spp.), a traditional South American drug, and its constituents. *Phytomedicine* 1995;2:17–22.

Pisha E, Chai H, Lee I-S, Chagwedera TE, Farnsworth NR, Cordell GA, Beecher CW, Fong HH, Kinghorn AD, Brown DM. Discovery of betulinic acid as a selective inhibitor of human melanoma that functions by induction of apoptosis. *Nat Med* 1995;1(10):1046–1051.

Priya KS, Gnanamani A, Radhakrishnan N, Babu M. Healing potential of *Datura alba* on burn wounds in albino rats. *J Ethnopharmacol* 2002;83(3):193–199.

Priya KS, Arumugam G, Rathinam B, Wells A, Babu M. *Celosia argentea* Linn. leaf extract improves wound healing in a rat burn wound model. *Wound Repair Regen* 2004;12(6):618–625.

Robson MC, Heggers JP, Hagstrom WJ. Myth, magic, witchcraft or fact? Aloe vera revisited. *J Burn Care Rehabil* 1982;3:157–163.

Ryan TJ. Traditional health knowledge: integration of Western and Asian Medicine. In: Niimi H, Xue RJ, Sawada T, Zheng C (eds.) *Microcirculatory Approach to Asian Traditional Medicine.* Amsterdam: Elsevier Science, 1996, pp. 1–16.

Ryan TJ. Global curriculum for wound management. *Trop Doct* 1997; 27(Suppl 1):31–35.

Ryan TJ. Antibacterial agents for wounds and burns in the developing world: report of a workshop. *J Trop Med Hyg* 1992;95:397–403.

Ryan TJ. Commentary on Biswas TK & Mukherjee B, 'Plant medicines of Indian origin for wound healing activity: a review.' *Low Extrem Wounds* 2003; 2:40–41.

Ryan TJ. The First Commandment: oil it! An appreciation of the science underlying water and emollients for skin care. *Commun Dermatol* 2004; 1:3–5.

Sachs M, von Eichel J, Asskali F. Wound management with coconut oil in Indonesian folk medicine. *Chirurg* 2002;73:387–392.

Sander P, Kiesling A, Litscher G, Voit-Augustin H, James RL, Schwarz G. Laser Doppler flowmetry in combined needle acupuncture and moxibustion: a pilot study in healthy adults. *Laser Med Sci* 2001;16:184–191.

Satimia FT, McBride SR, Leppard B. Prevalence of skin disease in rural Tanzania and factors influencing the choice of health care, modern or traditional. *Arch Dermatol* 1998;134(11):1363–1366.

Saunders CF. *Edible and Useful Plants of the United States and Canada.* New York: Dover Publications, 1976. Reprint of a work formerly published as *Useful Wild Plants of the United States and Canada,* revised edn., by R.M. McBride & Co., New York, 1934.

Shirwaikar A, Somashekar AP, Udupa AL, Udupa SL, Somashekar S. Wound healing studies of *Aristolochia bracteolata* Lam. with supportive action of antioxidant enzymes. *Phytomedicine* 2003;10(6–7):558–562.

Simpson EL, Basco M, Hanifin J. A cross-sectional survey of complementary and alternative medicine use in patients with atopic dermatitis. *Am J Contact Dermatitis* 2003;14(3):144–147.

Stepanovic S, Antic N, Dakic I, Svabic-Vlahovic M. *In vitro* antimicrobial activity of propolis and synergism between propolis and antimicrobial drugs. *Microbiol Res* 2003;158(4):353–357.

Tahara E, Satoh T, Toriizuka K, Nagai H, Nunome S, Shimada Y, Itoh T, Terasawa K, Saiki I. Effect of Shimotsu-to (a Kampo medicine, Si-Wu-Tang) and its constituents on triphasic skin reaction in passively sensitized mice. *J Ethnopharmacol* 1999;68(1–3):219–228.

Tatsumi T, Yamada T, Nagai H, Terasawa K, Tani T, Nunome S, Saiki I. A Kampo formulation: Byakko-ka-ninjin-to (Bai-Hu-Jia-Ren-Sheng-Tang) inhibits IgE-mediated triphasic skin reaction in mice: the role of its constituents in expression of the efficacy. *Biol Pharm Bull* 2001;24(3):284–290.

Thioune O, Khouma B, Diarra M, Diop AB, Lo I. [The excipient properties of shea butter compared with vaseline and lanolin]. *J Pharm Belg* 2003;58(3):81–84.

Tian B, Hua YJ, Ma XQ, Wang GL. [Relationship between antibacterial activity of aloe and its anthaquinone compounds]. *Zhongguo Zhong Yao Za Zhi* 2003;28(11):1034–1037 (article in Chinese).

Tjioe *et al. Acta Derm Venereol* 2002;82:299–301.

Ugur A, Arslan T. An *in vitro* study on antimicrobial activity of propolis from Mugla province of Turkey. *J Med Food* 2004;7(1):90–94.

UNAIDS. *Ancient Remedies, New Disease: Involving Traditional Healers in Increasing Access to AIDS Care and Prevention in East Africa.* UNAIDS/02.16E. Geneva: UNAIDS, 2002.

Vanherweghem LJ. Misuse of herbal remedies: the case of an outbreak of terminal renal failure in Belgium (Chinese herbs nephropathy). *J Altern Complement Med* 1998;4(1):9–13.

Van Hien T, Hughes MA, Cherry GWC. *In vitro* studies on the antioxidant and growth stimulatory activities of a polyphenolic extract from *Cudrania cochinchinensis* used in the treatment of wounds in Vietnam. *Wound Repair Regen* 1997;5:159–167.

Vaqas B, Ryan TJ. Lymphoedema pathophysiology and management in resource poor settings — relevance for filariasis control programmes. *Filaria J* 2003;2–4 (http://www.filariajournal.com/content/2/1/4).

Voegeli D. Skin hygiene practices, emollient therapy and skin vulnerability. *Nurs Times* 2005;101(4):57, 59.

Wampold BE, Minami T, Tierney SC, Baskin TW, Bhati KS. The placebo is powerful: estimating placebo effects in medicine and psychotherapy from randomized clinical trials. *J Clin Psychol* 2005;61(7):835–854.

Wang JS, Lan C, Chen SY, Wong MK. Tai Chi Chuan training is associated with enhanced endothelium-dependent dilation in skin vasculature of healthy older men. *J Am Geriatr Soc* 2002;50(6):1024–1030.

Watt JM, Breyer-Brandwijk MG. *The Medicinal and Poisonous Plants of Southern and Eastern Africa*, 2nd edn. Edinburgh: Livingstone, 1962.

Williams HC. Dermatology. In: Stevens A, Raftery J (eds.) *Health Care Needs Assessment*. Oxford: Radcliffe Medical Press, 1997, pp. 261–348.

Williams LR, Home VN, Zang X. The composition and bactericidal activity of oil of *Melaleuca alternifolia*. *Int J Aromather* 1988;1:15–17.

Xu Y. Treatment of facial skin diseases with acupuncture — a report of 129 cases. *J Tradit Chin Med* 1990;10(1):22–25.

Yan D, Masashi K, Kozue T, Yoshiyuki K, Anwarul A, Khaled H, Haruhiko S, Izumi N. T-cell-immunity-based inhibitory effects of orally administered herbal medicine *Juzen-taiho-to* on the growth of primarily developed melanocytic tumors in RET-Transgenic mice. *J Invest Dermatol* 2001;117:694–701.

Yokosuka A, Mimaki Y, Kuroda M, Sashida Y. A new steroidal saponin from the leaves of *Agave americana*. *Planta Med* 2000;66:393–396.

Yuan R, Lin Y. Traditional Chinese medicine: an approach to scientific proof and clinical validation. *Pharmacol Ther* 2000;86(2):191–198.

Zerehsaz F, Salmanpour R, Handjani F, Ardehali S, Panjehshahin MR, Tabei SZ, Tabatabaee HR. A double blind randomized clinical trial of a topical herbal extract (Z-HE) versus systemic meglumine antimoniate for the treatment of cutaneous leishmaniasis in Iran. *Int J Dermatol* 1999; 38:610–612.

Zhang W, Leonard T, Bath-Hextall F, Chambers CA, Lee C, Humphreys R, Williams HC. Chinese herbal medicine for atopic eczema. *Cochrane Database Syst Rev* 2004;(4):CD002291.

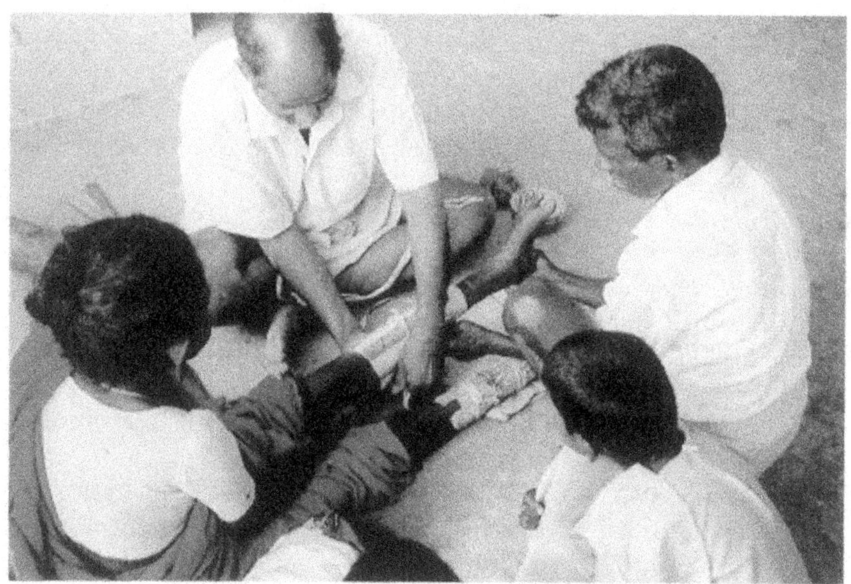

An Ayurvedic orthopaedic specialist in rural Tamil Nadu, India, uses flexible bamboo splinting in the management of leg fractures. [*Source*: Foundation for Revitalization of Local Health Traditions, Bangalore, India (www.frlht.org.in).]

CHAPTER 14

TRADITIONAL ORTHOPAEDIC PRACTICES: BEYOND 'BONESETTING'

Gemma Burford, Gerard Bodeker and Jonathan Cohen

14.1. Introduction

The World Health Report for 1999 attributes over 21 million disability-adjusted life years to the effects of musculoskeletal disease globally (World Health Organization, 1999). Malnutrition and infections, including tuberculosis, contribute heavily to musculoskeletal disease, along with congenital physical disabilities, trauma, and degenerative/destructive disease. The estimated burden due to injuries — much of which is attributable to war, including land mines, and road traffic accidents — is over ten times this figure, and constitutes one-sixth of the total global disease burden (Murray & Lopez, 1996). A 1984 study in rural Nepal showed that in 53.5% of households, one or more people had some form of active bone or joint problem (Anderson, 1984).

Although WHO has designated chronic disease as one of its highest priorities (World Health Organization, 1997), national services to reach those afflicted with musculoskeletal conditions are typically assigned a lower priority than services targeting endemic disease, fertility regulation and immunisation. In the non-industrialised world, Western-style orthopaedic surgery and rehabilitative services are usually unavailable to all but the urban elite (Anon, 1973a). For example, the Sudan — a country of 24 million inhabitants — had, in 1996, only six modern orthopaedic surgeons, of whom four were practicing in Khartoum (El-Tom, 1996). Traditional orthopaedic practitioners, often known as bonesetters, tend to be responsible for the primary care of patients suffering from chronic musculoskeletal conditions such as arthritis, post-polio residual paralysis and congenital deformities as well as those with acute injuries. The perception of their services as cheaper than hospital treatment, and the fact that they tend to be well known in their communities, are also factors in their enduring popularity (Thanni, 2000).

In industrialised regions, such as Western Europe, North America and Australasia, the situation is very different. Local traditions of orthopaedic treatment have been largely replaced by formal systems of 'complementary and alternative medicine' (CAM), namely osteopathy and chiropractic, for treating musculoskeletal complaints. These are widely accepted by the public. The evolution of these systems of manipulation from traditional practices is outside the scope of this chapter, since it has a dedicated journal of its own (*Chiropractic History*) and is well documented in the journals of national chiropractic and osteopathic associations. It is, however, an excellent historical example of what Last (1990) has called 'the professionalisation of indigenous healers'. Osteopaths and chiropractors are now officially recognised as health care professionals in several European countries, with legal requirements for training and registration as shown in Table 14.1, while in the United States the degree of 'Doctor of Osteopathy' (D.O.) is regarded as equivalent in status to a conventional medical degree.

The globalisation of health care systems, and the plurality of treatment options in many regions of the world, has tended to blur the boundaries between 'complementary and alternative medicine' (CAM) on the one hand and 'traditional medicine' on the other. Treatments for musculoskeletal conditions are no exception. Chiropractic and osteopathy, with their high level of acceptance in industrialised countries, fall neatly into the 'complementary and alternative' category; conversely, bonesetting as practiced in many developing countries is clearly 'traditional'. Confusion arises with the diversity of practices that are utilised, in one form or another, throughout the world for the treatment of musculoskeletal pain. These include massage, acupuncture, moxibustion, cupping, and the administration of oral and topical herbal preparations within the context of orthopaedic care.

Table 14.1. Regulation and Official Recognition of Chiropractic and Osteopathy in Selected European Countries.

Country	Regulatory Situation
Denmark	Chiropractors regulated by 1992 law: must inform the patient's practitioner of their diagnosis and treatment, unless referred by another allopathic physician. Public health insurance provides partial reimbursement of the cost up to five chiropractic consultations per year.
Finland	1994 decree gave registered chiropractors, naprapaths and osteopaths full professional status. They must complete at least four consecutive years of approved training to qualify for registration and the right to use the title 'Trained Chiropractor' or 'Trained Osteopath'. Unregistered practitioners are not forbidden to practice, but cannot use the title 'Trained'.
Italy	Chiropractic is recognised as a profession, but not licensed. Chiropractors considered medical auxiliaries, rather than specialists, and must work under the supervision of an allopathic physician.
Netherlands	Chiropractors and osteopaths have a similar legal status to allopathic paramedics: they can practice independently, but may not perform specific medical acts (including radiography).
Norway	Chiropractors officially recognised as health care professionals since 1990. The title 'chiropractor' is restricted to licensed members of the Norwegian Association of Chiropractors. To be licensed, a practitioner must complete an approved course and a year of practical training.
Sweden	Chiropractors completing an approved course have the right to obtain a license and be registered under the National Health Service. No Swedish training programme has yet been approved, and currently all registered practitioners have been trained abroad.
Switzerland	Chiropractic is an independent medical profession that is federally regulated (unlike other CAM therapies, which are regulated at the provincial level). Practitioners must study at least four years in a college accredited by American Council on Chiropractic Education, pass American and Swiss examinations, and complete a one-year internship with a Swiss-authorized chiropractor.
United Kingdom	The 1993 Osteopath Act and 1994 Chiropractor Act recognised both types of practitioners as professionals. Use of the titles is restricted to persons registered with the General Osteopathic Council and the General Chiropractic Council respectively. They are not recognised as official health care providers, and may not work in National Health Service hospitals.

It is not our goal, in this chapter, to provide a comprehensive overview of all the possible ways in which bone, joint and muscle problems can be treated. In particular, we have not reviewed the extensive literature on the use of traditional Chinese medicine in the treatment of musculoskeletal problems. Acupuncture, moxibustion and Chinese herbalism are all well documented in both ancient and modern texts, and are increasingly being adopted in Western biomedical settings. A number of countries, especially in Europe, have developed national legislation to regulate the practice of these disciplines (c.f. Bodeker *et al.*, Chapter 1 of this volume; Shia *et al.*, Chapter 4 of this volume). Conversely, there are many traditions of orthopaedic practice — such as bonesetting, traditional splinting, manipulation and massage — which have been overlooked by official health policies, and remain largely undocumented, but are often the primary source of orthopaedic care in rural areas of developing countries. Our goal, in this chapter, is to draw attention to these some of these practices.

We will present a general overview of practices worldwide, together with a critical review of prospective studies identified from the medical and anthropological literature, and attempt to set out a potential research and policy agenda for this neglected field of health care. As will be discussed, the study of these 'hands-on' healing modalities requires an innovative and inter-disciplinary approach to research and training, distinct from the methodologies used to date in the study of herbal medicine.

14.2. Global Overview of Traditional Orthopaedic Practices

In a literature search using the bibliographic databases MEDLINE, AMED, EMBASE, SOCIOFILE, Sociological Abstracts and the RAI Anthropological Index, we identified several distinct categories of relevant material. The majority of the material consisted of descriptive anthropological studies of traditional orthopaedic practice in contemporary rural communities — often including case studies, with varying degrees of clinical observation by the researchers. These descriptions have been summarised and combined here, in order to give a broad overview of practices around the world. Other types of research described in the literature, such as prospective studies and case studies, are discussed in Section 14.4 below.

The overview is organised regionally, using the current World Health Organisation classification of countries: the European and Eastern Mediterranean Regions have, however, been combined, as there is relatively little data available for the latter. Due to the preliminary nature of this work, we have focused on material available in English and French, and published in peer-reviewed journals cited in the above-named bibliographic databases: thus, there is an inherent bias towards Anglophone and Francophone countries. Online publications that do not form part of the mainstream literature, such as newsletters, bulletins and the websites of selected organisations, are cited only where they add significantly to the understanding of practice.

14.2.1. *Africa*

The reduction and subsequent immobilisation of fractures is described in several accounts of traditional orthopaedic practice in Africa, which illustrate considerable variation in the construction of splints. In Upper Volta (now Burkina Faso) strips of animal skin, bandages, rags, string, cardboard, bamboo, stones and *Azadirachta indica* (neem) twigs have all been used, while the Maasai of East Africa prefer strips of cow hide (Steinmetz, 1982). In Liberia, splints are woven from the split leaf stem of the oil palm, *Elaeis guineensis*, and the bark of *Xylopia* sp. (Harley 1941: 94). Among the Yoruba of Nigeria, splinting is done with 'pieces of raffia woven into a sheet big enough to wrap round the affected limb [and] tied into place with a rope' (Oyebola, 1980: 314). This is the same as the method used by the Akan bonesetters of Adweso, Ghana (Appiah-Kubi, 1981: 59). Elsewhere in Nigeria, bamboo stick splints are frequently used to immobilise fractures (Ofiaeli, 1991; Oguachuba, 1986; Onuminya *et al.*, 2000), and the use of cardboard has also been documented (Maclean, 1971). El-Tom (1996: 98) relates a more complex construction of splints from 'carved wood … with a layer of cotton wool, bars of wood, cotton cloth and an outer layer of adhesive plaster' in the Sudan.

Herbal preparations, believed to speed healing, are often applied to fractured limbs before immobilisation. Several of the interviewed healers were reluctant to disclose any details, describing the recipes as 'the secret of their success' (Oyebola, 1980: 318; c.f. Appiah-Kubi, 1981). A few, however, consented to name the plants used. The practitioner studied by Steinmetz (1982) in Burkina Faso used just two species: *Tamarindus indica* for its anti-inflammatory properties, and *Butyrospermum parkii* for its antiseptic action. By contrast, Harley (1941) describes three separate concoctions used sequentially in treating fractures and sprains in Liberia, each containing four ingredients (Table 1). In South Africa, the sedative plant *Dioscorea dregeana* was historically used as an anaesthetic during manipulation and stabilisation of limb fractures (van Wyk & Gericke, 2000).[1]

Heat may also be used to speed healing, either by burying the fractured limb in the earth and lighting a fire above it, or by holding the limb itself over a fire. The former method has been documented among two ethnic groups in Tanganyika (now Tanzania): the Yao (Steinmetz, 1982) and the Banyamwezi (Livingstone, n.d., cited in Harley, 1941). The latter is described by Oguachuba (1986) as a popular, although dangerous, practice among traditional orthopaedic practitioners (TROPs) in Plateau State, Nigeria.

Much less information is available on African traditional treatments for other musculoskeletal complaints. El-Tom (1996: 99–100) describes the treatment of dislocated joints, sprained ligaments, muscle cramps and spinal pains by a practitioner in the Sudan, using massage (with or without oil) and cauterisation with a heated needle. The explanation given for the latter process is that it 'creates an exit for pain'. In a contrasting example, Hewson (1998) describes a treatment for leg pains in Maputo, Mozambique. The practitioner firstly interviewed the patient about his life, then 'threw the bones for him' (actually a mixture of bones and other small objects, such as shells, nuts and dice) several times in order to divine the cause of the affliction before prescribing herbal mixtures.

14.2.2. *Europe and Eastern Mediterranean*

For centuries, manipulative techniques for treating disorders of the joints and spine were a popular treatment option for both trained physicians and

---

[1] Elsewhere in Africa, such operations are often performed without anaesthesia or analgesia, causing severe pain to the patients (Oguachuba, 1986; Oyebola, 1980; El-Tom, 1996).

folk practitioners[2] throughout Western Europe. In England, the medical establishment had largely abandoned these methods by the early 19th century, perhaps due to recognition of the dangers of manipulation in a population prone to tuberculosis, which can cause joint weakening (Anderson, 1983). Nonetheless, lay bonesetters continued to practice well into the 20th century, successfully treating many cases of stiff and immobile joints by breaking down adhesions, but also causing harm to some of their patients (Cotterell, 1885; Romer, 1915). Their treatments often included 'enveloping in linseed poultices and rubbing with neat's-foot oil' for a week before manipulation (Hood, 1871: 29). Some of the more renowned 19th century bonesetters, such as Hugh Owen Thomas, 1834–1891, and Robert Jones (1895) influenced the development of Western orthopaedic surgery (Cope, 1995; Strach, 1986).

In northern Europe, these methods have been largely replaced by osteopathy and chiropractic on the one hand, and professional hospital-based orthopaedics on the other: only Finland has maintained a separate tradition of massage and bonesetting within the 'folk medicine' sector. In 1989, a survey showed that folk medicine — which also includes sauna, cupping, shamanism, herbalism and various methods of water treatment — was still utilised by around 10% of the Finnish population, in combination with other systems of health care (Vaskilampi, 1991).

Traditional orthopaedics has retained a higher profile in the Mediterranean, and there is a strong tradition of bonesetting in Saudi Arabia (Abdullah, 1993), Malta (World Health Organization, 2001) and Turkey. The 'folk physicians' who are known in Turkish as *ocakli* specialise in treating fractures and dislocations (Ceylan *et al.*, 2002). Hatipoğlu & Tatar (1995) have interviewed 12 bonesetters and 20 clients in the Gaziantep Province of Turkey, and found that the most common procedure for treating fractures is to bathe with lukewarm water, pull the bone into line, and fix it with cotton and cardboard. Other common methods of holding the bone in place involve

---

[2]It is not only in recent years that the relationship between professional doctors and folk healers has been a difficult one. The surgeon Daniel Turner (1695) subtitled his *Apologia chyrurgica* as follows: 'A vindication of the noble art of chyrurgery, from the gross abuses offer'd thereunto by mountebanks, quacks, barbers, pretending bone-setters, with other ignorant undertakers. Wherein their fraudulent practices are plainly detected by several remarkable observations, their fair promises prov'd fictions, their administrations pernicious, their confident pretences injurious and destructive to the welfare of the people'.

the use of eggs mixed with flour or soap powder, strips of wood, various kinds of bandage, and in one case plaster. In addition, bonesetters use 'various tablets and ointments' to alleviate pain and relax muscles, although no details of these preparations are given.

14.2.3. *The Americas*

In North America, as in Western Europe, chiropractic and osteopathy are popular for treating musculoskeletal disorders. The profession of osteopathy is responsible for more than 10% of the total health care delivered in the United States. There are laws relating to the registration of practitioners in the USA and in at least nine Canadian provinces. In Canada, aboriginal practitioners providing traditional medicine services to members of their own communities are exempt from these requirements, while in the US the practice of traditional Native American medicine is regulated under the Self-Determination Act (World Health Organization, 2001).

In the case of Latin America, a World Health Organization review (2001) mentions 'bonesetting' as an important traditional medical specialty in four countries, namely Chile, Guatemala, Mexico and Peru. In Chile, the Mapuche Community Hospital — affiliated with Mapuche University and supported by the Ministry of Health — employs both bonesetters and allopathic doctors, although the extent of collaboration is not described. Massage is listed as an important specialty in Nicaragua.

Huber and Anderson (1996) interviewed eight traditional orthopaedic practitioners, *hueseros* (translated as 'bonesetters') in San Andrés Huyapan, a rural community in the Sierra Norte de Puebla, Mexico. The practitioners reported that they treated 'uncomplicated fractures, dislocated joints, musculoskeletal pain and sprains, simple cuts and bruises' (*ibid*, 28). They used visual examination and palpation in diagnosis, then treated patients with manipulation, massage, the movement of bones where necessary, and usually the application of heated medicines. These included preparations of elder and several other plants (for which the botanical names are not listed), as well as iodine, rubbing alcohol, and an inexpensive rum called *aguardiente*. Five of the eight TROPs had treated uncomplicated fractures by immobilising with reed splints, held in place by wrapping in a cloth smeared with heated pine resin. Elsewhere in Mexico, Werner (1999) observed another method of immobilising fractures: 'the juices of certain plants, boiled into a thick syrup and soaked into a cloth, will harden into a cast'. The plants are unfortunately not named.

Another type of traditional orthopaedic practitioner popular in Mexico is the *sobador*, variously translated as 'bonesetter', 'masseur' or 'folk healer who massages'. Anderson (1987) observed the practice of an individual *sobador* working in Ciudad Juárez, Chihuahua, treating boxers at the municipal gymnasium. Practice was limited to the treatment of cuts, bruises, musculoskeletal pain and stiffness. In addition to massage — often with the use of commercially available anodyne (rubifacient) liniments and lotions, whose mild counter-irritant effect appears to temporarily relieve pain — the *sobador* used more complex techniques of mobilization and manipulation, as practiced by chiropractors and osteopaths.

Detailed anthropological accounts of traditional orthopaedic practice are also available for two separate Highland Maya communities in Guatemala: San Pedro la Laguna (Paul, 1976) and San Juan Comalapa (Hinojosa, 2002). The first of these illustrates a clear distinction between the physical acts performed by the practitioner and the local explanatory model of treatment, as follows:

> *'From the outsider's point of view, the healer resets bones by means of adroit manipulation, massaging the area with marrow extracted from beef bones, placing heated tobacco leaves against the bare skin, and applying a tight bandage. A splint of cardboard or slats may be used to immobilise the injured area. But the bonesetters and their clients see the process differently. In their view the work is not done by the human practitioner but by a special little bone concealed in the hand of the healer... When the travelling bone finds the critical juncture it comes to a halt and stays clamped to the spot long enough to correct the break or dislocation' (Paul, 1976: 78).*

The Maya bonesetters of Comalapa have more empirical and secular assumptions, relying exclusively on their hands to diagnose and treat. They work mainly with *heridas*, a term referring to both deep tissue bruises and joint sprains, as well as more serious joint problems such as dislocations. Not all of them will attempt to reduce fractures; those who do so may use cardboard or sticks for immobilisation, or simply wrap the area with a cloth.

They generally check the injury site several days after reduction to examine its progress (Hinojosa, 2002).

14.2.4. *South-East Asia*

In the Indian subcontinent, orthopaedics — termed *Bhagna* — is an important aspect of the Ayurvedic medical system (Radhika, 2000). In the tenth century BCE, the writer Susrutha described 12 types of fracture, six types of dislocation, and the steps involved in treatment: traction, manipulation by local pressure, opposition and stabilisation, and immobilisation. Vedic literature also describes the aetiology and treatment of rheumatoid arthritis in detail: poor digestion, causing the accumulation of toxins, is said to be the underlying cause, and is treated by dietary restriction and oral herbal tonics. Herbal oils, steam treatment, splinting and intensive massage may also be used (Wilson, 1998).

Many specialist centres offer traditional orthopaedic treatment, especially in South India (Radhika, 2000; Nandakumar & Ghosh, 2000), and some have become highly renowned. Examples are the 'Coimbatore treatment' for club foot, involving a herbal oil and traction, and 'Ankola oil', effective against certain paralytic conditions (Shankar & Majumdar, 1997).

There is widespread use of plants in the treatment of musculoskeletal disorders in India. Oudhia (2003a) estimates that in the state of Chhattisgarh alone, traditional orthopaedic specialists utilise about 150 different species, while Varghese *et al.* (1993) have identified 24 separate species utilised by the Kharia in the treatment of joint disorders. Specifically, *Cissus quadrangularis*, used both orally and topically in the treatment of fractures and dislocations, has been shown to contain active ketosteroids and to hasten the healing of fractures in both pre-clinical and clinical studies (e.g. Udupa & Prasad, 1962; Udupa & Prasad, 1964; Sen, 1964). The related species *C. quadrangula* is known locally as *hadjod* (*had* = bone; *jod* = to fix) because of its utility in the treatment of fractures (Oudhia, 2003a). Other plants described as especially useful for TROP practitioners include *Terminalia arjuna* (Oudhia, 2003b), *Ampelocissus latifolia*, *Anetemisia lacniata* and *Banbase ceiba* (Radhika, 2000). Post-polio residual paralysis has been effectively treated with Ayurvedic preparations containing, among other ingredients, *Withania somnifera* and *Sida retusa* (Nair *et al.*, 1997).

While other countries in South-East Asia may not have codified systems of traditional health care comparable to Ayurveda, they maintain strong traditions of orthopaedic treatment. In Myanmar, where traditional medicine has its roots in Ayurveda, there is a strong tradition of local orthopaedic practice which has been evaluated by researchers in the Yangon Medical School. Flexible bamboo splinting has been found to lead to fractures healing more quickly and completely than with conventional fixed splinting procedures from modern medicine (personal communication from the Dean of Yangon Medical School to G. Bodeker, January 2004) The Tibetan treatments for rheumatoid arthritis and osteoarthritis — consisting of herbal tablets, dietary restrictions and behavioural advice — have been evaluated in a small prospective study (Ryan, 1997; see Section 14.4.1.1).

In Indonesia, a 1995 Ministry of Health survey estimated that there were 8781 bonesetters and 25,077 traditional masseurs/masseuses (World Health Organization, 2001). Village bonesetters are known as *dukuns*, and treat primarily gross fractures of the limbs by the application of splints and powders (Bleck, 1998).

In Thailand, a national survey of treatment for orthopaedic and arthritic cases suggested that there could be twice as many folk healers as qualified medical practitioners in the country (Vajcharadulaya *et al.*, 1984). The WHO review (2001) does not list bonesetting *per se* as a traditional specialty. Rather, it describes traditional Thai medicine as based principally on herbal saunas, herbal steam baths, hot compresses, massage, acupressure and reflexology — all of which could be beneficial for musculoskeletal problems. The Ministry of Health has a National Institute of Thai Traditional Medicine, which offers informal courses at primary and secondary levels, and a university-level program in Thai massage. In Chiang Mai in northern Thailand, there is a hospital of traditional medicine, The Old Medicine Hospital, which offers training in Thai traditional massage for practitioners as well as offering introductory courses for visitors.

14.2.5. *Western Pacific*

Traditional orthopaedic practices, including massage, bonesetting and the use of herbal medicines, are an integral part of martial arts culture in countries such as Japan, Korea and China (Ma, 1999; World Hwa Rang Do

Association, 1995). The practice of Chinese manipulation evolved from the 'Five Animal' play, an exercise created by Hwa To (known as the 'Father of Surgery') over 1700 years ago, which mimicked the movements of the tiger, bear, deer, wolf and bird. Treating low back pain with manipulation had become routine practice by the time of the Tang Dynasty, 618–907 CE, and remains popular today (Kuo & Loh, 1987).

In China, traditional orthopaedics is well accepted within the formal health care system. Smith observed, in 1974, the use of a classical traditional method of fracture reduction in the orthopaedic departments of smaller hospitals. This entailed the use of short wooden splints bandaged over soft paper padding, with the aim of maintaining motility in the muscles and joints around the fracture. Urban hospital-based orthopaedic practice involved a combination of modern and traditional methods: splinting for uncomplicated fractures with a good prognosis, and plaster for all others, with reduction performed under regional nerve block (Smith, 1974). A specific integrated method, combining traditional Chinese and Western techniques, has been developed for treating fractures of the forearm bones. This involves closed reduction by manipulation, immobilisation with thin wooden splints, and functional exercises (Fang *et al.*, 1963; Shang *et al.*, 1987).

While not specifically orthopaedic practices, acupuncture and traditional Chinese herbal medicine are widely used in the treatment of chronic musculoskeletal disorders, especially arthritis (Arichi *et al.*, 1983; Arnold & Thornbrough, 1999; Berman *et al.*, 2000; Chou & Kuo, 1995; Lin *et al.*, 1995; Tsung & Hsu, 1987). Moxibustion (Fang *et al.*, 1998) and cupping (Smith, 1974) are also popular.

Chimpa (1999) gives an account of traditional orthopaedic practice in Mongolia by *bariachi* (bonesetters), who treat fractures and dislocations without medicine, instruments or rituals. The practitioner '*just holds the fractured or dislocated part of the sufferer's body with his or her own hands, twisting it here and there … without any pain on the patient*'. Traditional orthopaedic practitioners are also known to exist in Malaysia (Karim, 1990), but no information is available about their methods.

Chiropractic, osteopathy and Traditional Chinese Medicine are all widely practiced in Australia and New Zealand, as in other industrialised countries, and are regulated by law in most states (World Health Organization, 2001). In indigenous Aboriginal communities, 'bush medicine' — the healing knowledge possessed by all adults — incorporates massage, herbal preparations and external treatments such as ochre, smoke, steam and heat (Maher, 1999). Self-medication is the norm for most 'natural' ailments, such as those caused by physical trauma.

14.3. Socio-Cultural Contexts of Practice

14.3.1. *Recruitment and Training*

Some TROPs are recruited to the profession by virtue of being the son or, more rarely, daughter of a practitioner; others voluntarily undertake an apprenticeship or formal training; and others develop their skills through instinct as a result of necessity. A fourth category represents the practitioners who receive a supernatural 'calling' to the profession, usually in the form of dreams, accompanied by physical suffering if they deny their vocation. All of these categories are represented in the available case studies, as illustrated in Table 14.2, but in the majority of cases recruitment is by inheritance — usually through the male line.

14.3.2. *Explanatory Models of Musculoskeletal Complaints and Their Treatment*

Mellado *et al.* (1994) and Huber & Anderson (1996) comment on the distinction between the naturalistic assumptions made by Mexican bonesetters and the supernatural beliefs of 'curers' and shamans, who perform divination and rituals: '*People go to bonesetters only because they are careless. If a person gets hurt, is it God's punishment or because they were bewitched? No, it is because of carelessness… They fall, trip or stumble.*' (Huber & Anderson, 1996: 30.)

Green (1999) notes that 'the rather obvious features of traumatic accidents' lead even religious and superstitious peoples to take a naturalistic view of musculoskeletal complaints and their treatment. This is true in some societies (El-Tom, 1996; Hinojosa, 2002). There are, however, notable exceptions. The San Pedro Maya, with their 'sacred bone' (Paul, 1976) constitute one example of a supernatural explanatory model. Elsewhere in highland Guatemala, the Quiché people regard dislocated bones and some other incapacitating injuries as a call to serve the gods and ancestors, necessitating special offerings and prayers at shrines (Schuster, 1997).

Table 14.2. Recruitment and Training of Traditional Orthopaedic Practitioners.

Location	Means of Recruitment	Type of Training	Reference
China (Kwangchow)	Personal choice	Formal training at a traditional medical college	Smith (1974)
England (rural areas, early 20th century)	Inheritance	Apprenticed to father or other close relative	Romer (1915)
Ghana (Adweso)	Inheritance	Apprenticed to father or other close relative	Appiah-Kubi (1981)
Guatemala (Highland Maya, Comalapa)	Urgent circumstance, often after own injury	None; practitioner's hands instinctively 'know' the patient's body	Hinojosa (2002)
Guatemala (Highland Maya, San Pedro)	Supernatural vocation via dreams	None; practitioner is perceived as merely the instrument, not the healer	Paul (1976a)
Mexico (Ciudad Juarez)	Personal choice	Apprenticed to unrelated practitioners	Anderson (1987)
Mexico (Hueyapan)	Urgent circumstance	None; self-taught through trial and error	Huber & Anderson (1996)
Mongolia	Inheritance	Apprenticed to father	Chimpa (1999)
Nigeria (Plateau State)	Inheritance	Apprenticed to father	Oguachuba (2000)
Nigeria (Yoruba)	Inheritance	Apprenticed to father	Oyebola (1980)
Sudan (Bagadi)	Inheritance	Apprenticed to father	El-Tom (1996)
Turkey (Gaziantep)	Inheritance or personal choice	Eight out of 12 apprenticed to father, uncle or mother-in-law; the rest learnt from someone outside the family	Hatipoglu & Tatar (1995)

14.4. Existing Research: A Critical Review

We conducted literature searches, using bibliographic databases as discussed in Section 14.2, to identify existing research on traditional treatments for musculoskeletal disorders. Where prospective studies could be identified, their methodology was examined in terms of sample size, randomisation, blinding and the relative objectivity of outcome measures. In this review, we chose to focus on the clinical assessment of holistic treatments, rather than *in vitro* pharmacological or toxicological investigations of specific plants. This is not intended to imply that plants are unimportant in the treatment of bone, joint and muscle problems, or that their pharmacological properties are irrelevant to the outcome of such treatments. Rather, it is an attempt to redress the balance between ethnopharmacology, to which substantial research funding has already been dedicated, and the hitherto neglected field of manual therapy in traditional orthopaedic practice.

Only a few prospective studies have been found for traditional treatments of bone, joint or muscular disorders (Ryan, 1997; Nair *et al.*, 1997; Anderson, 1987; Arichi *et al.*, 1983; Steinmetz, 1982). The scarcity of such material reflects a lack of interest in researching traditional manual therapies, as well as the practical difficulties inherent in ethnomedical research (Anderson, 1991). Traditional orthopaedic practice tends to be considered within the discipline of medical anthropology, rather than medical research *per se*, as if it merited descriptive study only. Other categories of research identified in the literature were case studies, mainly reporting complications of treatment; a single socio-demographic study, relating to the factors influencing patronage of TROPs; and a number of clinical studies of standard traditional Chinese medicine (TCM) treatments, such as acupuncture and moxibustion, for treating orthopaedic conditions. The latter will not be covered in detail here, as the TCM techniques used for these conditions have been well documented in standard texts, and the methodological issues involved in researching such techniques are discussed elsewhere (e.g. Ahn & Kaptchuk, 2005; White, 2004; Birch, 2004; Dincer & Linde, 2003). However, a study by Arichi *et al.* (1983), in which acupuncture was combined with manual therapy, has been included in the review.

14.4.1. *Prospective Studies*

14.4.1.1. Efficacy of a Tibetan Traditional Treatment for Arthritis (Ryan, 1997)

This is an open randomised controlled trial of the Tibetan and Western treatments for arthritis among Tibetan refugees in northern India. Fifteen matched pairs of arthritis patients were identified, with one of each pair randomly chosen to receive the Tibetan treatment (herbal tablets, dietary restriction and behavioural advice) and the other, what is described as 'the standard Western treatment (ibuprofen and indomethecin [sic])'. The study focused on limb mobility, which was quantified by the author and an Indian assistant, using a scoring system developed and used by Danish physiotherapists (Helin, 1994). For rheumatoid arthritis pairs, the experimenters focused on the movement of the hands, and for osteoarthritis pairs, on the knees. It was concluded that the Tibetan treatment worked better than the Western treatment for the improvement of limb mobility in both types of arthritis (P = 0.0005).

The author explains that the openness was inherent in the aim of the study — namely, to compare Tibetans' sensitivity to traditional treatment versus Western treatment. The investigation aimed to determine which treatment was more effective at improving limb mobility in Tibetan subjects, without considering whether the traditional treatment worked through a psychological (placebo) effect, a physiological effect, or a combination of the two. Thus, blinding the patients would have been both difficult, given the nature of the traditional treatment, and counterproductive. She does not, however, explain convincingly why hand and knee mobility was not assessed by an independent clinician — stating only that 'the fieldwork situation in a small town makes blind studies impractical'. The scoring system for knees is largely quantitative, referring to the angles of flexion and stretch defect, but that for hands is more qualitative and has some subjective aspects. It may be difficult, for example, to make a clear distinction between 'a handshake with a strong grip' and 'a handshake [that is] distinguishable but not as strong', if one has nothing against which to compare them. Thus, there is a possibility that researcher bias may affect results. The sample size is also very small. It should further be noted that the use of medication alone as a control is not a fair comparison, as 'Western' treatment for arthritis often involves physiotherapy, and may also include orthopaedic surgery if indicated.

14.4.1.2. Management of Post-Polio Residual Paralysis with Certain Ayurvedic Formulations (Nair *et al.*, 1997)

This is a randomised trial of two separate Ayurvedic treatments, both consisting of an internal and an external application, for the treatment of post-polio residual paralysis in children. There was no control or blinding, and only 14 patients were assigned to each treatment group. An assessment chart consisting of 12 symptoms — including muscle power, muscle wasting, straight leg raising test, muscle tone, various reflexes, etc. — was compiled and an apparently arbitrary numerical value assigned to each symptom. It is unclear whether this is a standard protocol, as no reference is given. The methods of assessing patients are not described, nor is any detailed description of the treatments given; it is clearly assumed that Ayurvedic physicians will recognise the names.

The results show an overall significant improvement in the numerical score ($P < 0.01$) after both treatments relative to the pre-treatment score, and over 75% improvement in the numerical score for seven cases. However, the small sample size and failure to describe assessment methods cast substantial doubt on the reliability of the conclusions, particularly as the study was not blinded. The absence of a control group might be justified with the argument that post-polio paralysis is very unlikely to improve without treatment, but the question should nonetheless have been raised.

14.4.1.3. The Treatment of Musculoskeletal Disorders by a Mexican Bonesetter (*sobador*) (Anderson, 1987)

This paper describes the work of a single Mexican bonesetter (*sobador*) in Ciudad Juarez, Chihuahua, Mexico. The investigator, a medical anthropologist and qualified chiropractor, visited the practitioner daily for ten weeks to record patient contacts, and witnessed at least part of the treatment for more than 20 individuals. The planned format, completed in only 11 cases, consisted of a pre-treatment clinical evaluation of the patient's chief complaint; documentation of the mode of treatment in terms of muscle and bone anatomy; and a brief post-treatment re-examination. The results were necessarily qualitative rather than quantitative, due to the small sample size.

The author notes that on the whole, the *sobador* is a safe practitioner who provides at least some relief to nearly all of his patients at little or no cost to the sufferer. Although he does not treat major orthopaedic disease, he does well in meeting medical standards of practice in the treatment of minor disorders, which may nonetheless be painful and incapacitating. According to the author's criteria, two of the 11 patients obtained 'excellent results', four more showed good improvement, four were slightly improved, and one showed no improvement. The major difficulty with this study is that the assessment criteria are not stated, and there is no way of knowing whether or not the author made any attempt at objectivity.

14.4.1.4. Effects of Acupuncture on Osteoarthritis Deformans and Rheumatoid Arthritis of the Knee, and on Disorders in Motility of the Knee Joint (Arichi *et al.*, 1983)

This is a study of the use of five treatment protocols, involving different combinations of acupuncture and flexion-extension exercises, for patients with knee problems (Table 14.3). Each protocol was tested on three groups of patients, each consisting of ten men and ten women: one group with osteoarthritis deformans, the second with rheumatoid arthritis and the third with disorders in motility of the knee joint after cerebral haemorrhage or thrombosis.

The treatment was evaluated as effective when the flexible angle was improved by more than ten degrees, relative to that measured immediately before treatment. The first protocol (acupuncture on the normal side and flexion-extension exercises on the affected side) proved to be effective in 80% (16/20) of osteoarthritis cases, while groups 2 and 3 had a 40% success rate, and groups 4 and 5 a 20% success rate, respectively. Groups 1 and 2 had a 30% success rate for rheumatoid arthritis, but no other treatment had any effect. None of the treatments were rated as effective for disorders of knee motility after cerebral haemorrhage or thrombosis.

As in the study by Ryan *et al.* (1997), blinding of patients would have been impossible due to the nature of the treatment. It is unclear whether the physician carrying out the measurements of flexible angle was aware which patients had been assigned to which treatment group, but the chosen

Table 14.3. Treatment Protocols Used by Arichi *et al.*, 1983.

Group	Acupuncture	Flexion-Extension Exercises
1	Healthy knee	Affected knee
2	Affected knee	Affected knee
3	Healthy knee	None
4	Affected knee	None
5	None	Affected knee

measure of outcome assessment is objective and well defined. The study could have been improved by increasing the sample size and recording the flexible angle in degrees for each patient, before and after treatment (rather than merely asking whether or not a ten-degree improvement was achieved). This would have permitted the assessment of statistical significance, using a paired Student's t-test.

14.4.1.5. Traditional Traumatology in Upper Volta [Burkina Faso] — Study of the Techniques of a Bonesetter in Yatenga District (Steinmetz, 1982)

This is another study of the practice of a single traditional orthopaedic practitioner, performed in Yatenga District, Burkina Faso, over the course of a year. The study was based on clinical observation, a register of patients, and X-rays where possible. No more than four specific case histories are listed, and 'time to full healing' (17, 29, 30 and 37 days, respectively) is the only outcome measure.

It is assumed that the practitioner saw more than four patients during the course of the year, and there is no explanation of why only these particular cases were recorded, nor any general discussion of the outcomes of other consultations. The author does provide a list indicating the usual duration of immobilisation required for six types of fracture, but it is unclear whether this was provided by the practitioner or derived from observations. An indication of expected healing times for similar cases under an orthodox Western-style treatment regime would have been useful for comparative purposes, but is not given. No complications of treatment were recorded during the period of the study, but the author did not make any attempt to assess the clinical efficacy of treatment in terms of parameters such as shortening or stiffness of the set limbs.

14.4.2. *Case Reports*

Individual case studies from Saudi Arabia (Abdullah, 1993), Turkey (Hatipoğlu & Tatar, 1995), Nigeria (Adebule, 1991; Eze, 1991; Garba & Deshi, 1998; Katchy *et al.*, 1991; Ofiaeli, 1991; Oguachuba, 1986; Onuminya *et al.*, 1999 and 2000) and Taiwan (Huang, 1986) describe the mismanagement of orthopaedic conditions by traditional practitioners.

Most are concerned with the inappropriate or excessively tight application of bamboo stick splints for fractures, leading to gangrene and in some cases necessitating amputation. Other reported errors by TROPs include the failure to set a dislocated elbow correctly (Hatipoğlu & Tatar, 1995) and the neglect of fractures of the femoral neck (Huang, 1986).

At first sight, these case studies imply that traditional orthopaedic practice is intrinsically dangerous, and the situation would seem to be worse in Nigeria than anywhere else. There is, however, an inherent selection bias in such a literature review. Those who have the interest and capacity to report cases to professional journals rarely see successful treatments: of the many patients treated by TROPs, only those who have been failed will seek hospital care. A study by Onuminya *et al.* (2000) illustrates how such bias can provoke an unjustified emotional response against TROPs. Of 100 major amputations performed on 96 patients in two regional Nigerian hospitals over a ten-year period, 60 were iatrogenic, resulting from fracture mismanagement by traditional practitioners. When considered in the context of the likely number of patients seen by such practitioners in the two regions over a ten-year period, however, an average of six failures per year does not seem so horrifying. It is claimed that 'the catchment areas for these regional hospitals include the states in the middle belt and eastern regions of Nigeria, respectively' — presumably serving huge numbers of people. The authors do not state how the 96 patients were selected, and it seems unlikely that exactly 100 amputations were performed at the two hospitals during the ten years: there may be an inherent bias even in the inclusion and exclusion of cases for this report.

It appears likely that the publication of the first study of fracture mismanagement by Nigerian traditional orthopaedic practitioners (Oguachuba, 1986) sensitised the medical community to such cases, and encouraged the practice of reporting them to journals. The publication of three separate articles on this subject in the *Nigerian Medical Journal* in 1991 alone (Eze, 1991; Katchy *et al.*, 1991; Adebule, 1991) may be more indicative of a fashion in publishing than a crisis in Nigerian traditional orthopaedics. This is illustrated by the invention of the terms 'bone setters elbow' (Adebule, 1991) and 'traditional bonesetter's gangrene (TBSG)' (Onuminya *et al.*, 1999).

Trained medical personnel are also not immune from human error, and the above situation is sometimes reversed: traditional methods may be successfully used to treat patients failed by hospitals. For example, Oyebola (1980) describes a case of a patient with fractures of the left tibia and fibula, admitted to the Ado-Ekiti State Hospital. The patient took a voluntary discharge when, after six weeks, the broken bones failed to unite, and subsequently received successful treatment from a Yoruba traditional orthopaedic practitioner. Such 'dealing with the other's mistakes' does little to foster communication between the two parties. Ofaieli (1991), in an attempt to bridge the divide, admits that it is not unusual to come across patients for whom either orthodox or traditional orthopaedic treatment has been carried out with good intentions and disappointing results.

14.4.3. *Factors Influencing Patronage of Traditional Orthopaedic Services*

Thanni (2000) carried out a random survey of 180 adults and adolescents at several locations ('a major motor park, a herbal maternity home, two private health clinics and out patient departments of the study centre') to determine their opinions about traditional bonesetters and orthodox orthopaedic services. The authors do not state how many people were interviewed at each of these locations. The survey was performed by means of an interviewer-administered questionnaire, in which respondents were asked questions such as whether they considered traditional bonesetters to be 'indispensable' (37%), 'desirable' (32.8%), 'undesirable' (8.9%), or 'nuisances/fraudsters' (11.1%). In response to a question on the competence of traditional bonesetters, 43% of respondents rated them as competent or very competent, 24% as satisfactory, and 23% as either incompetent or very incompetent. Education did not have a statistically significant effect on these beliefs.

Unfortunately, the survey did not include questions on whether the respondents had themselves used, or would consider using, traditional orthopaedic services. However, 57.2% of respondents said that traditional bonesetters were cheaper than modern orthopaedic services; 49.4% that they were well known in their communities; and 48.9% that traditional practitioners achieved faster healing.

14.5. Towards a Global Research and Policy Agenda

The lack of any cohesive global research strategy in traditional orthopaedics is clearly evident from the literature: existing research is fragmented, and follows no apparent priorities. Aside from the absence of analysis of biomedical efficacy — a problem identified by Anderson (1991) as applicable to all ethnomedical research — there have been no systematic epidemiological studies examining the patterns of use of traditional and modern orthopaedic care. Neither risks nor benefits have been adequately documented, with the exception of the risk of gangrene from inappropriate splinting of fractures. Furthermore, there have been no studies of the economics of traditional orthopaedic care, such as cost-benefit ratios.

The development of a global research agenda would bring a number of benefits. Firstly, it would identify best and worst practices within the field of traditional orthopaedics: this would empower patients to make informed decisions about their orthopaedic care, as well as highlighting training needs for TROPs. Secondly, it would identify areas of potential collaboration and cross-referral between traditional and Western-trained orthopaedic practitioners, as well as areas in which the Western-trained orthopaedic specialists can learn from TROPs, as discussed briefly by Steinmetz (1982) and El-Tom (1996). This would be a significant contribution to the provision of safer and more effective orthopaedic treatment by both categories of practitioners.

At the international level, a strong research base would act as a foundation for establishing appropriate policy guidelines — both for the orthopaedic profession and for health ministries throughout the developing world — on collaboration, training and formal recognition. Several countries are now establishing legislation regarding the licensing of traditional health practitioners: the development of specific government guidelines for licensing TROPs, combined with training, may help to eliminate unsafe practices such as those described in the Nigerian case studies. State recognition of traditional orthopaedic care should make it more difficult for incompetent or fraudulent practitioners to exploit vulnerable patients, thereby improving the safety of the treatment. It could be enforced, for example, through requisite membership of practitioners' associations in which a suitable expert examines all applicants.

With these aims in mind, there is an urgent need for multi-disciplinary international research collaboration in the field of traditional orthopaedics. Possible priorities for such an initiative are set out below.

14.5.1. *Maintaining the Knowledge Base: The Challenge of Documentation*

Despite their importance in rural societies, traditional orthopaedic specialists are not only invisible in national health policy arenas, but also largely absent from the international discourse on 'indigenous knowledge'. This is in part due to the focus on herbal aspects of traditional medicine (Ellen & Harris, 2000; Plotkin, 1993; also c.f. Schultes & Raffauf, 1990). Traditional orthopaedic specialists have been largely overlooked. Partly due to disapproval of their procedures by mainstream surgeons and in part due to the assumption that they have no patentable products to offer industrialised countries, investment in research has been almost non-existent.

Another likely reason for the lack of documentation of traditional orthopaedic practice is that while plant-based treatments can usually be summarised in writing to a large extent, manipulation and immobilisation techniques can be acquired only through observation or instinct. The skills die with their practitioners, unless the profession acquires new members: the existence of a written record cannot compensate for the absence of hands-on experience. Factors such as rural-urban migration, Westernisation, the increasing marginality of non-cash economies and the influence of religious groups may dissuade young people from taking up apprenticeships, resulting in a cumulative loss of traditional orthopaedic knowledge and skills. In Mongolia, for example, the family line of bonesetters is said to be in decline, leading to concern that the tradition may become extinct (Chimpa, 1999).

There is an urgent need to develop new research methodologies for better documentation and evaluation of traditional orthopaedic practices, and to promote efforts to revive the interest of younger generations in learning these techniques, so that the skills do not die with their elderly practitioners over the course of the next few decades. Audio-visual materials such as documentary films, videos and CD-ROMs may be helpful, both for training purposes and in providing a permanent archive. Care must be taken, however, to ensure that such records are not misused in creating a static system of practices that is unresponsive to circumstances. As Richards (1993) has highlighted, so-called 'indigenous knowledge systems' usually involve a significant element of improvisation. Traditional orthopaedic techniques are deeply embedded in their specific socio-cultural contexts, and every episode of treatment is contingent on personal and political factors. When a practice is documented in a permanent form, there is an increased risk that it will be promoted as 'the' correct treatment at the expense of all others, even in cases where it is not the most appropriate. The flexibility and personal nature of the services provided by traditional health care practitioners are among their greatest assets (c.f. Oyebola 1980), and should not be sacrificed in the name of preserving knowledge for posterity.

14.5.2. *Utilisation and Cost-Effectiveness*

Preliminary research by one of the authors (J. Cohen) has indicated that in The Telugupalayam Siddha Clinic in Coimbatore, Tamil Nadu, India, the most common reasons for seeking traditional orthopaedic care include chronic problems such as post-polio paralysis, cerebral palsy and club foot, as well as more acute conditions such as fractures and dislocations. Further research is needed to determine whether these are also the most common reasons elsewhere, and what other factors influence utilisation of TROPs. In areas where Western-style orthopaedic care is available, do patients use traditional treatment for social, cultural or economic reasons, or a combination of these factors? How cost-effective are traditional orthopaedic services? Also, are there pockets of excellence which draw people, and what are the reasons given for choosing this type of service?

14.5.3. *Measures of Success*

It is important to note the conditions for which traditional orthopaedic treatment appears to be most successful: this will require a definition of what constitutes 'success', which will differ according to the condition being researched. Clearly, patient satisfaction is an important criterion, as parameters such as pain are difficult to measure objectively: visual analogue scales may be helpful, together with standard 'quality of life' instruments such as the SF-36 and SF-12. Anderson (1991) notes, however, that self-evaluation by patients is a very limited measure of success if the concern is with biomedical evaluation of changes in the disease process. A balance should be sought between these two criteria.

In the case of fractures, successful 'bonesetting' can be measured by the absence of complications, such as shortening and stiffness: X-rays can be helpful for evaluation purposes. For arthritis, the functional disability scoring system described by Ryan (1997) is useful, as is the more straight-forward measurement of flexible angle used by Arichi *et al.* (1983).

A useful starting point for a global research strategy would be the development of guidelines or standard operating procedures for controlled clinical trials and cohort studies appropriate to the evaluation of traditional orthopaedic practices. These will need to be different for each condition being evaluated. Ideally, trials should be at least single-blind — the physicians carrying out the assessment of disability should be unaware which patients have received which treatment, although in practice it will often be impossible to have double blind for the patients. Statistically valid outcome assessment calls for a large sample size, and random assignment of patients to the treatment and control groups (Anderson, 1991). It may not always be appropriate to use orthodox Western treatment as a control, as Ryan (1997) has done; this will depend on whether Western treatment is normally available to the population concerned. If the patients' usual choice is between traditional orthopaedic care and no treatment at all, then the design of trials should reflect this choice, with an untreated control group showing the natural history of the disease or injury. In the study of conditions for which spontaneous improvement has been demonstrated to be rare, such as fractures, difficult questions may be raised with regard to the ethics of withholding treatment. Even in other conditions, patients may not consent to participate if they will receive a placebo or no treatment. The inclusion of untreated controls may not always be necessary if the sample size is sufficiently large to give a high statistical probability that any observed effect is due to the treatment.

14.5.4. *Best Practice*

It should not be assumed that within a particular category of treatment, such as bone setting or Ayurvedic therapy, all practitioners do the same job: as in orthodox Western medicine, best and worst practice can be identified within any specialty. An important role for a working group on traditional orthopaedics, incorporating practitioners, would to identify and document existing best practice. This could allow for (i) the development of guidelines for practitioners; (ii) training workshops aimed at promoting best practice and eliminating unsafe methods; and ultimately (iii) the development of a regulatory framework, e.g. criteria for membership of a specialist practitioners' association.

14.6. Possible Frameworks

14.6.1. *International Research Collaboration*

A useful model may be the Research Initiative on Traditional Antimalarial Methods (RITAM: Bodeker & Willcox, 2000), an international partnership that is already addressing several of the issues described above. RITAM is collaboration between clinicians, pharmacologists, traditional health practitioners, ethnobotanists, anthropologists and entomologists, and currently has over 200 members from 30 countries (Willcox & Bodeker, Chapter 10 of this volume). It addresses mosquito control and repellence, as well as the use of plants for the prevention and treatment of malaria. Since its inaugural meeting in Moshi, Tanzania in December 1999 — funded by the Rockefeller Foundation, the Nuffield Foundation and WHO's Special Programme for Research and Training in Tropical Diseases (TDR) — RITAM has held parallel sessions at several international conferences on tropical medicine, and maintained regular e-mail discussions. Its specialist working groups include Preclinical Studies; Clinical Studies; and Policy, Advocacy and Funding. Guidelines or standard operating procedures for pre-clinical and clinical studies have already been developed, and literature reviews compiled (Willcox *et al.*, 2004).

The proposed traditional orthopaedics research initiative may differ from RITAM, in needing to be established from a more limited knowledge base than has been the case with the malaria initiative. While many isolated researchers and institutions are already concerned with plants used in the treatment of malaria — and there is a significant body of work relating to 'CAM' modalities, such as acupuncture, osteopathy and chiropractic, used in treating musculoskeletal disease in industrialised countries — very little research has been conducted on traditional orthopaedic techniques, such as bonesetting and massage, in their original contexts. While it would clearly be of central importance to unify and coordinate any existing projects, a global traditional orthopaedics initiative could also develop and support new programmes of targeted research, aimed at comparing various aspects of practice between and within countries.

Such an analysis would be complicated by the vast diversity of diseases and injuries that can be considered as musculoskeletal problems. One starting point might be to choose specific conditions — such as traumatic injuries, polio, cerebral palsy and club foot — and launch a large-scale attempt to determine the level of utilisation of TROPs by sufferers in several countries. This could be achieved through a combination of methods. Firstly, patients attending hospitals and primary health care clinics could be interviewed about their use of traditional health care for orthopaedic conditions. It should be recognised that this would almost certainly lead to under-reporting, as some patients may feel that it would be disrespectful to medical staff to admit that they use traditional treatment (Dabis *et al.*, 1989). Further, the highest utilisation of TROPs is likely to be in rural areas with no formal Western health facilities, or where the staff at local health centres are not trained or equipped to deal with trauma.

Secondly, practitioners themselves could be asked about their patients — in some countries, traditional health practitioners' associations may be able to help by providing contact details. Thirdly, and perhaps most importantly, random community surveys could be carried out by an interviewer who is perceived as indifferent to the response — preferably a member of the community concerned (A/Rahman *et al.*, 1995). These should include not only hypothetical questions ('*would* you use TROPs?') but also questions about past experience ('*have* you used TROPs?'). Cohorts of patients should be followed prospectively to see which treatments are actually used (Willcox & Bodeker, 2004).

A practical challenge to this kind of endeavour is that the practitioners themselves are often excluded from global communication networks. Language can be a major barrier to participation, as can the lack of access to electronic resources in rural areas of the developing world. The problem may be compounded for traditional orthopaedic practitioners,

who are often of lower social status than herbalists or shamans (Huber &
Anderson, 1996) and are thus less likely to belong to associations that
can adequately represent their interests. High-profile practitioners' associations such as ZINATHA in Zimbabwe, THPAZ in Zambia and GHAF-
TRAM in Ghana undoubtedly have some members who practice traditional
orthopaedics, but at the international level these organisations may be more
concerned with advocacy for herbal medicine. Non-governmental organisations such as the Foundation for the Revitalization of Local Health Traditions (FRLHT: http://www.frlht-india.org) can play a major role in bridging
the gap between grassroots community groups and international agencies.

14.6.2. *Integrative Clinical Practice*

Collaboration between traditional and 'western' orthopaedic services could
do much to improve the safety of the former. Tragedies such as the Nigerian
iatrogenic amputations resulting from gangrene, for example, could have
been avoided by a follow-up visit to a doctor or medical assistant capable
of identifying the problem at an early stage.

In addition, there are undoubtedly cases in which collaboration with
skilled traditional practitioners could enhance the struggling discipline of
orthopaedics in the formal health care services of non-industrialised countries. Golding, a professor of tropical orthopaedics in the West Indies,
laments that *'the Third World has to face the situation where the techniques, equipment and maintenance [of orthopaedic technology] are
largely beyond their resources... and it is extremely difficult to cope using
antiquated methods which are so obviously inadequate'* (1988: 32). Traditional orthopaedic specialists may, over hundreds of years, have developed
parallel solutions to some of the problems for which Golding and his colleagues demand 'braces, appliances, surgical footwear, orthoses and pros-
theses' (*ibid.*). Even the most basic of western orthopaedic technology is
sometimes unsuitable for tropical contexts: plaster casts, for example, tend
to disintegrate in hot, damp climates (Steinmetz, 1982: 149). Integrating
appropriate traditional methods could improve the cultural appropriateness
and acceptability of clinical services: the Chinese methods of integrated
treatment of fractures (Fang *et al.*, 1963; Shang *et al.*, 1987) may be a
useful model for others to emulate.

As Wilson (1991: 138) has observed: '*it is unlikely that Third World medicine can do without the traditional healer. We [clinicians] must therefore make him [sic] our ally rather than our enemy*'.

14.6.3. *Regional Training Centres*

It has been debated in the past whether the West should provide more training for orthopaedic surgeons from developing countries, or train more paramedical personnel (Anon, 1973b). Aware of the need for sustainability, some have found more creative solutions than merely attempting to copy Western facilities. In Malawi, several hundred Orthopaedic Clinical Officers have been trained (Prof. J. Wilson, personal communication). These are nurses with a further 18 months of specialist training, who offer management of trauma — including some basic operative procedures, such as simple internal fixations — and can correct some deformities such as club foot. Trained by Western doctors, they are aware of the risks and complications of the procedures they perform, and recognise the limitations on their skills. A similar program has been developed in Uganda (Ofaieli, 1991). Such Clinical Officers remain dependent, however, on the training and support offered by Western orthopaedists. Even this more appropriate service remains expensive in the context of the resources available, and the cost of reproducing it countrywide would be inordinately high.

In attempting to address the educational needs of the developing world, orthopaedics could learn some helpful lessons from the profession of dermatology. The International Foundation for Dermatology, established in 1987, is committed to providing low-cost, sustainable skin care in rural areas of developing countries (Ryan, 2000; Ong & Ryan, 1994). The Regional Dermatology Training Centre (RDTC) at the Kilimanjaro Christian Medical Centre, Moshi, Tanzania, has so far trained 100 allied health professionals from all over sub-Saharan Africa as Dermatology Officers capable of advising universities and governments on skin care programs (see also Chapter 13). The RDTC's initiative goes further than the Orthopaedic Clinical Officer program in attempting to integrate safe and effective traditional remedies. A compounding facility donated by the Vancouver Rotary Club allows the students to practice making their own topical medicaments for skin conditions, for which medicinal plants and honey are available on site.

Consultation with traditional health practitioners is an important part of the curriculum, and joint workshops for students and traditional practitioners have been held at the centre.

Malawi, with its trained Orthopaedic Clinical Officers, would perhaps be one country which might begin an analogous attempt at greater integration between Western and traditional orthopaedic services. A 'Regional Orthopaedic Training Centre' based at a Western-style teaching hospital would also provide an ideal base for an international research network as discussed above.

14.7. Conclusions

A firm commitment, on the part of the profession of orthopaedics, to the developing world is urgently required. Western-trained orthopaedic specialists should recognise, as some dermatologists have done in recent years, that urban hospital-based practice cannot fulfil the needs of the rural areas of developing countries: addressing these needs calls for a new profession of 'public health orthopaedics'. Such a profession cannot but incorporate both allied health professionals, such as the Orthopaedic Clinical Officers trained in Malawi and Uganda, and traditional orthopaedic practitioners. Its success would be closely linked to the degree of trust and cooperation that can be established between its members. Its aims would be the promotion of simple, appropriate technology for the treatment of uncomplicated disease or injury, and the recognition of more serious or advanced conditions requiring specialist attention. Of course, specialists may not always be readily available, and in these circumstances practitioners should be trained to act according to the principle of *primum non nocere*.

An essential foundation for the establishment of public health orthopaedics is systematic research into the utilisation, safety and efficacy of traditional practices. This would be best achieved by the inauguration of an international research initiative, and requires a commitment of funding from international donor organisations — who, while they may be attracted to rehabilitation of war victims, are generally less excited by chronic and disabling musculoskeletal disease (Wilson, 2000). While specialist non-governmental organisations such as GIFTS of Health and

World Orthopaedic Concern have an important role to play in mobilising the necessary political will for such a programme, the primary responsibility may lie with larger agencies such as national Ministries of Health and the World Health Organization.

References

Abdullah MA. Traditional practices and other socio-cultural factors affecting the health of women and children in Saudi Arabia. *Ann Trop Paediatr* 1993;13:227–232.

Adebule GT. The bone setters elbow: the question of a justifiable but difficult moral dilemma for the orthopaedic surgeon. *Niger Med J* 1991;21:126.

Ahn AC, Kaptchuk TJ. Advancing acupuncture research. *Altern Ther Health Med* 2005;11(3):40–45.

Anderson R. The treatment of musculoskeletal disorders by a Mexican bonesetter (*sobador*). *Soc Sci Med* 1987;24(1):43–46.

Anderson R. The efficacy of ethnomedicine: research methods in trouble. *Med Anthropol* 1991;13:1–17.

Anderson RT. On doctors and bonesetters in the 16th and 17th centuries. *Chiropr Hist* 1983;3(1):11–15.

Anderson RT. An orthopedic ethnography in rural Nepal. *Med Anthrop* 1984;Winter:46–59.

Anon. Editorial: Orthopaedic training in developing countries. *B Med J* 1973a; 6 Oct:4–5.

Anon. Editorial: Orthopaedic training in developing countries. *Lancet* 1973b;2(834):890–891.

Anon. Notes and News: Orthopaedics in the Third World. *Lancet* 1989;23–30 Dec;1538.

Appiah-Kubi K. *Man Cures, God Heals: Religion and Medical Practice Among the Akans of Ghana*. New York: Friendship Press, 1981, pp. 58–61.

A/Rahman SH, Mohamedani AA, Mirgani EM, Ibrahim AM. Gender aspects and women's participation in the control and management of malaria in Central Sudan. *Soc Sci Med* 1995;42(10):1433–1446.

Arichi S, Arichi H, Toda S. Acupuncture and rehabilitation (III). Effects of acupuncture applied to the normal side on osteoarthritis deformans and rheumatoid arthritis of the knee and on disorders in motility of the knee joint after cerebral hemorrhage and thrombosis. *Am J Chin Med* 1983;11:1–4.

Arnold MD, Thornbrough LM. Treatment of musculoskeletal pain with traditional Chinese herbal medicine. *Phys Med Rehabil Clin North Am* 1999;10(3): 663–671.

Bannerman RH. *Traditional Medicine and Health Care Coverage.* Geneva: World Health Organization, 1983.

Beetham R. The history of World Orthopaedic Concern. *World Orthopaedic Concern Newsletter*; January 2000. Published on the Internet: http://www. worldortho.com/woc/woc_news80.html

Berman BM, Swyers JP, Ezzo J. The evidence for acupuncture as a treatment for rheumatologic conditions. *Rheum Dis Clin North Am* 2000;26(1):103–115.

Birch S. Clinical research on acupuncture. Part 2. Controlled clinical trials, an overview of their methods. *J Altern Complement Med* 2004;10(3):481–498.

Bleck EE. Letter: Comments on the medical and social models in rehabilitation. *Asia Pac Disabil Rehabil J* 1998;9:2.

Bodeker G. The GIFTS of Health Reports. *J Altern Complement Med* 1996;2(3):397–405, 435–447.

Bodeker G. Planning for cost-effective traditional health services. In: *Traditional Medicine, Better Science, Policy and Services for Health Development: Proceedings of a WHO International Symposium*, Awaji Island, Hyogo Prefecture, Japan, 11–13 September 2000. Kobe, Japan: WHO Center for Health Development, 2001.

Bodeker G, Kabatesi D, Homsy J, King R. A regional task force on traditional medicine and AIDS in East and Southern Africa. *Lancet* 2000;355:1284.

Bodeker G, Willcox M. New research initiative on plant-based antimalarials. *Lancet* 2000;355:761.

Ceylan S, Hamazaoğlu O, Kömürcü S, Beyan C, Yalçin A. Survey of the use of complementary and alternative medicine among Turkish cancer patients. *Complement Ther Med* 2002;10:94–99.

Chimpa L. On traditional Mongolian medicine. *AyurVijnana* 6, Spring 1999. Published on the Internet: http://www.kreisels.com/ittm/ittm48.htm

Chou C-T, Kuo S-C. The anti-inflammatory and anti-hyperuricemic effects of Chinese herbal formula danggui-nian-tong-tang on acute gouty arthritis: a comparative study with indomethacin and allopurinol. *Am J Chin Med* 1995;23:261–271.

Cope R. Hugh Owen Thomas: bone-setter and pioneer orthopaedist. *Bull Hosp Joint Dis* 1995;54(1):54–60.

Cotterell E. *On Some Common Injuries to Limbs: Their Treatment and After-Treatment Including Bone-Setting (so-called).* London: Lewis, 1885.

Dabis F, Breman JG, Roisin AJ, Haba F. The ACSI-CCCD team. Monitoring selective components of primary health care: methodology and community assessment of vaccination, diarrhoea, and malaria practices in Conakry, Guinea. *Bull World Health Org* 1989;67:675–684.

Dincer F, Linde K. Sham interventions in randomized clinical trials of acupuncture — a review. *Complement Ther Med* 2003;11(4):235–242.

Ellen RF, Harris H. Introduction. In: Ellen RF, Parkes P, Bicker A (eds.) *Indigenous Environmental Knowledge and Its Transformations: Critical Anthropological Perspectives*. Amsterdam: Harwood, 2000, pp. 1–33.

El-Tom AO. The bone setter: A case study from central Sudan. *African Anthropol* 1996;3(1):91–112.

Eze CB. Limb gangrene in traditional orthopaedic (bone setters) practice and amputation at the NOHE — facts and fallacies. *Niger Med J* 1991;21:125

Fang HC, Gu YW, Shang TY. The integration of modern and traditional Chinese medicine in the treatment of fractures. A simple method of treatment for fractures of the shafts of both forearm bones. *Chin Med J* 1963;82:493. Reprinted with commentary by L. Peltier: *Clin Orthop* 1996;323:4–11.

Fang JQ, Aoki E, Seto A, Yu Y, Kasahara T, Hisamitsu T. Influence of moxibustion on collagen-induced arthritis in mice. *In Vivo* 1998;12(4):421–426.

Garba ES, Deshi PJ. Traditional bone setting: a risk factor in limb amputation. *East Afr Med J* 75(9):553–555.

Golding JSR. The problem of orthopaedics in the Third World. *Curr Orthop* 1988;2:32–34.

Green SA. Orthopaedic surgeons: inheritors of tradition. *Clin Orthop* 1999; 363:258–263.

Hammond L. *The Need for Integrating Indigenous and Bio-Medical Health Care Systems: Case Study from Ada Bai Returnee Settlement*, Humera, Ethiopia. 1994 Thematic Monitoring Report UNDP Emergencies Unit for Ethiopia. Published on the Internet: www.africa.upenn.edu/eue_web/health94.htm

Harley GW. *Native African Medicine: With Special Reference to Its Practice in the Mano Tribe of Liberia*. London: Frank Cass & Co., 1941.

Hatipoğlu S, Tatar K. The strengths and weaknesses of Turkish bone-setters. *World Health Forum* 1995;16:203–205.

Helin P. *Funktionsbevarende Kontrolsystem ved Rheumatoid Arthritis. Manual for the Measurement of Limb Mobility in Rheumatoid Arthritis*. Copenhagen: Glostrup Hospital, 1994.

Hewson MG. Traditional healers in southern Africa. *Ann Intern Med* 1998;128(12):1029–1034.

                                    G. Burford et al.

Hinojosa SZ. "The hands know": bodily engagement and medical impasse in Highland Maya bonesetting. *Med Anthrop Quart* 2002;16(1):22–40.

Hood WP. *On Bone-Setting (So-Called) and Its Relation to the Treatment of Joints Crippled by Injury, Rheumatism, Inflammation.* London and New York: Macmillan and Co., 1871.

Huang C-H. Treatment of neglected femoral neck fractures in young adults. *Clin Orthop* 1986;206:117–126.

Huber BR, Anderson R. Bonesetters and curers in a Mexican community: conceptual models, status, and gender. *Med Anthropol* 1996;17(1):23–38.

Jones R. Discussion on the treatment of intractable talipes equinovarus. *Trans Br Orthop Soc* 1895;1:20

Karim WJ. *Emotions of Culture: A Malay Perspective.* Singapore: Oxford University Press, 1990.

Katchy AU, Nwankwo OE, Chukwu CC, Ukegbu ND, Onabowale BO. Traditional bone setters treatment of femoral fractures. How far? *Niger Med J* 1991;21:126.

Kuo PP-F, Loh Z-C. Treatment of lumber intervertebral disc protrusions by manipulation. *Clin Orthop* 1987;215:47–55.

Last M. Professionalization of indigenous healers. In: Johnson TM, Sargent CF (eds.) *Medical Anthropology: Contemporary Theory and Method.* New York: Praeger, 1990, pp. 349–366.

Lin C-C, Chen M-F, Chen C-F. The anti-inflammatory effects of Chinese crude drug preparations on experimental arthritis. *Am J Chin Med* 1995;23:145–152.

Lodha R, Bagga A. Traditional Indian systems of medicine. *Ann Acad Med Singapore* 2000;29(1):37–41.

Ma GX. Between two worlds: the use of traditional and modern health services by Chinese immigrants. *J Comm Health* 1999;24(6):421–437.

Maclean C. *Magical Medicine: A Nigerian Case Study.* London: Penguin Press, 1971.

Maher P. A review of 'traditional' aboriginal health beliefs. *Aust J Rural Health* 1999;7(4):229–236.

Mellado C, Sánchez RVA, Femia P, Navarro AM, Erosa ES, Bonilla DMC, Domínguez HM del S. *La Medicina Tradicional de los Pueblos Indígenas de México [The Traditional Medicine of the Indigenous Peoples of Mexico].* México D. F: Instituto Nacional Indigenista, 1994, p. 69

Murray CJL, Lopez AD. *The Global Burden of Disease: A Comprehensive Assessment of Mortality and Disability from Diseases, Injuries and Risk Factors in 1990 and Projected to 2020.* Cambridge: Harvard University Press, 1996.

Nair PRC, Vijayan NP, Madhavikutty P. Management of post-polio residual paralysis with certain Ayurvedic formulations. *J Res Ayurveda Siddha* 1997; 18(1–2):11–20.

Nandakumar N, Ghosh G. Herbs bind broken bones. *The Hindu Folio — Indian Health Traditions* 2000;October 8:42–43.

Ofiaeli RO. Complications of methods of fracture treatment used by traditional healers: a report of three cases necessitating amputation at Ihiala, Nigeria. *Trop. Doct* 1991;21:182–183.

Oguachuba HN. Mismanagement of elbow joint fractures and dislocations by traditional bone setters in Plateau State, Nigeria. *Trop Geogr Med* 1986;38: 167–171.

Ong C-K, Ryan TJ. *Healthy Skin for All.* Oxford: International Foundation for Dermatology, 1994.

Onuminya JE, Onabowale BO, Obekpa PO, Ihezue CH. Traditional bone setter's gangrene. *Int Orthop* 1999;23(2):111–112.

Onuminya JE, Obekpa PO, Ihezue CH, Ukegbu ND, Onabowale BO. Major amputations in Nigeria: a plea to educate traditional bone setters. *Trop Doc* 2000;30:133–135.

Oudhia P. *My Experience and Interactions with Herb Collectors and Growers of Chhattisgarh, India Associated with Medicinal Herb Hadjod (Cissus quadrangula)*, 2003a. Published on the Internet and accessed 20.05.2005 at 16:28. http://www.botanical.com/site/column_poudhia/43_hadjod.html

Oudhia P. *Traditional Medicinal Knowledge About Medicinal Herbs Koha (Terminalia arjuna) and Sarphonk (Tephrosia purpurea) in Chhattisgarh Plains*, India, 2003b. Published on the Internet and accessed 20.05.2005 at 16:30. http://www.botanical.com/site/column_poudhia/64_koha.html

Oyebola DDO. Yoruba traditional bonesetters: the practice of orthopaedics in a primitive setting in Nigeria. *J Trauma* 1980;20(4):312–322.

Paul BD. The Maya bonesetter as sacred specialist. *Ethnology* 1976;15(1):77–81.

Plotkin M. *Tales of a Shaman's Apprentice: An Ethnobotanist Searches for New Medicines in the Amazon Rain Forest.* New York: Viking, 1993.

Radhika M. A tradition of bone setting. *The Hindu Folio — Indian Health Traditions* 2000;October 8:38–41.

Richards P. Cultivation: knowledge or performance? In: Hobart M (ed.) *An Anthropological Critique of Development: The Growth of Ignorance.* London: Routledge, 1993, pp. 61–78.

Romer F. *Modern Bonesetting for the Medical Profession.* New York: Rebman, 1915.

Ryan M. Efficacy of the Tibetan treatment for arthritis. *Social Sci Med* 1997;44(4):535–539.

Ryan TJ. Dermatology in the developing world. *Deliv Dermatol Health Care* 2000; 18(2): 201–210.

Schultes RE, Raffauf RF. *The Healing Forest: Medicinal and Toxic Plants of Northwest Amazonia*. Portland, OR: Dioscorides Press, 1990.

Schuster AMH. Rituals of the modern Maya. *Archaeology* 1997;50(4):1–4.

Sen SP. Study of the active constituents (ketosteroids) of *Cissus quadrangularis* Wall. *Indian J Pharm* 1964;26(9):247–248.

Shang TY, Gu YW, Dong FH. Treatment of forearm fractures by an integrated method of traditional Chinese and Western medicine. *Clin Orthop* 1987;215:56–64.

Shankar D, Majumdar B. Beyond the Biodiversity Convention: the challenges facing the biocultural heritage of India's medicinal plants. In: Bodeker G, Vantomme P (eds.) *Medicinal Plants for Forest Conservation and Health Care. Non-Wood Forest Products Series, 11*. Rome: Food and Agriculture Organization, 1997.

Smith AJ. Medicine in China: best of the old and the new. *Br Med J* 1974;2(915):367–370.

Steinmetz JP. Traumatologie traditionelle en Haute-Volta. Étude des techniques d'un rebouteux du Yatenga. [Traditional traumatology in Upper Volta. Study of the techniques of a bonesetter in Yatenga district]. *Méd Trop* 1982;42(2):145–150.

Strach EH. Club foot through the centuries. *Prog Paed Surg* 1986;20:215–237.

Thanni LOA. Factors influencing patronage of traditional bone setters. *West Afr J Med* 2000;19(3):220–224.

Tsung P-K, Hsu H-Y. *Arthritis and Chinese Herbal Medicine*. Long Beach, CA: Oriental Healing Arts Institute, 1987.

Turner D. *Apologia Chyrurgica*. London: J. Whitlock, 1695.

Udupa KN, Prasad GC. *Cissus quadrangularis* in healing of fractures: a clinical study. *J Indian Med Assoc* 1962;38(11):590–593.

Udupa KN, Prasad GC. Further studies on the effect of *Cissus quadrangularis* in accelerating fracture healing. *IJMR* 1964;52(1): 26–35.

Vajcharadulaya Y, Vajchirapornthip A, Vajcharachaisurapol S. [Traditional healers who practice treatment of the diseases of bone and joint in Thailand.] In: *The 50th Anniversary of the Royal Academy of Thailand*, 31 March 1984, pp. 321–357 (in Thai). Cited in: Okanurak K, Sornmani S, Chitprarop U. *The Impact of Folk Healers on the Performance of Malaria Volunteers in Thailand*, TDR/SER/PRS/10. Geneva: World Health Organization Special Programme for Research and Training in Tropical Diseases, 1992.

Van Wyk B-E, Gericke N. *People's Plants*. South Africa: Briza Publications, 2000.

Varghese E, Jain SK, Bose N. A quantitative approach to establish the efficacy of herbal remedies: a case study on the Kharias. *Ethnobotany* 1993;5:149–154.

Vaskilampi T. The role of alternative medicine: the Finnish experience. In: Lewith G, Aldridge D (eds.) *Complementary Medicine and the European Community*. Saffron Walden, UK: The C W Daniel Company Ltd, 1991, pp. 101–112.

Werner D. *Disabled Village Children: A Guide for Community Health Workers, Rehabilitation Workers, and Families*, 2nd edn. Berkeley, CA: Hesperian Foundation, 1999.

White PJ. Methodological concerns when designing trials for the efficacy of acupuncture for the treatment of pain. *Adv Exp Med Biol* 2004;546:217–272.

Willcox ML, Bodeker G. Frequency of use of traditional herbal medicines for the treatment and prevention of malaria: an overview of the literature. In: Willcox ML, Bodeker G, Rasoanaivo P (eds.) *Traditional Medicinal Plants and Malaria*. Boca Raton: CRC Press, 2004.

Willcox ML, Bodeker G, Rasoanaivo P (eds.) *Traditional Medicinal Plants and Malaria*. Boca Raton: CRC Press, 2004.

Wilson JN. Editorial: Iatrogenic gangrene in the Third World. *Trop Doct* 1991;21(4):137–138.

Wilson JN. Whither then WOC — 2000 onwards? *World Orthopaedic Concern Newsletter*, January 2000. Published on the Internet, accessed 20.05.2005 at 16:59: http://www.worldortho.com/woc/woc_news80.html

Wilson JN. Reports from the field. *World Orthopedic Concern Newsletter*, January 1998. Published on the Internet, accessed 20.05.2005 at 17:00: http://www.worldortho.com/woc/woc_news74_1.html

World Health Organization. *World Health Report 1997: Conquering Suffering, Enriching Humanity*. Geneva: World Health Organization, 1997.

World Health Organization. *World Health Report 1999: Making a Difference*. Geneva: World Health Organization, 1999.

World Health Organization. *Legal Status of Traditional, Complementary and Alternative Medicine: A Worldwide Review*, WHO/EDM/TRM/2001.2. Geneva: World Health Organization, 2001.

World Health Organization, International Union for the Conservation of Nature and World Wide Fund for Nature (WHO/IUCN/WWF). *The Chiang Mai Declaration: Saving Lives by Saving Plants*. WHO/IUCN/WWF International Consultation on Conservation of Medicinal Plants, Chiang Mai, Thailand, 21–26 March 1988. Geneva: WHO, 1988.

World Hwa Rang Do Association. Hwa Rang Do: preserving a past, present and future. *Dojang Magazine*, Winter 1995. Published on the Internet and accessed 20.05.2005 at 17:02: http://www.hwarangdo.com/dojang1.htm

Zerner C. Telling stories about biological diversity. In: Brush SB, Stabinsky D (eds.) *Valuing Local Knowledge: Indigenous People and Intellectual Property Rights*. Washington DC: Island Press, 1996, pp. 68–101.

Zhuo D. Traditional Chinese rehabilitative therapy in the process of modernization. *Int Disabil Studies* 1988;10(3):140–142.

RESEARCH

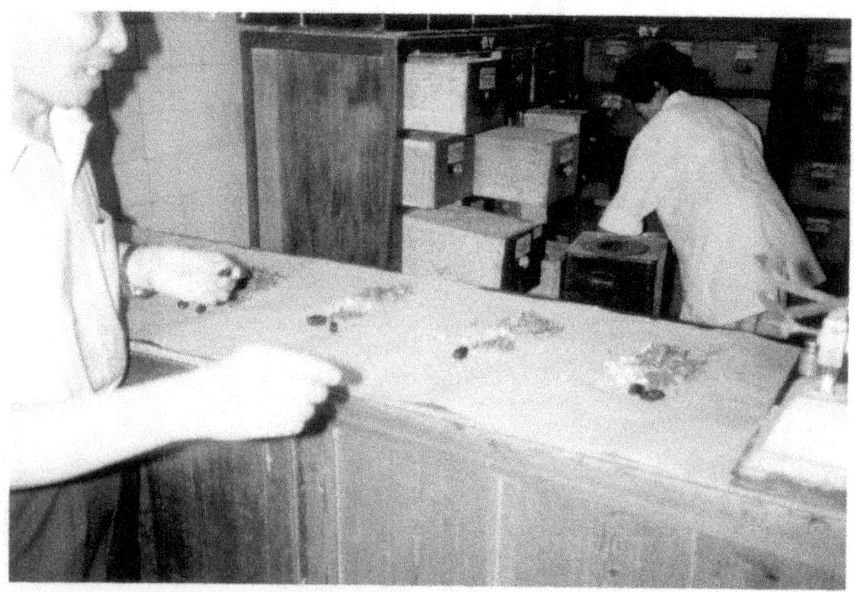

Complex mixtures of plants at the National Institute of Burns, Hanoi, Vietnam, used traditionally for managing severe burns. (*Photo courtesy of G. Bodeker.*)

CHAPTER 15

CLINICAL TRIAL METHODOLOGY

Ranjit Roy Chaudhury, Urmila Thatte and Jianping Liu

15.1. Introduction

Clinical studies on herbal medicines have, in the past, been carried out either by individuals with experience in clinical trial methodology of synthetic drugs but a poor background in traditional systems of medicine, or by traditional medicine practitioners who have less training in the conduct of clinical trials according to modern concepts of clinical pharmacology. In the age of evidence-based medicine, the results of such trials are often not acceptable to the wider scientific community and practitioners of allopathic medicine, who need clear-cut and high quality evidence of efficacy and safety before they can translate research findings to clinical practice.

The clinical evaluation of herbal remedies within the specific framework of rigorous clinical pharmacological principles, done without trampling on the concepts of traditional systems of medicine, is an important challenge (Chaudhury, 1992). It is also necessary for practitioners of traditional systems of medicine to accept the use of modern clinical trial methodology to evaluate herbal preparations they use (Chaudhury, 2001a).

The basic principles in the clinical evaluation of herbal remedies are, of course, the same as for a synthetic compound (Chaudhury & Chaudhury, 2002). However, there are also very important differences. In this chapter, the issues that arise during clinical development of herbal medicines because of these differences will be described with examples from the Indian programme, which has taken note of these differences and modified the clinical trial methodology accordingly.

15.2. Starting Material

The medicinal plant on which research is planned presents formidable challenges to a researcher. From correct identification through the method and site of harvesting, the part of the plant being used, the processing, standardisation, purity and to the final formulation; all have to be taken into consideration. The WHO publication *Quality Control Methods for Medicinal Plant Materials* (1998) describes all the precautions that have to be followed before any research is undertaken on a herb. With special consideration of tropical diseases, the UNICEF/UNDP/World Bank/WHO Special Programme for Research & Training in Tropical Diseases (TDR), has provided operational guidance on information needed to support clinical trials of herbal products (TDR, 2005). Special attention must also be paid to standardisation of the compound, using markers — if possible, bioactive markers (*Indian Herbal Pharmacopoeia*, 2002). Besides, the terminology of medicinal plants or herbs should comply with the WHO ATC guidelines using both pharmaceutical name and botanical Latin name in the documentation (Uppsala Monitoring Centre, 2004).

Traditional formulations, as described in ancient texts, are easier to work with in the existing regulatory and ethical scenario. However, research must also be conducted to identify more effective extracts (to reduce the dose) and newer dosage forms of herbal remedies. The work with *Tinospora cordifolia* is symbolic of this approach. Clinical studies were first initiated with the 'balguti', which is the formulation widely used in Ayurveda (Rege *et al.*, 1993). However, once initial studies indicated efficacy, a standardised film-coated tablet of the water extract was prepared and used for further studies (Dahanukar & Thatte, 1997).

Similarly, in initial exploratory studies conducted by the Central Drug Research Institute, Lucknow (http://www.cdriindia.org) with *Picrorhiza kurroa*, the whole extract was used. While these studies were going on, the active hepatoprotective extract, Picroliv, was identified and developed into a new drug, following the regulatory path for a new chemical entity. Now multi-centre clinical trials are being carried out with Picroliv.

The quality of the herbal medicine is crucial to the study — and if it is not determined prior to initiating the clinical study, precious resources may be wasted. For example, using samples obtained from the northeast state of Bihar, early phase II trials with *Vicoa indica* demonstrated its efficacy as an anti-fertility agent. In later studies, the drug obtained from the northwestern state of Madhya Pradesh proved ineffective.

In traditional medicine, importance is given to the vehicle, e.g. honey, ghee, ginger juice (Gogte, 2000), in which the active herbal medicine is administered. This enhances the effects of the medicine or counteracts side effects.

Finally, it is very common to have a formulation of many plants, which interact with each other — such as formulations containing Guggul (*Commiphora wightii*). Guggul has anti-inflammatory, analgesic and hypolipidemic properties. It is combined with other plants like Triphala (a combination of *Phyllanthus emblica*, *Terminalia chebula* and *Terminalia belerica*) to potentiate its actions and minimise its side effects. Guggul is combined with *Azadiracta indica*, *Tinospora cordifolia*, and *Adhatoda vasica*, in the formulation Panchtiktaghrit guggul, to treat skin disorders, or with *Boerhavia diffusa* (in Punarnava guggul) to treat oedema (Rajeshwardatashastri, 2001). Attempting to determine which of the many plants in the combination is responsible for the effect adds to the challenges of clinical research on herbal medicines.

15.3. Phases of Clinical Development

In classical clinical pharmacology the clinical development of a compound is divided into four phases. In principle, the same applies to a herbal medicine, with some specific differences.

15.3.1. *Phase I*

Phase I studies are done to determine the safety and maximum tolerated dose of the product, usually in healthy adults. With herbal medicines, there is a paucity of data from animal studies, and even if available, it is found that results in animals cannot be easily extrapolated to humans. Further, the choice of starting dose also poses a challenge although suggestions from traditional practices and literature may be useful.

If the plants under study have been in use in traditional medicine, classical phase I studies may not be needed and the need for animal toxicity is also considerably reduced. However, if a new formulation or combination of plants has been made, the safety and activity in normal human subjects has to be evaluated, as is currently being done with an Indian herbal anti-fertility agent (Chaudhury, 2001).

One aspect studied in phase I is pharmacokinetics. With herbal medicines, pharmacokinetic studies are difficult, due to difficulties in plasma estimation of 'active' molecules. Sometimes there is not only one active molecule, but many, and they may undergo further metabolic changes during absorption. Nonetheless, some such studies have been attempted (Bhattaram *et al.*, 2002). A study of 'effect kinetics' is an attractive option to assess the time course of action of herbs and gain an initial picture of their pharmacokinetic behaviour in the body.

15.3.2. *Phase II*

Phase II trials are exploratory studies conducted in a limited number of patients, at selected centres under strictly controlled conditions, to assess the effective dose range and safety of the product. Although blinded studies are advisable (see Section 15.5), they are not mandatory at this stage. Toxicity studies are not needed prior to phase II trials unless there are reports suggesting toxicity, or the herbal preparation is to be used for more than three months (DTAB, 2002).

It would be necessary to undertake at least a four- to six-week toxicity study in two species of animals when: (a) there are reports suggesting toxicity; (b) the herbal preparation is to be used for more than three months; or (c) a larger multi-centre phase III trial is subsequently planned, based on the results of the phase II study (DTAB, 2002).

15.3.3. *Phase III*

Phase III studies are confirmatory studies performed to assess the efficacy and safety of the drug in a larger number of patients, usually in multiple centres (see below). The study drug is compared with a standard drug and/or a placebo, if a standard drug does not exist for the disease under study.

15.3.4. *Phase IV*

After approval of the drug for marketing, phase IV studies are undertaken to obtain additional information about the drug's risks, benefits and optimal use. As the number of patients treated grows, side effects not recorded in strictly controlled trials are often discovered in this stage, which represents the 'real life situation'. Many herbal medicines are already in the market, and therefore most studies fall into this category.

15.4. Multi-centre Trials

Multi-centre studies are often necessary, but are not easy to conduct. All centres must use the same protocol; trained personnel to conduct the study, using common recruitment and laboratory methods and identical reagents; and procedures to assess safety and efficacy. A centralised laboratory and data management group is useful. When multi-centre studies are being done on herbal remedies, the mode of storage, transport and shelf-life/stability of the formulations have to be very carefully attended to.

The clinical trial of *Pipalliyadi vati*, a herbal contraceptive, is a good example of a multi-centre study. This was conducted under a National Task Force with representatives of many research organisations of the country. Standardisation of the three constituents (*Embelia ribes, Piper longum* and borax) led to an acceptable formulation. Teratology studies were performed (Chaudhury *et al.*, 2001) and clinical studies initiated. The multi-centre studies had to be terminated as the combination appeared to lose its activity after three months — illustrating the problems with coordinating multi-centre studies with herbal materials across a country as large as India. Now, fresh samples are prepared every two weeks with strict standardisation.

15.5. Blinding

Blinding (preferably double-blinding) in clinical studies increases confidence in the results, as it eliminates investigator bias. A double-blind study is one in which neither the investigator nor the participant is aware of the exact drug being given. In a single-blind study, either the investigator or the patient knows what is being given, while the other remains 'blind'.

With herbal medicines, it is indeed a challenge to plan double-blind randomized clinical trials. There are examples, however, in which this design has been successfully used. One of these was a double-blind flexible dose, randomized, multi-centre trial of Vijayasara (*Pterocarpus marsupium*), in diabetes mellitus (Chaudhury, 2001c). Another was a double-blind, placebo-controlled randomised study of *Tinospora cordifolia*, which confirmed its immunostimulant activity in patients with breast cancer, tuberculosis and obstructive jaundice (Dahanukar & Thatte, 1997).

It should be emphasised that the gold standard of double-blind, randomised clinical trials is not the only way to determine effectiveness, particularly in the case of herbal medicines. Very useful results can be obtained in single-blind studies, where either the patient or the doctor is aware of what medication is being used. One way to reduce bias of the investigator in this design is to use a team of two investigators — one administers the medicine, and the other assesses the response.

At an early stage in a drug's development, open studies are also useful. Thus, at one stage, an open trial of the plant *Pterocarpus marsupium* had to be carried out. This provided a vital link leading to the double-blind, flexible-dose, randomised clinical evaluation of the plant (Chaudhury, 2001c).

The clinical studies with ksharasootra (a medicated thread covered in the ashes of *Curcuma longa*, *Euphorbia nerifolia* and *Achyranthus aspera*, used to treat fistula-in-ano) are also illustrative of the usefulness of this approach. Four collaborating centres conducted controlled, randomised, multi-centre open (i.e. not blinded) studies with objective variables for assessment of efficacy, and showed that this medicated thread was as effective as surgery in treating anal fistula (Shukla *et al.*, 1991).

15.6. Use of a Placebo

A placebo is a formulation that looks, smells and (where relevant) tastes similar to a drug being assessed, but contains no active medication. It is unethical to assign patients to a placebo if an effective treatment of their condition is available (Rothman & Michels, 1994). For example, proven therapy may not be omitted in trials of new anti-retroviral treatments in patients with AIDS, or new thrombolytic drugs in patients with recent myocardial infarction (Ellenberg & Temple, 2000). Under these circumstances, the new drug under study should be compared to an available drug.

However, when evaluating herbal remedies that relieve minor symptoms or enhance quality of life, placebo-controlled trials would pose no greater risk and would be justified (Rothman & Michels, 1994). Placebo-controlled trials have proved the clinical value of herbs such as St. John's Wort in mild or moderate depression (Linde *et al.*, 1996), *Ginkgo biloba* for dementia (Ernst & Pittler, 1999) and saw palmetto in benign prostate hyperplasia (Wilt *et al.*, 1998).

The major challenge in research on herbal medicines is the preparation of a placebo whose colour, taste, odour, flavour and formulation exactly match those of the plant product. Investigators should ensure that in an attempt to match the placebo to the active compound, another plant extract or incompletely extracted plant material is not used as a placebo. The placebo should be truly inert, so that results are not compromised.

15.7. Other Study Designs

15.7.1. *Single-Case Studies*

In addition to the above designs, evidence from studies of individual cases is very useful for herbal medicines (WHO, 2000). To be meaningful, single-case designs should have a common protocol, which could be the basis of collaborative research between practitioners.

15.7.2. *Observational Studies*

In observational studies, the traditional medicine practitioner continues his treatment without modifying it in any way, and the clinical investigator records the clinical response (Vaidya *et al.*, 2003). These studies could provide a valuable model for studying both the efficacy and the safety of herbal medicines.

Observational studies cost less, allow for a wider range of patients to be studied, are closer to real-life situations, and provide valuable information. However, it is imperative that rigorous and standardised methods are used to record the observations, so as to make conclusions which are meaningful and can be generalised. These, like all studies, must adhere to the highest ethical standards.

15.7.3. *Add-On Studies*

The 'add-on' design is another useful design for herbal therapies. Here, the conventional treatment is given as usual, and the herbal medicine (or placebo in the control group) is added. This therefore does not compromise the conventional therapy. For example, when a study was conducted in patients of pulmonary tuberculosis (Rege *et al.*, 1999), *Tinospora cordifolia* or placebo (given in a randomised manner) were administered in addition to conventional anti-tuberculosis agents. Results indicated that *Tinospora cordifolia* hastened radiological clearance and sputum conversion rate. It also improved weight gain and appetite significantly, as compared to placebo.

15.7.4. *Qualitative Research*

Some aspects outside clinical studies affect the evaluation of herbal intervention, such as patients' preference, experience, attitude, knowledge, and expectation, as well as practitioners and researchers' perspectives. The importance and benefits of using qualitative research in the area of TCAM is increasingly being recognised. Qualitative methods aim to make sense of, or interpret, phenomena in terms of the meanings people bring to them (Greenhalgh & Taylor, 1997). They preserve the richness and variability of the subject and the interventions, which randomised trials may lose. The commonly used methods are documents, passive observation, participant observation, in-depth interviews, and focus group. The validity of qualitative methods can be improved by using a combination of methods (triangulation).

15.8. Randomized Controlled Trials (RCTs) for Herbal Medicines

It is accepted practice today that all clinical trials should be randomised to rule out bias. As far as possible this practice should be followed;

randomisation is possible in nearly every comparative clinical trial, including herbal clinical studies. However, herbal medicines derived from traditional medical systems involve complex interventions which are holistic in nature, focus on symptoms rather than well-defined diseases, involve intra- and inter-variation in responses, and require a long duration of therapy in order for the effect to be seen. This makes the use of RCTs challenging (Liu *et al.*, 2002).

Methodological flaws have been identified during last several years in RCTs related to Chinese herbal medicine (Tang *et al.*, 1999; Liu *et al.*, 2002). These included limited description of methodology such as the randomisation method, allocation concealment, double blinding, and withdrawal/drop-outs; small sample size; inadequate of controls used; and description of intervention regimens.

To adopt the characteristics of traditional herbal medicine, several designs of RCTs have been developed, such as stratified randomisation by practitioners or the syndrome complex ('Zheng' in traditional Chinese medicine), waiting list randomisation to differentiate the effect from natural history of disease, N of 1 trial, pragmatic trials to understand the system effect (not component efficacy), and expertise-randomisation to assess operational procedures for specific skills or expertise.

15.9. Selection of Patients

In any clinical trial, the right drug has to be given to the right patient. In traditional Indian systems of medicine, the *prakriti* (in Ayurveda) or *mijaj* (in Unani medicine) determines the effectiveness of a particular herbal medicine. Prakriti could be described as the temperament or the psychomotor character of the individual (Dahanukar & Thatte, 1989 and 1996). A person could have predominantly one of the following prakriti: *vata*, *pitta* or *kapha*, and the treatment varies according to the prakriti. Thus, although it is widely accepted that *Commiphora wightii* (guggul) is effective in the treatment of arthritis, Ayurveda recommends specific formulations for patients with different prakritis: a kapha prakriti individual will respond to Yograj guggul, Hingwashtak churna and Dashamool; a pitta prakriti person to castor oil and Sinhanad guggu; and a vata prakriti patient to Panchatiktaghruta guggul and Maharasnadiquath (Gogte, 2000). In another example, a study on sibutramine in patients with obesity showed that most of the responders to the drug had a pitta prakriti, while most of the non-responders were of the kapha prakriti.

Sometimes a herbal medicine useful for one type of patient is actually harmful when administered to a patient with the same disease but a different constitutional type. Kanaka is effective in patients of bronchial asthma with a kapha constitutional type, but will cause congestion in pitta patients. The fresh juice of *Momordica charantia* will be effective in diabetic patients who are kapha or pitta, but should be avoided by vata patients. Similarly, a hypertensive patient with vata or kapha constitutional type would respond to Samirpannaga rasa, but this will produce side effects in a pitta patient, who would do better with Tagaradi Churna. In malarial fever (Vishama jwara), a combination of the bark of *Azadirachta indica* (*neem*), *Zingiber officinale* (dried ginger, known in Sanskrit as 'sunti') and *Piper nigrum* (black pepper, known in Sanskrit as 'maricham') would be effective in the kapha type of individual, but not in the pitta or vata type, where side effects would manifest.

Hence, it is strongly recommended that the prakriti is assessed and used as an inclusion/exclusion criterion in clinical studies. Objective question-naires are available to assess this characteristic (Dahanukar & Thatte, 1996). Similar principles, using traditional taxonomies for classifying patients and diseases, would apply in the evaluation of traditional Chinese medicines.

Another issue to consider while researching herbal medicines is that the choice of therapy may vary according to concomitant symptoms. For example, an asthmatic patient with associated gastrointestinal disturbances will respond to one medicine, while another patient without gastrointestinal disturbances would need another medicine (Chaudhury, 1992).

15.10. Clinical End-Points and Efficacy Variables

In the case of safety end-points, no compromises can be made. However, with efficacy end-points, traditional descriptions of the medicine's effects on patients should be kept in mind. Innovative scoring methods and clini-cally meaningful, multi-dimensional quality-of-life scores must be devel-oped to evaluate herbal medicines. Any clinical end-point selected must be valid, reliable, objective and above all, clinically relevant to the health of patients, if it is to influence the decisions made by physicians and patients.

Just as patients are included on the basis of symptom complexes described in the traditional medicinal system, these symptom complexes must be used in developing efficacy variables, rather than using only conventional parameters (such as fasting and post-prandial blood sugar concentrations, or glycosylated haemoglobin, in diabetes trials) to judge efficacy.

15.11. Laboratory Support

As with other drugs, during development, ongoing communication with the laboratory is essential. Thus, as clinical trials are proceeding, new information may make the design of specific animal studies necessary to refine the clinical trials. The story of *Streblus asper* is illustrative. Initial exploratory clinical trials demonstrated a therapeutic effect of this plant in filariasis. However, there was some cardiac toxicity. Further detailed experimental work revealed the cause of the cardiac toxicity, and a new extract without cardiac toxicity was developed. New clinical studies will now be initiated.

15.12. Ethical Considerations

All the ethical considerations applicable to research on allopathic medicine also apply to planning and conducting clinical evaluations of herbal medicines. The principal investigator must take a traditional (e.g. Ayurvedic, Unani etc.) physician as a co-investigator when doing a trial on a herbal remedy. When a folklore medicine is ready for commercialisation after it has been found effective, the legitimate rights of the tribe or community from whom the knowledge was gathered should be addressed appropriately while applying for Intellectual Property Rights and Patents for the product (See also Bodeker, Chapter 17 of this volume).

As for allopathic medicines, informed consent must be obtained from patients when a trial is being conducted on herbal medicines. It is interesting that due to the strong cultural and social beliefs that traditional medicines are safe and effective, patients are often encouraged to choose these remedies. There appears to be a subconscious trend for patients to volunteer, with very few inhibitions, to participate in a study on a herbal medicine.

The Indian Council of Medical Research has Ethical Guidelines for Biomedical Research on Human Subjects (2000), which are a useful guide for those planning research on herbs.

15.13. Conclusions

This chapter has highlighted the complexities of evaluating medicinal plants in a clinical setting. It is hoped that it will help investigators to plan clinical trials of medicinal plants, which would respect both the concepts of the traditional systems of medicine and those of modern clinical trial methodology. There is an urgent need to develop, alongside herbal remedies, research methods that can be used to assess the value of traditional medicines. Thus, a higher level of evidence can be made available for traditional therapies that are of potential benefit to the wider public.

References

Bhattaram VA *et al.* Pharmacokinetics and bioavailability of herbal medicinal products. *Phytomedicine* 2002;Suppl III:1–33.

Chaudhury MR, Chandrashekharan S, Mishra S. Embryotoxicity and teratogenecity studies of an Ayurvedic contraceptive, *Pippalyadi vati. J Ethnopharmacol* 2001;74:189–193.

Chaudhury RR. *Herbal Medicines for Human Health.* New Delhi: World Health Organization Regional Office for South East Asia, 1992.

Chaudhury RR. Commentary: challenges in using traditional systems of medicine. *Br Med J* 2001a;322:164.

Chaudhury RR. In: Gupta CM, Chaudhury SR (eds.) *Proceedings of Symposium on Current Status of Fertility Regulation.* Lucknow: Central Drug Research Institute, 2001b, pp. 11–21.

Chaudhury RR. Antidiabetic effect of *Vijayasar Pterocarpus marsupium.* In: Gupta SK (ed.) *Pharmacology and Therapeutics in the New Millennium.* New Delhi: Narosa Publications, 2001c, pp. 355–356.

Chaudhury RR, Chaudhury M. Standardisation, preclinical toxicology and clinical evaluation of medicinal plants including ethical considerations. In: Chaudhury RR, Rafei UM (eds.) *Traditional Medicine in Asia*. New Delhi: World Health Organization Regional Office for South East Asia, 2002, pp. 209–226.

Dahanukar SA, Thatte UM. *Ayurveda Revisited*. Mumbai: Popular Prakashan, 1989.

Dahanukar SA, Thatte UM. *Ayurveda Unravelled*. New Delhi: National Book Trust, 1996.

Dahanukar SA, Thatte UM. Current status of Ayurveda in phytomedicine. *Phytomedicine* 1997;4:359–368.

DTAB. *Good Clinical Practices for Clinical Research in India*. Delhi: Director General of Health Services and Chairman, DTAB, 2002.

Ellenberg S, Temple R. Placebo-controlled trials and active-control trials in the evaluation of new treatments. Part 2: Practical issues and specific cases. *Ann Inter Med* 2000;133:464–470.

Ernst E, Pittler MH. *Ginkgo biloba* for dementia: a systematic review of double-blind, placebo-controlled trials. *Clin Drug Invest* 1999;17:301–308.

Gogte VM. *Uses of Medicinal Plants in Ayurvedic Pharmacology and Therapeutic (Dravyaguna)* 1st English edn. Bhartiya Vidya Bhavan's SPARC Publication, 2000, pp. 257–259.

Greenhalgh T, Taylor R. How to read a paper: papers that go beyond numbers (qualitative research). *Br Med J* 1997;315:740–743.

Indian Council of Medical Research. *Ethical Guidelines for Biomedical Research on Human Subjects*. New Delhi: Indian Council of Medical Research, 2000.

Indian Herbal Pharmacopoeia, revised edn. Mumbai, Indian Drug Manufacturers' Association, 2002.

Linde K *et al.* St. John's wort for depression: an overview and meta-analysis of randomised clinical trials. *Br Med J* 1996;313:253–258.

Liu J, Kjaergard LL, Gluud C. Misuse of randomization: a review of Chinese randomized trials of herbal medicines for chronic hepatitis B. *Am J Chin Med* 2002;30:173–176.

Rajeshwardatashastri (ed.). Amavatadhikar. In: *Bhaishajya Ratnavali*, 14th edn. Varanasi: Chaukhambha Publications, 2001, pp. 565, 632.

Rege NN *et al.* Immunotherapy with *Tinospora cordifolia*: a new lead in the management of obstructive jaundice. *Indian J Gastroenterol* 1993;12:5–8.

Rege NN, Thatte UM, Dahanukar SA. Adaptogenic properties of six *rasayana* herbs used in Ayurvedic medicine. *Phytother Res* 1999;13:275–291.

Rothman KJ, Michels KB. The continuing unethical use of placebo controls. *New Engl J Med* 1994;331:394–398.

Shukla NK *et al*. Multicentric randomized controlled clinical trial of *Kshaarasootra* (Ayurvedic medicated thread) in the management of fistula-in-ano. *Indian J Med Res* 1991;94(B):177–185.

Tang JL, Zhan SY, Ernst E. Review of randomised controlled trials of traditional Chinese medicine. *Br Med J* 1999;319:160–161.

TDR. *Operational Guidance: Information Needed to Support Clinical Trials of Herbal Products*. UNICEF/UNDP/World Bank/WHO Special Programme for Research & Training in Tropical Diseases (TDR), WHO, Geneva, 2005.

Uppsala Monitoring Centre. *Guidelines for Herbal ATC Classification*. WHO Collaborating Centre for International Drug Monitoring, 2004.

Vaidya RA, Vaidya ADB, Patwardhan B, Tillu G, Rao Y. Ayurvedic pharmacoepidemiology: a proposed new discipline. *J Assoc Physicians India* 2003;51:528.

Wilt TJ *et al*. Saw palmetto extracts for treatment of benign prostatic hyperplasia. *JAMA* 1998;280:1604–1609.

World Health Organization. *Quality Control Methods for Medicinal Plant Materials*. Geneva: World Health Organization, 1998.

World Health Organization. *General Guidelines for the Methodologies on Research and Evaluation of Traditional Medicines*. Geneva: World Health Organization, 2000.

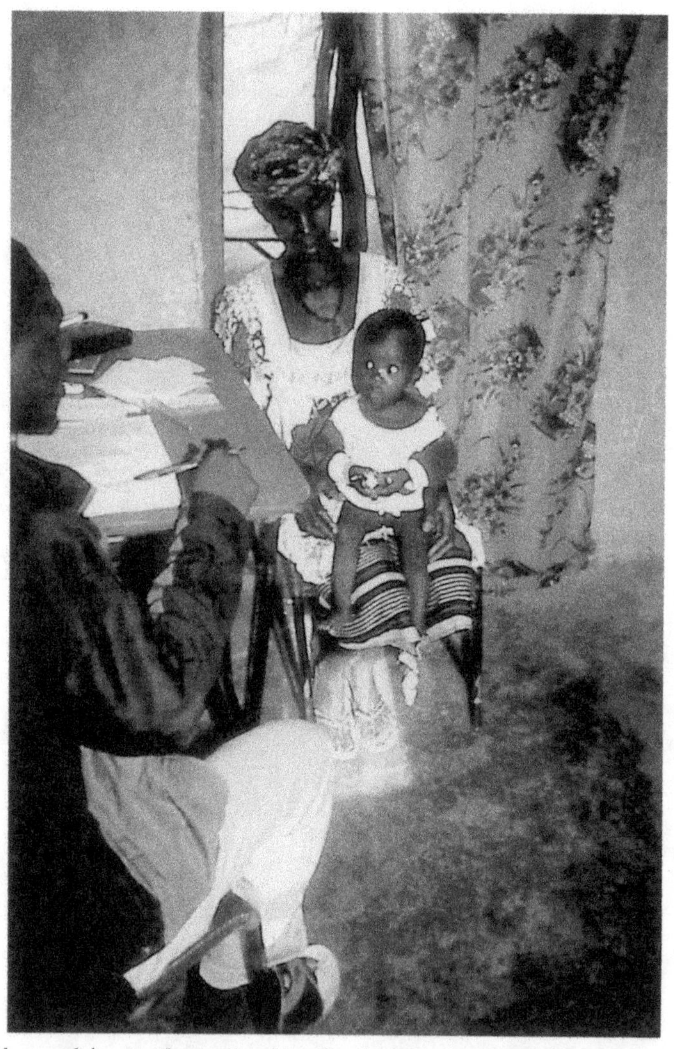

A researcher explains an observational study of a herbal anti-malarial plant, and obtains informed consent, to a patient and her mother in Missidougou, Mali. (*Photo courtesy of M. L. Willcox.*)

CHAPTER 16

ETHICAL ISSUES IN RESEARCH

Merlin L. Willcox, Gerard Bodeker and Ranjit Roy Chaudhury

16.1. Introduction

Traditional medicine is defined as '*the sum total of the knowledge, skills and practices based on the theories, beliefs and experiences indigenous to different cultures, whether explicable or not, used in the maintenance of health, as well as in the prevention, diagnosis, improvement or treatment of physical and mental illnesses*' (World Health Organization, 2000). Like modern medicine, it has evolved on the basis of observation, trial and error. Traditional medical systems also have underlying theories of health and disease, which help to determine which treatments will help a particular set of symptoms. Codified systems such as Ayurveda and traditional Chinese medicine have very elaborate written theories and prescriptions. Oral systems such as African traditional medicine are more fluid over time and space, as they are transmitted from generation to generation. Until recently, however, practitioners and patients of traditional medicine have not sought to prove its safety and efficacy by conducting scientific experiments in the same way as modern pharmaceutical medicine. For many patients in developing countries, it is the only type of treatment that they can access and afford. Others choose to use it in preference to pharmaceutical medicine for certain conditions, because they perceive it to be more effective, or have more trust in traditional healers than in doctors (Hahold & Kroeger, 1990).

Although general ethical issues on clinical trials are just as pertinent to traditional medicine as to conventional medicine, they have already been discussed in detail elsewhere (General Medical Council, 2001), and are outlined in the Declaration of Helsinki (World Medical Association, 2002).

This chapter aims to examine those issues specific to traditional medicine, according to the four cardinal principles of medical ethics as set out by Beauchamp & Childress (1989):

1. Autonomy (freedom of choice)
2. Non-maleficence (not doing harm)
3. Beneficence (doing good)
4. Justice (equal allocation of resources).

Ethical dilemmas raised by traditional medicine regulation and research in developing countries have been neatly summarised as follows by Kitua & Malebo (2004):

> *'It is difficult and will be unethical to stop any of the existing traditional medical practices in the absence of a better substitute, and yet it is equally unethical to let practitioners administer to individuals and populations medicines for which there is no scientific evidence of efficacy and safety'.*

This apparently self-contradictory statement will be dissected and discussed in detail below, from the viewpoints of the different ethical principles.

16.2. Autonomy

This principle is that a person should be allowed to act 'in accordance with a freely self-chosen and informed plan' (Beauchamp & Childress, 1989). In other words, patients should have the freedom to choose what treatment they take for their illness, and the freedom to choose whether or not to participate in a research study.

Eighty per cent of the world's population is said to rely on traditional medicine for primary health care (Bannerman *et al.*, 1983). To stop any existing traditional medical practices in developing countries would remove patients' freedom of choice, and so would not be ethical, unless there were good evidence that a particular practice was seriously harmful to patients. In this case the principle of autonomy may be overridden by the principles of non-maleficence and beneficence, which highlight the need to protect patients from harm and to do good. However in most cases, there is no reliable scientific evidence for or against the safety or efficacy of traditional medical practices. Therefore the principles of non-maleficence and beneficence cannot be applied. To prevent patients from using traditional medicines would contravene their autonomy. Yet it is unclear to what extent the decision to use traditional medicine is truly autonomous. Although some patients have a free choice whether to use this or modern medicine, in many cases, traditional medicine is their only option. In this circumstance, the way to improve patients' autonomy would be to provide an alternative, rather than to stop the use of traditional medicine.

Freedom of choice depends on the availability and affordability of different treatment options. Many patients in developing countries, especially those living in remote rural areas, do not have ready access to, let alone the means to afford, modern health care. Furthermore, the level of information available about traditional medicine is very limited. Very few traditional medicines have been evaluated pre-clinically, and even fewer clinically, as to their safety and efficacy. Therefore research on traditional medicine is needed in order to empower patients to make truly autonomous, informed decisions. Even for patients who do not have access to modern medicine, research can help to determine which forms of traditional medicine are the safest and most effective, thereby enabling them to make an informed choice between different traditional treatments.

However, participation in such research should also be autonomous, following the principles of informed consent. Patients should not be compelled or unfairly enticed to participate in a study, and should be fully informed about all important potential risks and benefits of participation, so that they can decide for themselves whether or not to take part. This can be difficult to achieve in a developing country context, where patients are used to health professionals telling them what to do, and where patients may not be able to read or sign consent forms. The challenge for researchers is to establish procedures that are both ethically sound, and culturally sensitive; this could be done, for example, through sustained community involvement in research (Lindegger & Bull, 2003).

16.3. Non-maleficence

The principle of non-maleficence is summed up by the dictum '*primum non nocere*' (first do no harm), and this raises the primary concern with traditional medicines: their safety. Some argue that traditional medicines should be subject to the same stringent toxicological tests as modern pharmaceuticals. However, these are very expensive and may therefore inhibit any research on traditional medicine. By definition, traditional medicine is not a new discovery which belongs to one person or company, so it cannot be patented. Therefore big pharmaceutical companies are not interested in funding research on it.

Furthermore, it does not seem logical to impose the same criteria on medicines that have been used for centuries as on newly synthesised chemical entities never before ingested by humans. Laboratory toxicity tests are designed to evaluate whether a novel chemical is safe to administer to humans. Traditional medicines, by definition, have already been used by humans for decades, centuries or even millenia. Oral and written traditions incorporate safeguards to prevent toxicity, such as cautions about the method of preparation, the safe dose to administer, and the use of additional measures to offset side effects (Lei & Bodeker, 2004). Often medicinal plants are also incorporated in the diet — for example, rhubarb, basil, ginger and mint. No one requires extensive toxicity tests before eating these in a meal — when the quantities ingested may be as large or even larger than those prescribed for medicinal purposes. WHO (1998) recognises this in its guidelines for appropriate use of traditional medicines. It maintains the position that there is no requirement for pre-clinical toxicity testing; rather that evidence of traditional use or recent clinical experience is sufficient. Pre-clinical toxicity testing is only required for new medicinal herbal products which contain herbs with no traditional history of use. Trouiller *et al.* (2002) argue: '*The global application of unduly and unnecessarily high standards of drug regulation may be contributing paradoxically to the disease burden and its costs in developing countries'.*

It could be postulated that human beings have evolved to avoid toxic plants. This is supported by the observation that deaths from plant poisoning are rare, except when people move to an unknown area (Reynolds & Cousins, 1993). In general, traditional herbalists inherit from their elders the knowledge of which plants are safe and which are unsafe to use. Although there are few reports of serious adverse effects of traditional medicines, some occurrences are undoubtedly unreported. Interestingly, many of the reports that do exist are concerned with alternative uses of the plants, such as food, other medical problems, or accidental ingestion (Willcox *et al.*, 2004).

In the absence of scientific evidence of efficacy and safety, it is impossible to label a treatment either as maleficent or as non-maleficent. Producing scientific evidence is a good reason for conducting research on such traditional medicines, because it will help patients and practitioners to decide whether a particular treatment is harmful or safe, ineffective or effective. Until such evidence is available, the ethical decision whether or not to use a treatment will depend on other principles, such as freedom of choice.

Therefore, if patients are freely choosing to take a particular traditional medicine, in the absence of good evidence for or against its safety and efficacy, it would be unethical to prevent them. WHO (2000) states that:

'If the product has been traditionally used without demonstrated harm, no specific restrictive regulatory action should be undertaken unless new evidence demands a revised risk-benefit assessment'.

A logical extension of this reasoning is that clinical observational studies can be undertaken on traditional medicines without first having formal evidence of safety. If patients taking traditional medicine give their informed consent to participate in a study, it is acceptable to observe the course of their disease and any adverse effects which may arise in the course of treatment. In such a study, it is not the investigators who are choosing to administer a traditional medicine to the patients; it is the patients themselves who are choosing to use it.

It is important to note that the above argument applies only to true traditional medicines, administered in their traditional form and dosage, rather than purified extracts or compounds which have not been used traditionally.

Likewise, it does not apply if the formula is altered from the textual or recorded version. The question of adjuvant treatment — adding a traditional drug to a conventional pharmaceutical regime — poses ethical and clinical challenges. Interactive effects could produce reduced potency in one or other drug and/or side effects could be intensified. Unless co-administration of the particular traditional and modern medicines is in common practice without reported adverse effects, further evidence of safety of the combination is necessary before proceeding to clinical studies.

The first and most important step when planning a clinical observational study is to establish good evidence of traditional use. A literature search is also necessary to see whether cases of toxicity have been reported for the preparation in question, or whether there is any other reason for conducting laboratory tests of toxicity. Pre-clinical safety data should not be viewed in isolation, but should be complemented by careful clinical observations in treated patients.

The information obtained from such preliminary observational studies can be used to plan further controlled clinical trials, in which investigators would be administering a traditional medicine to patients, often allocated to this treatment by randomisation. Before conducting a study of this sort, the principle of non-maleficence suggests that there should be good evidence of safety. If a practitioner is giving a particular treatment to a patient, who would not otherwise have taken it, they should be convinced that the risk of harm to the patient is low. Evidence of safety from observational studies in humans would be more useful than animal data, but may not always be sufficient on its own.

The principle of non-maleficence extends beyond humans to other animal species used in research. Animal models are often used without clear evidence of relevance to human health and disease. This has sometimes resulted in false negative and false positive results, for example when screening plants for their anti-malarial effect in the mouse *Plasmodium berghei* model (Rasoanaivo *et al.*, 2004). Where such tests will need to be repeated in humans regardless of the result of the animal experiments, there can be little justification for causing potential suffering and expending resources in this way. For these reasons, the British National Institute of Medical Herbalists (2001) does not advocate the use of animal experimentation for research in herbal medicine.

16.4. Beneficence

The principle here is that health care practitioners should not only avoid doing harm, but should actively do good for their patients. In practice, few treatments are without side effects, so benefits must be balanced against risks. There is much debate as to how this principle should be applied in a setting of limited resources, especially in developing countries. It could be argued, for example, that all patients should be offered the best available treatment for their diseases, regardless of cost. While this would be ideal, it is far removed from the real world of limited resources. Interpreted in this literal way, it would prevent clinical research on any unproven treatment, where an effective treatment already exists, and would prevent much research in developing countries (Benatar & Singer, 2000). It would also deny patients any freedom to choose their treatment.

On the other hand, the desire to do positive good to patients is one of the motivations for medical researchers in developing countries, including those researching traditional medicines. The ultimate aim is often to prevent mortality from potentially fatal diseases such as malaria, HIV/AIDS and TB, or to reduce morbidity, for example through pain relief, prevention of epileptic fits or asthma attacks. In the real world, while effective treatments for these conditions exist, they are often unavailable and/or unaffordable to patients in developing countries. It is easy and tempting for the armchair ethicist to idealise about what 'should' be. However, patients and practitioners in the field are powerless to change the global economy. They are faced with choices that are less than ideal, but are nevertheless real. Appropriate research can help them to choose the best option available in their daily situation (rather than in an idealised research setting, which will cease to exist as soon as the study is over, or at the very least will not be replicable on a large scale). Finding effective traditional treatments would be of great practical benefit, because these can often be cultivated and prepared locally at little or no cost (Hirt & M'Pia, 2001; Mueller *et al.*, 2000). This approach may be more sustainable, and reach more patients, than aid programmes to donate pharmaceuticals.

The local cultivation, preparation and use of traditional medicines discussed above contrasts with the commercialisation of 'traditional' medicines on a larger scale, often motivated by the lure of large profits.

In this context, the principle of beneficence requires that regulatory agencies and practitioners should prevent fraudulent claims about medicines, so that patients are not tricked into buying ineffective or harmful treatments. Recently, there is an increasing tendency for those importing traditional medicines from China, South Africa and elsewhere into African countries to claim that they are food additives and therefore may not require proof of efficacy. Many of these are making lucrative businesses by advertising that they heal more than 100 diseases, while others claim that they have a cure for HIV/AIDS and many other diseases (Kitua & Malebo, 2004). Such claims are not beneficent, unless substantiated by research. The adulteration of traditional medicines with steroids, antibiotics and other modern medical ingredients constitutes an area of medical ethics addressed in the chapter on Safety (Shia *et al.*, Chapter 4 of this volume), which also requires a regulatory response.

Research studies need to be carefully designed in order to ensure that participants are treated at least as well as those not participating in the study. The balance of benefit and risk of every study needs to be considered on a case-by-case basis. Ethics committees may understandably be uneasy about observational studies of patients treated for serious, or even potentially fatal conditions, by those who have access to drugs known to be efficacious. Such studies need careful planning, and safe protocols. For example, falciparum malaria is a potentially serious and fatal condition. Therefore in order to justify a study on a traditional treatment for malaria, there should be good ethnomedical and/or laboratory evidence of its efficacy. Then, the logical approach would be to start with a patient group who are at very low risk of severe disease. In malaria-endemic areas, patients over the age of five years rarely get severe disease (with the exception of pregnant women), so initial studies could include only this low-risk patient group. If controlled studies in these patients showed a treatment to be equivalent or better than other locally available treatment options, subsequent studies could evaluate its effectiveness in higher risk patients such as children under five years of age. In all such studies, whether with high or low risk patients, it is crucial to observe patients carefully for danger signs or deterioration. There need to be strict criteria for defining a 'treatment failure', so that patients who do not respond to the trial treatment are given timely alternative treatment. Thus the principle of beneficence must always be taken into consideration.

16.5. Justice

Justice is concerned with the fair allocation of resources. This applies both to financial resources for the provision and development of health care, as well as to intellectual resources and involvement in health care research.

Everyone has a right to a decent minimum standard of health care. However there is a huge disparity between developed and developing countries in expenditure on health care and health research. Ambitious targets of 'health for all' seem more elusive than ever, while the 'inverse care law' applies on a global scale. Less than 10% of global spending on health research is devoted to 90% of the world's health problems (Global Forum for Health Research, 2000). Furthermore, it would not be unrealistic to estimate that less than 1% of this 10% is spent on researching traditional medicines, upon which 80% of people in developing countries are said to rely, and that almost none of this research takes due consideration of the concepts and practices of traditional medical systems, or involves traditional practitioners as equal partners in the research team.

For example, some traditional medical diagnostic frameworks highlight different responses to a common drug by different types of patients (Chaudhury, 2002; Chaudhury *et al.*, Chapter 15 of this volume). Ayurvedic medicine delineates three major constitutional types, known as doshas — *vata, pitta* and *kapha* (Sharma & Clarke, 1999). The Ayurvedic medicine '*kanaka*' is considered effective in patients with the Ayurvedic body type of *kapha* who have bronchial asthma, but for patients of the *pitta* type, it is predicted to cause congestion. Such considerations should be taken into account in patient assignment and randomisation can be done, for example, taking into account traditional diagnostic categories. The Indian Council of Medical Research has developed two herbal drugs — a contraceptive and a treatment for diabetes mellitus — using randomised controlled trials (RCTs) guided by the clinical assumptions and diagnostic categories of India's Ayurvedic medical system. This requires that traditional medical practitioners be part of clinical research teams and that their perspectives be given serious and respectful consideration in designing appropriate RCTs of their medicines. Development of new products from traditional medicines and the commercialisation of privately held traditional medical knowledge represents an ethical area within the domain of intellectual property rights and is addressed in Bodeker (Chapter 17 of this volume).

The lack of biomedical interest and funding for research on traditional medicines, as well as the lack of involvement of traditional practitioners, has resulted in poor quality research in this area (Chaudhury, 1992). Allocation of research funding according to need rather than potential for profit, and equal involvement of traditional practitioners, would help to improve the quantity and quality of studies on traditional medicines, which could then improve health care for patients in developing countries.

16.6. Conclusions

Research on traditional medicine in developing countries raises issues relating to all four of the cardinal principles of biomedical ethics. Autonomy must be respected, by allowing patients to choose traditional treatments if they wish, by providing them with better information on traditional treatments through research, and by seeking their informed consent for participation in such research. Non-maleficence requires that safety of traditional medicines must be adequately evaluated, but this can be done through observation of patients who freely choose to take a traditional medicine. This sample of patients may be biased, but will at least provide some baseline safety data on the basis of which medicines can be selected for study in larger controlled trials. Beneficence often motivates researchers to find effective treatments for common diseases, but regard must be given to their availability and affordability; traditional medicine may be a more realistic and sustainable solution in developing countries than modern pharmaceuticals. Finally, justice in the allocation of research resources and in the involvement of traditional practitioners and health systems would result in greatly improved quality and quantity of research on traditional medicine in developing countries.

References

Bannerman RH *et al.* (eds.) *Traditional Medicine and Health Care Coverage.* Geneva: World Health Organization, 1983.

Beauchamp TL, Childress JF. *Principles of Medical Ethics*, 3rd edn. Oxford: Oxford University Press, 1989.

Benatar SR, Singer PA. A new look at international research ethics. *Br Med J* 2000;321:824–826.

Chaudhury RR. Standardization, preclinical toxicology and clinical evaluation of medicinal plants, including ethical considerations. In: Chaudhury RR, Rafei UM (eds.) *Traditional Medicine in Asia*. New Delhi: World Health Organization Regional Office for South-East Asia, 2002, pp. 209–225.

Chaudhury RR. *Herbal Medicine for Human Health*. New Delhi: World Health Organization Regional Office for South-East Asia, 1992.

General Medical Council. *Research: The Role and Responsibilities of Doctors*. London, 2001.

Global Forum for Health Research. *The 10/90 Report on Health Research 2000*. Geneva, 2000.

Hahold A, Kroeger A. *Superacion de la Enfermedad en las Alturas de los Andes del Peru: Resultado de una Encuestra Poblacional*. Quito: Ediciones Abya-Yala, 1990.

Hirt HM, M'Pia B. *Natural Medicine in the Tropics*. Winnenden: Anamed, 2001.

Kitua AY, Malebo HM. Malaria control in Africa and the role of traditional medicine. In: Willcox ML, Bodeker G, Rasoanaivo P (eds.) *Traditional Medicinal Plants and Malaria*. Boca Raton: CRC Press, 2004 (in press).

Lei SH, Bodeker G. Changshan (*Dichroa febrifuga*): ancient febrifuge and modern antimalarial: lessons for research from a forgotten tale. In: Willcox ML, Bodeker G, Rasoanaivo P (eds.) *Traditional Medicinal Plants and Malaria*. Boca Raton: CRC Press, 2004 (in press).

Lindegger G, Bull S. Ensuring valid consent in a developing country context. *Online J Sci Dev*, 22 May 2003.

Mueller MS *et al*. The potential of *Artemisia annua* L. as a locally produced remedy for malaria in the tropics: agricultural, chemical and clinical aspects. *J Ethnopharmacol* 2000;73:487–493.

National Institute of Medical Herbalists. NIMH ethical guidelines for evaluation of research in herbal medicine. *Eur J Herbal Med* 2001;7:special issue.

Rasoanaivo P *et al*. Guidelines for the non-clinical evaluation of the efficacy of traditional antimalarials. In: Willcox ML, Bodeker G, Rasoanaivo P (eds.) *Traditional Medicinal Plants and Malaria*. Boca Raton: CRC Press, 2004 (in press).

Reynolds P, Cousins CC. *Lwaano Lwanyika: The Tonga Book of the Earth*. Washington DC: Panos Books, 1993.

Sharma H, Clarke C. *Contemporary Ayurveda*. New York: Churchill Livingstone, 1999.

Trouiller P *et al.* Clinical trials and pharmaceutical needs in developing countries. *Good Clin Pract J* 2002;9:28–33.

Willcox ML *et al.* Guidelines for the pre-clinical evaluation of the safety of traditional herbal antimalarials. In: Willcox ML, Bodeker G, Rasoanaivo P (eds.) *Traditional Medicinal Plants and Malaria*. Boca Raton: CRC Press, 2004 (in press).

World Health Organization. *Guidelines for Good Clinical Practice (GCP) for Trials on Pharmaceutical Products*, WHO Technical Report Series, No. 850, Annex 3. Geneva: World Health Organization, 1995.

World Health Organization. *General Guidelines for Methodologies on Research and Evaluation of Traditional Medicine*. Geneva: World Health Organization, 2000 (WHO/EDM/TRM/2000.1).

World Health Organization Regional Office for the Western Pacific. *Guidelines for the Appropriate Use of Herbal Medicines*. Manila: World Health Organization Regional Office for the Western Pacific, 1998.

World Medical Association. *World Medical Association Declaration of Helsinki, 2002* (http://www.wma.net/e/policy/b3.htm), accessed 4 May 2004.

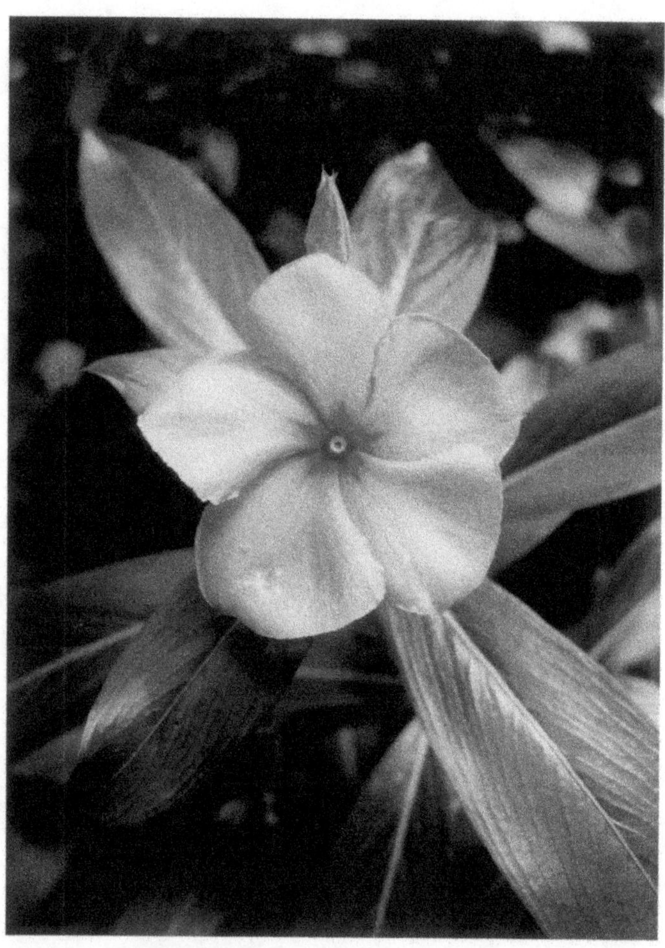

The rosy periwinkle (*Catharanthus roseus*) of Madagascar, a patented source of the anti-cancer drugs vincristine and vinblastine. (*Source*: National Tropical Botanical Garden, Hawaii, USA.)

CHAPTER 17

INTELLECTUAL PROPERTY RIGHTS[1]

Gerard Bodeker

17.1. Introduction

The last decade of the twentieth century saw increasing international debate and legal challenge over the patenting of traditional knowledge (TK) and its products. There have been two broad positions in this debate. The first is the attempt by non-indigenous individuals and organisations to claim ownership of indigenous knowledge for commercial gain. The second is the attempt by indigenous representatives and developing countries to prevent this from happening, and either to take ownership of such products themselves or to engage in partnerships with fair sharing of benefits for the commercial development of their knowledge, products or processes (Dutfield, 2001). This dynamic has taken place against the backdrop of two international legal frameworks that, until the present, have stood in apparent contradiction to one another. These are the Convention on Biological Diversity (CBD), and the World Trade Organization's Trade-Related Aspects of Intellectual Property Systems (TRIPS).

---

[1]This chapter draws on Bodeker G. Traditional medical knowledge, intellectual property rights and benefit sharing. *Cardozo J Int Comp Law* 2003;11:785–814. With permission of the *Cardozo Journal of International and Comparative Law*, New York.

17.2. The Convention on Biological Diversity (CBD)

The Convention on Biological Diversity (1993) is the only major international convention that assigns ownership of biodiversity to indigenous communities and individuals, thereby giving them the right to protect this knowledge. Article 8(j) declares that State Parties are required to:

> *'... respect, preserve and maintain knowledge, innovations and practices of indigenous and local communities embodying traditional lifestyles relevant for the conservation and sustainable use of biological diversity and promote the wider application with the approval and involvement of the holders of such knowledge, innovations and practices and encourage the equitable sharing of the benefits arising from the utilisation of such knowledge, innovations and practices'.*

Article 18.4 states that Contracting Parties should *'encourage and develop models of co-operation for the development and use of technologies, including traditional and indigenous technologies'.*

17.3. Trade-Related Aspects of Intellectual Property Rights (TRIPS)

The CBD competes for influence with the far more powerful Agreement on Trade-Related Aspects of Intellectual Property Rights (TRIPS), which is Annex 1C of the Marrakesh Agreement Establishing the World Trade Organization, 1994. TRIPS, now the key international agreement promoting the harmonisation of national IPR regimes, covers four types of intellectual property rights: patents, geographical indications, undisclosed information (trade secrets), and trademarks. TRIPS makes no reference to the protection of traditional knowledge and it proposes 'protection of plant varieties either by patents, by an effective *sui generis* system or by any combination thereof' (Article 27.3(b)). *Sui generis* systems are those that are developed according to the needs of a country or region. They are unique to that country and region.

Essentially, the CBD takes the view that if a product or process has existed in a culture for a long period of time, it is owned and hence protected under intellectual property law. By contrast, the view under TRIPS is that if it is not patented it is not owned. If it is not owned, it represents knowledge that is part of a global commons available for exploitation by all who so wish. The CBD has published a summary of cases on access to genetic resources and benefit sharing (Convention on Biological Diversity, undated electronic document).

17.4. The Doha Declaration and the Harmonisation of CBD and TRIPS

In November 2001, the declaration of the Fourth Ministerial Conference of the World Trade Organization in Doha, Qatar, mandated a review of TRIPS provisions and called for harmonisation between the CBD and TRIPS. The Doha Declaration specifically requested the Council for Trade-Related Aspects of Intellectual Property Rights to address the protection of traditional knowledge and folklore, with reference to Article 27.3(b) of TRIPS.

17.4.1. *Review of TRIPS Provisions*

At the time of writing, this review is still in progress. Some early recommendations from member countries include the following.

- Patents inconsistent with Article 15 of the Convention on Biological Diversity should not be granted.
- Article 27.3(b) should be implemented five years after the present review ends.
- Technology transfer should be provided on fair and mutually advantageous terms.
- Article 27.3(b) should be amended in the light of the CBD, and the present review should clarify that the following are not patentable: all living organisms (including whole or parts of plants and animals, and including gene sequences), biological and other natural processes for producing plants, animals and their parts.

Other comments have focused on benefit sharing based on prior informed consent (a provision of the CBD, and a counter to so-called 'biopiracy') and whether TRIPS should be amended to take this into account. A number of countries, have raised questions about the international enforceability of proposed *sui generis* provisions.

A number of test cases (Bodeker, 2003) have illustrated that, in the absence of effective consensus development, protocols and regulatory procedures, neither national governments nor inter-governmental treaties are in a position to guarantee the integrity of any bioprospecting contract. Equally, there is no adequate mechanism to date, including the CBD, which is capable of safeguarding the rights and interests of local communities. The TRIPS Council's review exercise is being watched closely for how it will offer solutions to such challenging situations.

17.5. From International to National Challenges

There is an international focus on issues surrounding the patenting of traditional knowledge, centred on the commercial interests of the pharmaceutical industry. However, there is a current global trend for large pharmaceutical companies to move away from natural products research and development, and to re-focus on genetically based drugs as the source of future therapy. While multinational pharmaceutical companies have largely reduced their interest in traditional medicine as a source of leads for new drugs, smaller national-level pharmaceutical companies have retained an interest. This may have the effect of relocating the IP challenge to within domestic borders. The key figures become local pharmaceutical companies or government agencies, aiming to commercialise the national pool of traditional medical knowledge for the purposes of drug development. The question then arises as to whether the knowledge is owned by the nation or by the traditional medical sector and its community-based custodians. This issue has not been resolved internationally, although under the IPR frameworks of many countries, it is the state that holds ultimate ownership — a situation that is by no means acceptable to indigenous groups or traditional medicine societies and tradition holders.

17.6. The Role of the Herbal Sector

A further challenge to intellectual property rights can be found in the burgeoning market in traditional medical knowledge within the herbal medicine sector. The World Bank has predicted that botanical medicines will constitute a substantial international industry, and thus a role for developing country producers (Lambert *et al.*, 1997). Much of this market is based on products derived in part from traditional knowledge about the use of plants for medicines. The herbal sector tends to operate on the assumption that a global commons prevails and that traditional medical knowledge is available for any and all to commercialise, frequently without consideration of benefit sharing or customary ownership rights.

One important reason for this trend is that the herbal sector places little emphasis on patenting, as it does not currently have the same regulatory requirements to conduct research on the safety and efficacy of its products, as does the pharmaceutical industry. The high cost of this investment for pharmaceutical development — often estimated to be in the vicinity of US$300 million — means that pharmaceutical companies understandably wish to protect their investment from exploitation by competitors, hence the role of patent protection. However, in the absence of this research and development requirement in the herbal sector, patenting is of low priority, although its importance is now increasing.

17.6.1. *Traditional Knowledge, Benefit Sharing and the Herbal Industry*

The concept of benefit sharing in the development of herbal medicines has only recently begun to find its place in the intellectual property sphere. One well-known example from India is that of a partnership between the Kani tribe and the Tropical Gardens Botanical Research Institute (TGBRI), Trivandrum, India (Dutfield, 2000). TGBRI holds the patent on *Trichopus zeylanicus*, or 'Jeevani' as it is known locally. Indigenous knowledge of the plant resides with the Kani tribe in the Western Ghat forests. Through customary use and, more recently, in laboratory studies, Jeevani has been found to be an immunomodulator, hepatoprotective and an aphrodisiac. TGBRI, the sole patent holder on Jeevani as an immunomodulator, signed a commitment to share royalties with the Kani. In turn TGBRI issued a seven-year license to an Ayurvedic herbal pharmacy which produces herbal extracts from Jeevani. Despite this being an important and new model of patenting and benefit sharing within the herbal sector, there are still some difficulties with this approach. Yet, in the Jeevani case, the benefit sharing dimension highlights a way forward for partnerships between traditional knowledge holders and herbal manufacturers.

17.7. IPR Models for the Protection of Traditional Knowledge

The following are some potential IPR models for the protection of traditional knowledge.

17.7.1. *Certificates of Origin*

Certificates of origin could be used to illustrate that all obligations to the country and indigenous people or local community had been fulfilled, e.g. prior informed consent and equitable benefit sharing. Patent applications would need to include these certificates. Without them, the applications would automatically be rejected.

17.7.2. *Transforming Traditional Knowledge into Trade Secrets*

Knowledge from communities wishing to participate in a project would be catalogued and deposited in a restricted access database. Each community would have its own file in the database.

17.7.3. *Local Innovations Databases*

The Society for Research and Initiatives for Sustainable Technologies and Institutions (SRISTI), India, has developed databases of traditional knowledge and innovations in close collaboration with local community members (Gupta, 1999). The plan advocates a global registration system of local innovations. Individual and collective innovators would receive acknowledgement and financial rewards for commercial applications of their knowledge, innovations and practices. Links would then be built between small investors, entrepreneurs and innovators for mutual financial benefits. In turn, individuals or communities could seek IPR protection in such forms as inventor's certificates and petty patents. (The intellectual property law of Kenya was amended in 1989 to provide for a petty patent for traditional medicinal knowledge.) Under this plan, all national patent offices would be able to access local innovation databases when carrying out prior art searches and examinations. SRISTI founder Professor Anil Gupta argues that disclosure should provide that the source material has been rightfully and lawfully acquired (Ghate *et al.*, 1999).

In addition to the above community-based initiatives to protect local TK with respect to indigenous medicine, there are two new and important database initiatives, designed to establish prior art as a pre-emptive measure against patenting of indigenous medical products and applications of plants. One of these, in India, operates internationally for the defence of national TK, and the other, established by the Science and Human Rights Program of the American Association for the Advancement of Science (AAAS), operates internationally for the defence of TK globally.

17.7.3.1. National Database to Establish Prior Art on Indian Medicinal Heritage

Following its high profile challenge to a turmeric patent filed in the United States of America, and subsequent challenges to patents on neem (*Azadirachta indica*) and basmati rice, India has now embarked on a national programme to establish prior art on all Indian traditional knowledge relating to patent applications for medicine. The Government of India in October 2003 released a set of CD–ROMs containing all of India's Ayurvedic medicinal plant knowledge. Subsequent CD–ROMs will add data from other Indian systems of medicine as well as records of folk applications of plants as medicines. The Indian database is intended to be distributed to patent offices worldwide to provide a record of prior art in Indian traditional medicinal knowledge. The Government of India is also continuing with its legal strategy to seek revocation of non-Indian patents on Indian life forms (Government of India, undated electronic document).

17.7.3.2. International Database to Establish Prior Art on Traditional Knowledge

The Science and Human Rights Program of the American Association for the Advancement of Science (AAAS) has established a new international project on traditional knowledge. The AAAS established the Traditional Ecological Knowledge Prior Art Database (T.E.K.*P.A.D.) with the aim of 'protecting indigenous knowledge against inappropriate patents based on this knowledge' (AAAS, undated electronic document).

The AAAS characterises T.E.K.*P.A.D. as operating on the principle of 'defensive disclosure'. As with the other database models for recording and publicising traditional knowledge, T.E.K.*P.A.D. aims to establish a record of prior art by means of publication. T.E.K.*P.A.D. has issued an offer to traditional knowledge holders to submit their knowledge to the database if they wish for it to be placed in the public domain.

17.8. Is Patenting by Customary Knowledge Holders a Solution?

In response to the IP challenges of databases and the international trend towards unacknowledged use of traditional knowledge as the basis for patents by corporations and research institutes, some have argued that a solution would be for knowledge holders and indigenous communities to seek patents themselves. Graham Dutfield (2000) has argued, however, that for various reasons patents are not a viable option for most indigenous communities or custodians of traditional knowledge. Traditional knowledge is collectively held and generated, whereas patent law refers to the inventiveness and achievement of individuals, and patent applications must supply evidence of a single act of discovery. Furthermore, patent specifications must be written in a technical way that examiners can understand, and applying for patents and enforcing them when they have been awarded is prohibitively expensive.

17.9. Working Towards an Equitable Future: Some *Sui Generis* Models

TRIPS calls for the development of *sui generis* models for traditional knowledge protection, a position also promoted by the United States. The challenge is what form a *sui generis* system should take and how it is best enforced, given the failure of the prevailing IP regime to adequately protect traditional knowledge.

Paul Kuruk (1999) has argued that as IP laws are generally inadequate as a means of protecting, a *sui generis* regime to protect TK need not be consistent with IP criteria. Kuruk argues for community ownership and rights over TK, rather than individual ownership and rights. He also proposes that traditional or customary owners should have rights to products developed from their TK, whether or not IP rights over them have been obtained over them in other countries.

These principles are reflected in a recent Organization of African Unity (OAU; now the African Union) Model Law (undated electronic document), which proposes the establishment of a regional *sui generis* system to recognise, protect and support the 'inalienable rights' of local communities over their biological resources, knowledge and technologies. Central to the OAU model law is the requirement of consultation and written Prior Informed Consent (PIC) from both the national competent authority and the concerned local community. PIC is defined as:

'the giving by a collector of complete and accurate information, and, based on that information, the prior acceptance of that collector by the government and the concerned local community or communities to collect biological resources, or indigenous knowledge, or technologies'.

The OAU model assumes that governments and traditional communities have common interests and objectives. However, if both community and government dispute ownership of TK, this will affect the OAU model's provisions for PIC and benefit sharing, to the possible disadvantage of traditional knowledge holders.

Central to the debate over national and regional *sui generis* systems is whether they have any enforceability outside the national or regional legislative system. Reichmann has called attention to the fact that the problems of protecting computer and biogenetics innovations 'have been worsened by the lack of any credible *sui generis* alternative to correct the manifest defects of stretching the patent and copyright paradigms beyond their traditional boundaries' (Kaiser, 2002). If economically and politically powerful sectors such as the computer industry and biogenetics have failed to evolve effective and enforceable *sui generis* systems, it is reasonable to ask whether there is genuine hope for an equitable *sui generis* system developing for the international protection of such a historically marginalised field as traditional knowledge.

17.10. A Broad-Based Agenda for TK/IP Protection

The preceding review of instruments for IP protection does not offer a single clear protective track for traditional medical knowledge holders. In response, the global context is evolving the diverse forces of grassroots lobbying and action, international legal review (such as the WTO/WIPO effort to harmonise TRIPS and CBD), case law and the ever-evolving scenario of partnerships on the ground between TMK holders and those interested in commercialising this knowledge. In order to ensure an equitable future for customary knowledge holders and TK within the international IPR regime, three broad issues will need to be addressed: research, advocacy and partnerships.

17.10.1. *Research*

In order to guide communities and countries, non-governmental organisations and companies in developing fair and equitable arrangements for sharing traditional knowledge and its benefits, it is proposed that a comprehensive information resource is needed. Such a resource should:

- gather data on what is happening globally in this field;
- identify best practice;
- document case law;
- highlight problematic areas;
- provide model contracts for use and adaptation to local conditions;
- record cases of dispute resolution, and the methods used to achieve this;
- provide a current bibliography of reference material and research in the field of IPR and traditional knowledge;
- provide an advocacy service by making information available that can inform the development of policy and fair partnerships between industry and communities, countries and traditional knowledge holders.

17.10.2. *Advocacy*

To date, advocacy on behalf of the rights of individual and community holders of TK has come primarily from the NGO sector and its supporters. India has established a track for the national redress of abuse of TK rights in its challenges to the turmeric, neem and basmati patents.

A higher profile for advocacy is now needed in view of the 2001 WTO Ministerial Declaration WTO/MIN(01)/DEC/1, and the subsequent review of the CBD and TRIPS clauses dealing with TK. A higher degree of international funding and support is necessary if a solid body of legal precedent is to be established in this field and if a consistent response to patent violations of TK is to be established to support *sui generis* forms of protection. This could be funded by international agencies responsible for the legal dimensions of this field — such as WIPO and WTO, both wealthy agencies. There is a need for the promotion of dialogue leading to the establishment and enforcement of an ethical international IP and traditional knowledge regime.

17.10.3. *Partnerships*

In order for significant advances to be made in the protection of the rights of TK holders in the medicinal field, there is a need for active partnerships among the central actors involved in the field. These partnerships would involve the local community and the NGO sector to promote development of the sector; the local community and the private sector for commercial benefit; the public/private/community for new legal directions and protection; and the public sector/NGO sector to ensure equity and oversight.

17.11. Conclusions

The debate on IP and traditional knowledge has reached new levels of review and new prospects for TK protection since the adoption of the WTO Ministerial Declaration WTO/MIN(01)/DEC/1 in Doha in November 2001, and the resulting process for the harmonisation of TRIPS and CBD with respect to traditional knowledge.

The growth of the herbal sector, and the constant demand for new and marketable traditional medical products, is new in the field of IP and traditional medical knowledge. This trend will clearly grow and should become a primary focus of IPR development. Of fundamental importance is the need for the herbal industry to become more proactive and responsive to this dimension. The herbal and traditional medicine industry should, of its own accord, develop industry standards that are based on ethical practice. These standards should be overseen by monitoring groups including representatives from industry, government, NGOs and indigenous communities.

To provide new models for development, information needs to be gathered on current practice. This, in turn, needs to be analysed according to principles of best practice in benefit sharing and IPR. *Sui generis* systems alone may or may not be the way forward. They offer unique local means of protecting traditional knowledge that work for the local context, but at the same time, are at risk of being unenforceable outside the country or region of origin and hence creating vulnerability to the biopiracy that they are designed to prevent. For *sui generis* systems to work, there will need to be reciprocity among countries to respect one another's local *sui generis* regimes — a prospect that would seem somewhat distant in the prevailing international IP political environment.

Such developments as those outlined above require backing and enforcement within the context of national and international IPR regimes. If this can be achieved, the health benefits offered to the world through the globalisation of traditional medical knowledge also stand to benefit many communities and countries.

References

Bodeker G. *Cardozo J Int Comp Law* 2003;11:785–814.

Convention on Biological Diversity, 1993 (http://www.biodiv.org/convention/articles.asp), accessed 24 February 2004 at 21:47.

Convention on Biological Diversity, Access to Genetic Resources and Benefit-Sharing Case Studies (http://www.biodiv.org/programmes/socio-eco/benefit/case-studies.asp), accessed 24 February 2004 at 21:52.

Dutfield G. *Case W Res J Int L* 2001;13:239–291.

Dutfield G. *Intellectual Property Rights, Trade and Biodiversity: Seeds and Plant Varieties.* London: Earthscan, 2000.

Ghate U, Gadgil M, Sheshagiri Rao PR. *Curr Sci* 1999;77:1418–1425.

Government of India, Council of Scientific Research and Central Council for Research in Ayurveda and Siddha. *Globalisation of Ayurveda: Traditional Knowledge Digital Library* (http://indianmedicine.nic.in/html/ayurveda/ ayurveda.htm#glo), accessed 25 February 2004 at 12:57.

Government of India, Ministry of Health and Family Welfare, Department of Ayurveda, Yoga and Naturopathy, Unani, Sidda and Homeopathy (AYUSH) (http://indianmedicine.nic.in), accessed 25 February 2004 at 12:59.

Gupta AK. *Indian J Agric Econ* 1999;54:340–369.

Kaiser J. NIH to limit scope of foreign patents. *Science* 2002;296:2316.

Kuruk P. Protecting folklore under modern intellectual property regimes: a reappraisal of the tensions between individual rights and communal rights in Africa. *Am L Rev* 1999;48:769–849.

Lambert J *et al. Medicinal Plants: Rescuing a Global Heritage*, World Bank Technical Paper No. 355 (Washington D.C.: World Bank, 1997).

Organisation of African Unity (OAU) Scientific, Technical and Research Commission. *African Model Legislation for the Protection of the Rights of Local Communities, Farmers and Breeders, and for the Regulation of Access to Biological Resources* (http://www.grain.org/docs/ova-modellaus-2000-en.doc), last visited 3 March, 2003.

Traditional Ecological Knowledge Prior Art Database, 2004 (http://ip.aaas. org/tekpad), accessed 25 February 2004 at 13:01.

World Trade Organization. *Annex 1C of the Marrakesh Agreement Establishing the World Trade Organization: Agreement on Trade Related Aspects of Intellectual Property Rights (TRIPS).* World Trade Organization, 1994 (http://www.wto.org/english/docs_e/legal_e/27-trips.pdf), accessed 24 February 2004 at 21:45.

World Trade Organization. *Doha WTO Ministerial 2001, Ministerial Declaration adopted on 14 November 2001, WT/MIN(01)/DEC/1.* Geneva: World Trade Organization, 2001, Article 19 on Trade-related aspects of intellectual property rights (http://www.wto.org/english/thewto_e/minist_e/ min01_e/mindecl_e.htm), accessed 24 February 2004 at 21:59.

EPILOGUE

Gerard Bodeker and Gemma Burford

What has been offered in this volume is a first attempt to gather a set of perspectives that address public health and policy dimensions of traditional, complementary and alternative medicine. Most of the collected works to date have been on anthropological or biomedical research perspectives.

While many forms of traditional medicine are now becoming globalised, as shown in the WHO Global Atlas on TCAM — such asTraditional Chinese Medicine, acupuncture and Ayurveda — our emphasis has been on the role played by traditional health systems in their countries of origin. It is here that they are most widely used, and frequently serve as the first and last resort for health care for the majority of the population, particularly in rural areas.

It is clear that much more is needed, in order to give a truly comprehensive view of both the policy and the public health dimensions of the TCAM sector. Some of the necessary work for the future would include:

- National data collection systems to track the levels of use, the modalities used, and the outcomes of TCAM.
- Economic analyses — both microeconomic and macroeconomic — to determine the effects of traditional medicine use on family income as well as on costs and savings for the nation. Comparative economic analyses

across countries and regions could highlight different ways of maximising the cost-effectiveness of the sector.

- Epidemiological and public health mapping exercises are not a feature of research in this field, as yet. They offer the potential of shedding light on the population-based outcomes of TCAM use, as well as for mapping the presence and quality of service of TCAM providers, especially in areas where there is limited biomedical care.

- Gender specific medicine. One demographic fact that has become clear from studies around the world is that women are the majority users of TCAM — as they are of health services generally. In traditional societies, cultural knowledge of health care is frequently passed from grandmothers to their daughters and granddaughters for the care of the family. This gender dimension merits much greater documentation and understanding, as do the approaches that are present in TCAM systems for women's health conditions and needs. Furthermore, in the context of the new field of gender-specific medicine (Legato, 19 ... , Elsevier), a wider focus on gender differences is warranted to understand, for instance, the services that are used by men and by women; the differing ways in which TCAM may be applied; different TCAM approaches for men and for women for common medical conditions; and the contributions to men's health and women's health from relevant TCAM specialities.

- In the areas of epidemics and communicable diseases, a research agenda for malaria, HIV, and emerging diseases such as avian flu and SARS, Ebola virus and necrotising faciitis, is warranted.

Clearly, the last of these — evaluating the contribution of TCAM to managing major diseases — will require an experimental methodology leading to randomised controlled clinical trials. However, there is a need to broaden the research agenda beyond the RCT focus that has dominated national and international debates on evidence-based TCAM (Bodeker, 2000). A body of high quality public health and policy research on TCAM is long overdue. It can potentially make a significant contribution towards the development of the services and national frameworks required to give a formal home to what is already an informal reality for most people in most countries of the world.

Yet, in promoting an expanded TCAM research agenda, it is also worth noting that many models of effective TCAM practice and services do exist.

Based on popular demand for TCAM and, in many instances, higher public expenditures than on biomedicine, it would seem that the time has come for development agencies to move beyond the stage of simply supporting more and more 'demonstration' or 'pilot' projects. As has already been noted, the public has moved far beyond this position of experimentation. Implementation of known best practice is now needed to meet the global demand for quality TCAM services.

The underlying issue for all of this work is the combination of political will and resource allocation. While the WHO Global Atlas on TCAM does appear to show evidence of increased political will in support of this sector, as evidenced by the widespread growth of policy development and standard-setting for the TCAM sector, there remains chronic under-funding. The consequence is that much important research and applied work is either neglected altogether, or carried out at minimal levels of effectiveness. This maintains a biomedical control of resources for health care research and service provision, even when growing numbers of the public are clearly spending more of their own resources on TCAM use than on biomedicine.

In developing integrated health care services and policy — combining the best of biomedicine with the best of TCAM, within a common system — attention must be paid to the risk that imposition of biomedical standards of practice and evaluation may override indigenous theoretical assumptions and methods of identifying, preparing and individualising herbal and other traditional medicines. This, in turn, could impact on some of the distinctive features of TCAM services, which are factors in their enduring popularity, such as their holism, cultural familiarity and patient-centred approach. The biomedicalisation of TCAM has already become a subject of discussion in the context of standard-setting exercises by regulatory agencies in North America and Europe, and has been an ongoing debate in India for some decades. Care should also be taken to ensure TCAM services remain affordable and accessible to the poorest members of society, especially those with inadequate access to biomedical systems of health care.

In developing integrated health care services and policy — combining the best of biomedicine with the best of TCAM, within a common system — care should be given to developing culturally sensitive research methodologies that draw on indigenous theoretical assumptions and methods of identifying, preparing and individualising herbal and other traditional medicines. Care should also be taken to ensure TCAM services remain affordable and accessible to the poorest members of society, especially those with inadequate access to biomedical systems of health care.

It is our hope as editors, shared by the many contributors to this volume, that this book will contribute to expanding the view of TCAM within policy and public health circles and will be a part of ensuring that the public does, in the future, have access to safe and effective integrated health care services of their choice.

Index

CPSIA information can be obtained
at www.ICGtesting.com
Printed in the USA
FSHW010836230320
68370FS